The Quokka protocol

Immediacy in modern implantology

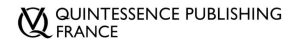
QUINTESSENCE PUBLISHING
FRANCE

62 boulevard de La Tour-Maubourg
75007 Paris - France
www.quintessence-international.fr

© Quintessence International 2023
ISBN : 978-2-36615-078-0

All rights reserved. This book or any part thereof may not be reproduced, stored in a retrieval system, or transmitted in any form or by any means, electronic, mechanical, photocopying, or otherwise, without prior written permission of the publisher.

Production and design: Quintessence International, France
Editor: Quintessence Publishing United Kingdom
Illustrations: Laurent Baudchon
Printed in Croatia

The Quokka protocol
Immediacy in modern implantology

Hervé Buatois | Nicolas Guillon

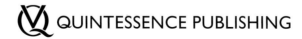

Berlin | Chicago | Tokyo
Barcelona | London | Milan | Mexiko City | Paris | Prague | Seoul | Warsaw
Beijing | Istanbul | Sao Paulo | Zagreb

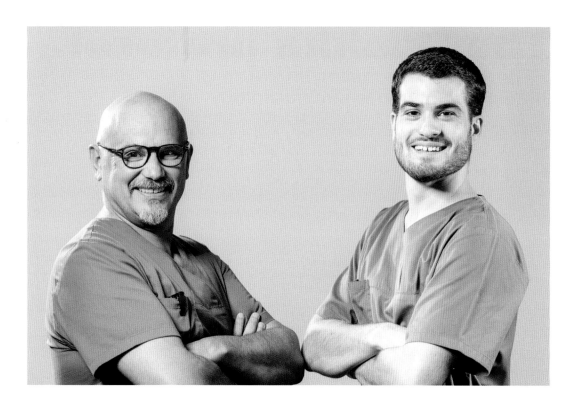

Hervé Buatois

Doctor of Dental Surgery, Claude-Bernard University, Lyon 1.

Postgraduate in implantology, New York University (NYU), USA.

Co-director of CampusHB continuing education center, Grenoble.

Private practice in implantology and esthetic prosthetic rehabilitation, Grenoble.

Author of the book "L'implantologie supra crestale" published in 2016 by Editions Quintessence.

Nicolas Guillon

Doctor of Dental Surgery, Claude-Bernard University, Lyon 1.

Postgraduate in implantology, EAO (2025).

Co-director of CampusHB continuing education center, Grenoble.

Private practice in implantology and esthetic prosthetic rehabilitation, Grenoble.

Foreword

The idea for this book emerged gradually, driven by the repeated success of our immediate implant treatments and immediate loading assisted by a digital workflow in our practice.
This book, based on more than 200 documented cases, analyzed and broken down into single, multiple, and full edentulous cases, is at the root of our thinking and the standardization of our approach. Our approach has always been based on research and the application of clinical protocols validated by the literature. This was the driving force behind the genesis and writing of our previous book, *L'implantologie supra crestale*. This book aimed to develop a form of implantology based on the consideration of the periodontal environment and the relevance of its reconstruction to the durability of implant treatments by appealing to evidence-based dentistry.

Underpinned by this solid foundation, we asked ourselves how we could take into account the wishes of patients, who are always asking for shorter treatment times and optimal physical and psychological comfort during our therapeutic treatments. If we analyze how implantology has evolved since the end of the 1980s, its metamorphosis has often been induced by the demands of our patients.

This is the case with the development of single-tooth edentulism in esthetic areas, immediate implantation, and immediate loading in the 1990s and 2000s. As a social phenomenon that inexorably affects our specialty, is immediacy compatible with esthetic and durable implantology? Clinical protocols still need to be developed and scientific evidence confirmed in order to integrate immediacy into our daily therapeutic arsenal. We must resolve to forget about transitional removable prostheses, which are simple to insert for the practitioner but so destabilizing for our patients.
Can we offer immediate implantation and loading on a daily basis while standardizing our results?

The literature is advancing, as are the therapeutic tools, to move towards immediate implantation and loading. Implant designs, implant surfaces, guided bone regeneration (GBR), and periodontal reconstructive techniques are leading us in this direction. The advent of digital options and tools in dentistry, as in many other professional and personal activities, brings new perspectives.

What about implant treatment? Will these new tools change the approach towards implant therapy and facilitate the procedure? As with any technological evolution, it is important to examine its impact on our practice and the clinical benefits that it can offer in a sustainable manner. Our initial view of the digital workflow was in no way technological and even less passionate with regard to the integrated circuit! Our questions related more to the potential ergonomic tool. Can the digital solution help us to address some of our limitations in the planning and management of procedures? Can it improve the reproducibility and quality of our results?

We have identified several areas for reflection based around:
- the fusion of biological and theoretical prosthetic rules in implantology;
- ergonomic management of restorations and immediate loading by way of:
  - a shorter operating time;
  - improvement of the esthetics and integrity of the tooth or the fixed or removable partial denture;
  - precise management of the emergence profile in its anatomy as well as its surface condition.

The purpose of this book is to share our experience in this evolution that has allowed us, for the past 6 years, to no longer manage temporary removable prostheses, to develop reproducible clinical protocols based on our knowledge and by integrating an ergonomic tool that is the digital workflow, and to propose immediate loading with temporary prostheses connected to the prosthetic bases before surgery. In addition to saving time and providing peace of mind, this significant development enables us to define GBR and guided tissue regeneration (GTR) and perform suturing techniques guided by the prosthesis. We would like to help you understand this approach by sharing fundamental guidance and innovative clinical protocols, illustrated using numerous cases treated in our office.

This introduction would not be complete without thanking Jérôme Vaysse from Laboratoire High Tech Dental in Toulouse, France and Dr. Dimitri Pascual, both of whom have done pioneering work. Their innovative experience has encouraged us to embrace this philosophy and allowed us to develop our protocol over the past 6 years.

We hope you will enjoy reading this book as much as we enjoyed imagining, structuring, and creating it.

Hervé Buatois, Nicolas Guillon

CONTENTS

Foreword V

Chapter 1   **Immediate implant placement** 1

       Fundamental reminders 3

       Decision-making criteria 6

       Positioning protocol 7

       Hard and soft tissue management in the Quokka protocol 9

Chapter 2   **Restoration and immediate loading** 17

       Interest 19

       Conditions for success 21

       Emergence profile, the essential guide 27

Chapter 3   **Presentation of the Quokka protocol** 31

       Introduction 33

       The prosthetic project 34

       Implant-prosthetic planning 49

       The surgical guide 52

       Guided surgery and immediate loading 55

       Transfer of the project to the final prosthesis 62

Chapter 4	**Single-unit clinical applications**	73
	Alveolus intact, vestibular bone wall preserved – Single-unit cases 1 to 5	75
	Alveolus with narrow vestibular dehiscence (< 1/3 of root exposure volume) – Single-unit cases 6 to 9	113
	Alveolus with medium vestibular dehiscence (1/3 to 2/3 of root exposure volume) – Single-unit cases 10 and 11	141
	Alveolus with large vestibular dehiscence (> 2/3 of root exposure volume) – Single-unit cases 12 to 15	155
Chapter 5	**Clinical applications for partially edentulous patients**	183
	Two to three anterior teeth – Plural-unit cases 16 and 17	185
	Two to three posterior teeth – Plural-unit cases 18 and 19	199
	Four anterior teeth – Plural-unit cases 20 and 21	211
	Six teeth or more – Plural-unit cases 22 to 24	231
	One implant for two teeth – Plural-unit case 25	259
Chapter 6	**Full-arch clinical applications**	269
	Toothed unimaxillary – Full-arch clinical cases 26 to 37	273
	Edentulous unimaxillary – Full-arch clinical cases 38 and 39	393
	Maxillomandibular – Full-arch clinical cases 40 and 41	417

Immediate implant placement

Fundamental reminders 3

Decision-making criteria 6

Positioning protocol 7

Hard and soft tissue management in the Quokka protocol 9

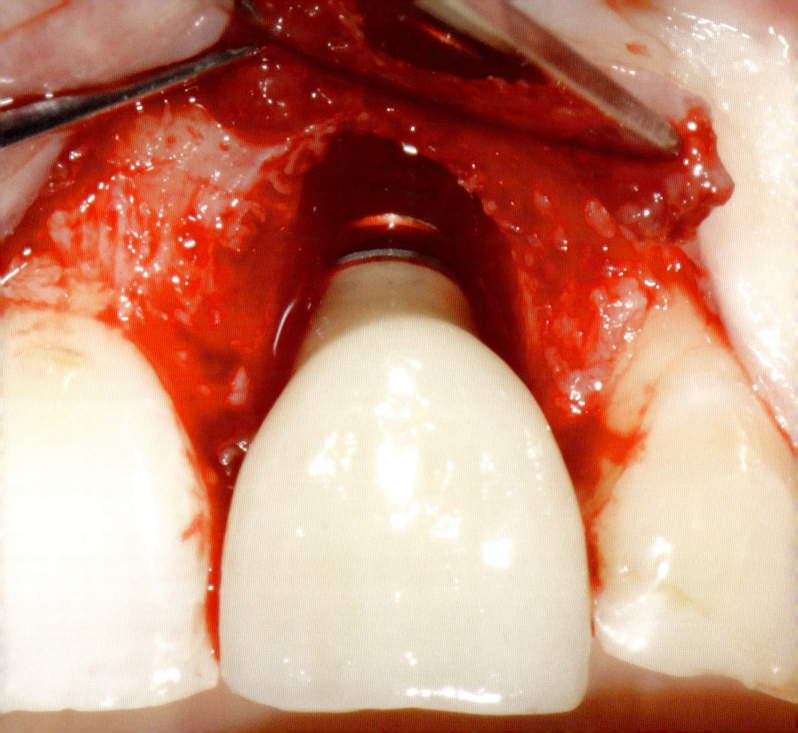

Fundamental reminders

Immediate implant placement represents the ultimate evolution of implant dentistry. This technique was developed to control the bone resorption inherent in any extraction[1]. From implantation in a previously edentulous bone site, clinical validation has made it possible to reduce the amount of time required for immediate implant placement, i.e., placement that is performed at the same time as the extraction. The terminology had to be adapted to reflect this evolution: the Third International Team for Implantology (ITI) Consensus Conference that took place in 2003 proposed new terminology, modified in 2008 by Chen and Buser, when the ITI Treatment Guide Volume 3 on immediate implant placement was published[2]. It now refers to four types of implantation:

type 1: immediate implant placement, which occurs on the day of extraction without prior bone or gingival healing;

type 2: early implant placement that occurs 6 to 8 weeks after soft tissue healing has taken place in the extraction site, but without significant bone healing;

type 3: early implant placement that occurs 12 to 16 weeks later once partial bone healing has taken place, with significant soft tissue and bone healing;

type 4: late implant placement, which takes place more than 6 months after extraction, once the alveolus has healed completely.

Immediate implant placement is recognized as a validated procedure in current implantology[3-6]; however, it is still associated with a higher risk of gingival recession during the initial healing phase than early implantation in esthetic areas[3-5]. The implantation time should not alter the rules for the 3D positioning of the implant in accordance with the surrounding tissue biology, which must adapt to this procedure. Replacing a tooth with an implant implies the reconstruction and **repositioning** of the optimal coronal volume lost following the avulsion of the tooth and the associated tissue modifications.

Our approach involves focusing on the positioning of the prosthetic implant platform, which we consider to be the guiding element of implant-prosthetic rehabilitation as it supports the emergence profile. Without optimal support, it will not be possible to achieve an anatomically and color-matched coronal volume through ceramic layering **(Fig 1-1)**.

Of course, this support must be integrated seamlessly into a stable periodontal volume

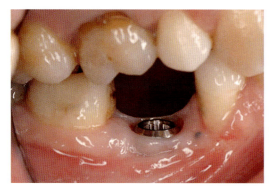 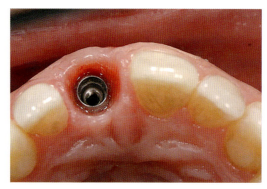 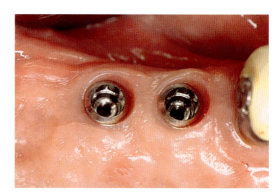

Fig 1-1 The location of the prosthetic platform is the guiding element of the emergence profile.

while taking into account the anatomic and biologic differences that exist between implants and natural teeth[6,7]. This philosophy implies the reconstruction of bone and gingiva in many clinical situations to restore a peri-implant bone architecture that is compatible with both horizontal and vertical periodontal stability (biologic distance), in accordance with the implant design. The emergence profile is managed through the mesiodistal and bucco-lingual positioning of the implant and not burying the implant. Vertical positioning based on the implant design only achieves periodontal integration through relevant hard and soft tissue reconstructions[8,9] (Fig 1-2).

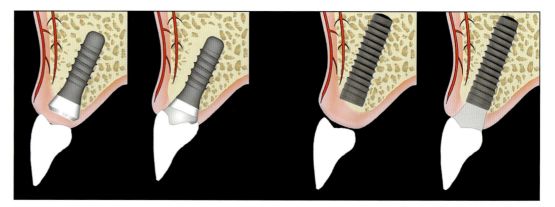

Fig 1-2 The emergence profile is managed by the mesiodistal and vestibulolingual/palatal positioning of the implant and not by the burying of the implant. The vertical positioning facilitates the periodontal integration.

Regardless of the implantation time, the choice must allow for an optimal functional and esthetic result for the patient. This is a crucial element in the therapeutic decision tree. Early implantation remains the reference procedure in the esthetic zone[3]. The relevance of this work is to describe an immediate approach that makes it possible to achieve similar results to other timed approaches. In our method, we have identified three master biologic rules that guide us during the surgical phase. These are as follows:

- The presence of a 2-mm native or reconstructed bone wall is the recognized standard for achieving stability of the vestibular wall around an implant[8,10,11];
- Constant bone remodeling by resorption leads to the formation of the biologic space and brings the bone level 2 mm more apical to the prosthetic hiatus[12,13];
- A minimum of 3 mm keratinized gingiva with a minimum gingival thickness of 2 mm is recommended. A minimum gingival thickness of 2 mm is an important factor in restructuring the biologic space[14,15].

To understand these biologic rules, it is essential to know the main principles of bone resorption following extraction. The literature is clear on this point. Within 1 year after extraction, vertical bone loss of 2 to 3 mm and horizontal bone loss of 50% of the initial bone volume are observed. Two-thirds of this resorption occurs during the first 3 months[12,16]. These figures refer to situations where the alveolus is intact following extraction (Diagrams 1-1 and 1-2).

The figures will be higher in the presence of unfavorable architecture (dehiscence or natural fenestration of the vestibular bone) or the existence of an apical infectious pathology (granuloma, cyst) or periodontal pathology (angular bone defect). Vestibular vertical resorption is affected by the initial bone thickness: it is twice as important when the initial thickness is less than 2 mm[12]. This notion is significant when referring to a study conducted by Huynh-Ba et al on a sample of 93 patients where measurements of vestibular bone wall thickness were less than or equal to 1 mm in 87.2% of cases and greater than 2 mm in only 2.6% of cases[17]. The thin vestibular bone wall (less than 2 mm), often referred to as the vestibular bone lamina, receives most of its vascularization from the periodontal ligament and is therefore tooth-dependent. Avulsion of the tooth removes this vascular supply, so this bone layer is lost after extraction, regardless of the filling procedures performed. The reduction in healing time is motivated by the desire to minimize postextraction bone resorption and thus bone reconstruction procedures; however, in many cases (where the bone wall thickness is less than 2 mm), this resorption will occur as an inexorable consequence of biologic rules. Reconstruction is therefore necessary to compensate for the bone loss resulting from this remodeling. A study by Chen and Darby on a sample of 34 patients who had undergone flapless extraction of a maxillary central or lateral incisor with the adjacent teeth present showed that 16 patients had an intact socket, 9 had dehiscence, and the remaining 9 exhibited fenestration after 1 day[18]. At 8 weeks, 57% of the sites that were intact after extraction and 56% of the sites with fenestration had dehiscence[18]. The immediate implant placement procedure must therefore incorporate an implant positioning and bone and gingival reconstruction protocol that is able to neutralize this remodeling to ensure a predictable outcome for the patient[19-21]. Various studies have validated this technique and given it its place in the therapeutic arsenal. This is true in terms of implant survival rates as compared to delayed protocols since the first publication was written on this topic by Lazzara in 1989[22]. Since then, this procedure has been validated by numerous studies[23-26].

Immediate implantation, like any other treatment option, presents advantages and disadvantages that must be kept in mind when developing treatment plans[19,27].

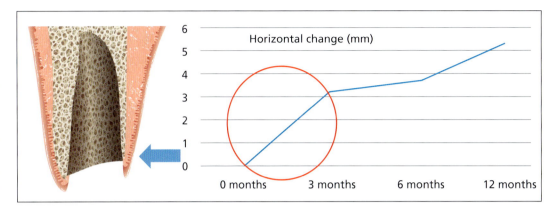

Diagram 1-1 Diagram of horizontal bone resorption over time.

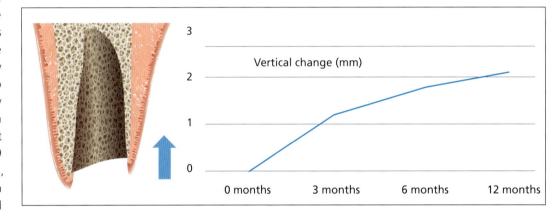

Diagram 1-2 Diagram of vertical bone resorption over time.

The advantages are as follows:
- it involves a single surgical procedure;
- the treatment period is reduced;
- the residual walls of the cavity are favorable to filling (three- or four-wall defect).

The disadvantages are as follows:
- bone architecture, depending on bone loss and initial dental axes, can be an unfavorable guide;
- the size of the cell may compromise primary stability;
- more invasive apical drilling may be necessary;
- there is a decrease in the height of keratinized tissue due to the absence of gingival closure during alveolar healing, and therefore a more frequent need for connective tissue grafting;
- there is an increased risk of vestibular recession of the marginal gingiva;
- the procedure is generally more complex than for early implantation (types 2 and 3).

Decision-making criteria

As with any therapy, knowledge of the favorable and unfavorable conditions for the optimization of a procedure is essential. In view of the literature and the recommendations of the ITI Consensus, a number of points must be understood before immediate implantation can be selected.

FAVORABLE CONDITIONS (Fig 1-3)
These include areas of low esthetic risk according to the ITI Esthetic Risk Assessment (ERA) classification[28]:
- thick periodontal phenotype;
- low smile line;
- unitary edentulism;
- intact alveolus with a minimum vestibular wall thickness of 1 mm and a vestibular marginal margin that is no more than 3 mm more apical than the prosthetic platform of the implant neck;
- presence of unaltered proximal bone peaks;
- monoradicular tooth socket;
- site without acute phase infection;
- apical and palatal or lingual bone volume compatible with primary stability.

UNFAVORABLE CONDITIONS (Fig 1-4)
These include areas of high esthetic risk according to the ITI ERA classification[28]:
- fine periodontal phenotype;
- thin vestibular wall (less than 1 mm);
- high smile line;
- vestibular dehiscence (bone edge located more than 3 mm apical to the ideal position of the future implant neck);
- multiple missing teeth;
- pluriradicular tooth;
- significant apical bone defect compromising primary implant stability;
- site with an acute infection;
- limited apical bone volume in relation to an anatomic obstacle.

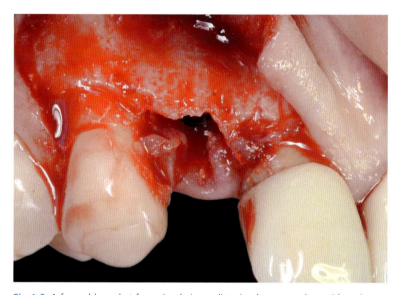

Fig 1-3 A favorable socket for a simple immediate implant procedure with an intact buccal wall with a thickness greater than 1 mm, with intact proximal bone peaks, thick gingival tissue, and sufficient keratinized gingiva.

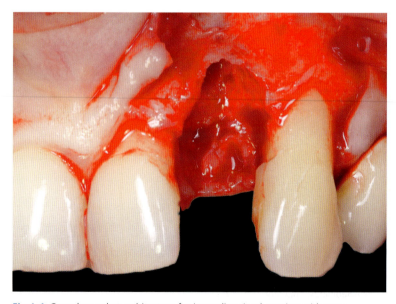

Fig 1-4 Complex socket architecture for immediate implantation with more than 3 mm vestibular bone loss from the optimal bone level for collar alignment. Proximal bone loss and alteration of the palatal wall can be observed; however, the gingival context is favorable.

To complete our review of the factors impacting the choice of therapy, a study by Kan et al of 100 patient CBCTs analyzed the bony environment of 600 teeth, and the authors derived a classification based on the root–cortex ratio[29]:

Class 1: roots in contact with the vestibular cortex (81.1% of sites);
Class 2: roots in the middle of the alveolus not in contact with the cortices (6.5% of sites);
Class 3: roots in contact with the palatal cortex (0.7% of sites);
Class 4: two-thirds of the roots in contact with both cortices (11.7% of sites).

As will be discussed in detail in Chapter 3, Class 1 is most favorable for immediate implantation, followed by Class 2 and Class 3. Class 4 is the least favorable anatomic ratio for immediate implantation. This option is contraindicated if the apical bone site at the socket is not sufficient to achieve primary implant stability (Fig 1-5).

Positioning protocol

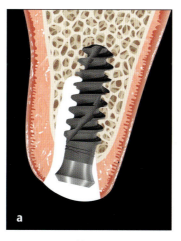 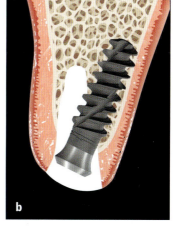 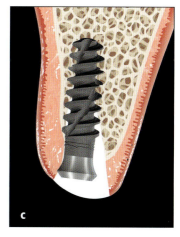

Fig 1-6 a to c (a) Suitable position for immediate extraction-implantation, combining implant positioning and primary stability. (b) Implant neck position too buccal. (c) Implant position in line with the bone socket, leading to overly buccal positioning of the implant neck and unstable primary implant stability.

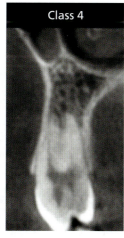

Fig 1-5 Radiologic appearance of the two root relationships in relation to the vestibular and palatal bone walls. Class 1 corresponds to the most favorable situation for immediate implantation, whereas Class 4 is the most unfavorable situation for such a procedure.

Simple procedure

Because each technique needs a learning curve, as a beginner it is important to learn how to perform immediate implantation in a favorable context, namely a site with:
- a thick periodontal phenotype;
- a thick vestibular bone wall (greater than 1.5 mm);
- sufficient bone apically, palatally, and lingually to ensure primary stability;
- the absence of acute infection (chronic silent infections are not a contraindication)[30-33];
- the possibility of opting for flapless surgery.

The procedure involves perforating the palatal or lingual cortical bone of the alveolus in its limit corresponding to the middle or apical third using a ball bur or pointing drill. The first drill will penetrate this perforation with a 45-degree vestibular angulation, then its axis will be straightened as it is driven in to finish drilling in an axis parallel to the axis of the extracted tooth. The final position of the implant should be 2 mm more palatal to the vestibular inner wall and 1 mm more apical to the desired 3D position. The space left between the implant body and the vestibular wall will be filled with a slow-resorbing bone substitute[34,35]. In the case of a tissue-level (TL) or tapered tissue-level (TLX) implant, a 2-mm space must be left between the implant neck and the vestibular inner wall. The purpose of this drilling is to exploit the bone triangle that is frequently present in the anterior maxilla between the tooth socket, often in a very vestibular position, and the palatal cortex. For premolars and molars, the principle is the same, relying on the area corresponding to the middle and apical thirds of the palatal wall of the vestibular alveolus of the maxillary premolars, the lingual wall of the mandibular premolars, the vestibular wall of the palatal alveolus of the maxillary molars, and the interradicular bony septum of the mandibular molars (Fig 1-6).

Advanced procedure

This is another step in the learning curve that should make it possible to treat more complex cases that present with:
- a thin alveolar bone wall (less than 1 mm);
- dehiscence of the buccal wall exposing the coronal third of the root volume;
- unaltered proximal bone peaks;
- a fine phenotype;
- an apical granuloma without fenestration;
- a combination of the above factors.

To validate such a procedure, it is necessary to ensure that the residual surrounding bone volume will allow primary stability in the modified 3D position as described above. In addition, a minimum of 3 mm keratinized gingival height around the tooth to be extracted is required[14,15]. If these two conditions are met, immediate implantation is possible. Periodontal reconstruction of the implant environment will then be required to enable stability of the gingival level around the implant emergence profile. It will also ensure the buccal gingival margin is in a position similar to that of the contralateral tooth, or at least with a change in vertical positioning (recession) of less than 1 mm. Recession greater than 2 mm will be considered an esthetic failure[36]. In this clinical context, buccal recessions are more frequent and associated with three times the risk of vertical bone resorption (mean 2.1 mm)[34,37-39]. It will therefore be necessary to overcorrect the defects to compensate for the tissue shrinkage that occurs during soft tissue healing and associate it with partial regeneration of the bone tissue, particularly in the medial zone of the defect, which is the furthest from the cellular sources of regeneration. This will involve use of guided bone regeneration (GBR) techniques with a graft consisting of a slow-resorbing bone substitute (deproteinized bovine bone mineral [DBBM]) by filling in the thin vestibular bone wall or overcorrecting the bone defect horizontally[20,38,40-42]. The latter will be covered with a resorbable collagen membrane. A dense connective graft of the tuberosity type will complete this correction in the vestibular region in cases with a thin phenotype, making it possible to minimize the occurrence of gingival recession and achieve more similar results between thin and thick phenotypes[42-45].

Complex procedure

This represents the highest level of complexity in immediate implantation: its implementation therefore requires skills acquired through routine practice of the two previously described procedures. Sites may exhibit:
- an alveolus with dehiscence and/or fenestration exposing two-thirds or more of the coronal volume;
- gingival recession on the tooth to be extracted;
- loss of proximal bone peaks;
- proximal angular defects;
- an attack on the lingual or palatal wall;
- vestibular keratinized gingiva of less than 3 mm.

Of course, the bone volume, regardless of its alteration, must allow for primary implant stability in the optimal prosthetic axis. It must also allow for bone and gingival reconstruction, leading to a 3D environment similar to that required in the literature on healed crests. Overcorrection is even more important in this case, since the risk of partial bone regeneration is correlated to the distance from cellular and vascular sources. This complex context poses several contentious issues to which appropriate answers must be found.

Insufficient keratinized gingiva

The soft tissues will need to be corrected not only by thickening, but also by increasing the keratinized gingiva. This means that a connective graft must be performed, not on the tuberosity but rather on the deep palate, which is more vascularized but less fibrous, to be able to expose part of this graft and induce keratinized healing in this area[46]. The difficulty often lies in being able to combine the thickness and the increase in the quantity of keratinized tissue. As such, large connective tissue grafts are required.

Major bone loss but proximal peaks not altered

The increase in the size of the bone defect will complexify the predictability of GBR over the entire volume. As the size increases, the distance between the vascular and cellular sources becomes greater and the mechanical stabilization of the graft becomes more random. It is therefore necessary to provide the graft with greater osteoinductive activity by adding autogenous bone to the DBBM and/or by using growth factors such as plasma rich in growth factors (PRGF)[47,48]. For the sake of standardization, the use of PRGF has been systematized according to the Anitua protocol during immediate implantation, regardless of the level of complexity[49-51]. The rules of GBR are more applicable than ever with a collagenous resorbable membrane stretched and stabilized using pins. A nonresorbable membrane may be a solution for this type of defect, but the need for its eventual removal is more questionable in the context of immediate implantation with unburied implants. Complementary surgery should be evaluated in terms of the benefits and risks it presents for the management of the surrounding soft tissue. Supplementation with a tuberosity (bulky and fibrous) graft will secure the result in the event of partial failure of GBR[52].

Altered proximal bone peaks

In this context, we have reached the limit of the capabilities of vertical GBR. As such, it is necessary to review the 3D positioning of the implant according to a modified prosthetic axis with a more apical vertical position of the implant towards the altered proximal bone peaks, implying a more apical emergence profile. This can be minimized by adding a tuberosal fibrous connective graft, but will inevitably have an esthetic impact of which the patient must be informed. Such situations are often encountered in the sequelae of periodontal disease, which frequently leads to alteration of the neckline[53]. In the case of a patient with no alteration of the surrounding gingival levels but with attachment loss affecting the adjacent teeth, performing pre-implant or peri-implant vertical bone reconstruction would be biologically impossible, except if performing strategic extractions to avoid altering the proximal bone peaks.

Buccal gingival recession

In addition to the previously described GBR procedures associated with connective tissue grafting, the esthetic impact of coronal positioning in terms of repositioning the mucogingival junction line and therefore determining the pink esthetic score for the final result must be evaluated. In such contexts, if recession is associated with reduced or absent keratinized gingiva (Miller class 2), the type 2 (early implant placement) procedure should be preferred. The practitioner may also choose to maintain the indication for immediate implantation provided that the patient is clearly warned of the esthetic risk of a 2-mm gingival lift.

Hard and soft tissue management in the Quokka protocol

The notion of immediacy has a temporal justification and aims to shorten the duration of implant-prosthetic treatment. From the present authors' point of view, it is primarily of biologic interest as it limits the number of interventions. This makes it possible to work with the soft tissues in their full vascular and elastic capacity during implant placement. Conversely, increasing the number of interventions will lead to tissue that is increasingly scarred and therefore less easily mobilized and less vascularized in theory[54]. We combine immediate implantation with immediate restoration to offer patients a certain psychological comfort; they arrive at the office and then leave with their tooth having been fixed. From a clinical perspective, this immediate restoration also makes it possible to guide the volume of GBR that is required through the presence of the coronal volume, as well as the volume of soft tissue adapted, which, associated with adequate 3D positioning, will help to obtain an optimal emergence profile. This has become a real comfort in daily practice.

A screw-retained prosthesis, finalized and connected to a titanium baseplate before surgery, is the clinical ideal that guided us in our intellectual path. It offers several significant advantages: a much smoother surface than that achieved after relining in the mouth, a more finished esthetic of the tooth, and, above all, the possibility of an operative time that will make it possible **to suture the soft tissues around the provisional prosthesis**. This is an important development that allowed us to achieve optimal maturation of the emergence profile at 3 months post-implantation **(Figs 1-7 and 1-8)**. From this point of view, the digital workflow will make it possible to standardize these possibilities in cases of single- and multiple-tooth and complete edentulism thanks to planning and CAD/CAM. This workflow will be detailed later in this book.

The therapeutic tools used are:
- creation of a flap through tunnelling;
- elevation of a full-thickness flap with or without releasing incision;
- GBR with a bovine inorganic bone substitute (Bio-Oss; Geistlich, Wolhusen, Switzerland) incubated in PRGF phase F2 (Endoret; BTI Biotechnology Institute, Vitoria, Spain);
- fibrin membrane from PRGF phase F1 (Endoret);
- a non-crosslinked bilayer collagen membrane (Bio-Gide; Geistlich);
- grafting of tuberous connective tissue;
- palatal connective tissue grafting;
- a half-thickness incision for tension-free coronal traction;
- an anchored suspended advanced flap (ASAF) suture **(Fig 1-9)**;
- a papillary suture.

The Quokka protocol

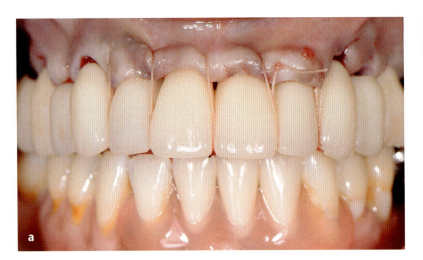
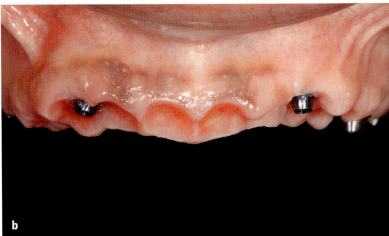

Fig 1-7 a and b (a) Immediate (instantaneous) loading of a provisional fixed/removable partial denture of twelve teeth connected to six implants. Note the sutures hanging vertically from the vestibular flap after coronal repositioning following a half-thickness incision, and the plunging pattern of the pontics in the non-implant extraction sites. (b) Scar situation 3 months after GBR-induced surgery, GTR, and placement of provisional prosthesis-guided sutures.

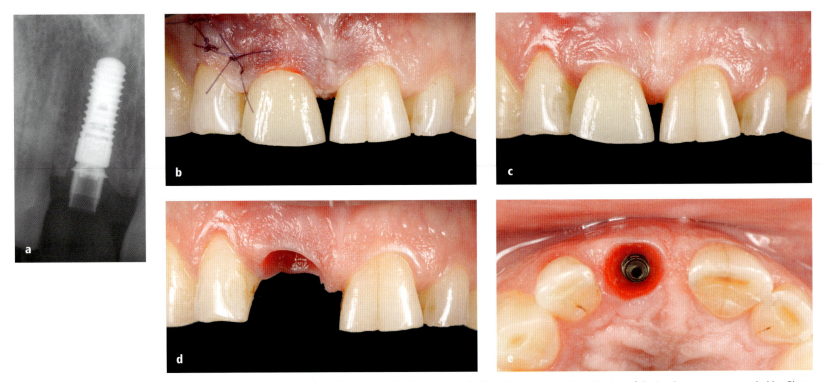

Fig 1-8 a to e (a) Radiologic view of the BL RC implant with a Variobase (Straumann, Basel, Switzerland). Note the more apical positioning of the implant as recommended by Chen et al. (b) Immediate loading of a screw-retained provisional tooth connected to a titanium baseplate on a bone-level (BL) implant with an ASAF suture. (c) Clinical appearance at 3 months postoperatively. Note the absence of inflammation. (d and e) Appearance after removal of the temporary tooth. Note the quality of soft tissue support and 3D periodontal volume and emergence profile architecture consistent with a provisional tooth–induced central incisor, GBR, and sutures.

Chapter 1 - Immediate implant placement

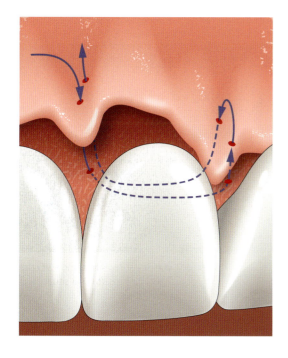
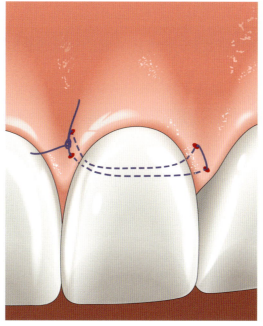

Fig 1-9 An anchored suspended advanced flap (ASAF) suture.

Treating more than 200 cases in total has allowed us to streamline our clinical approach to hard and soft tissue management during immediate implantation. Depending on the clinical situation at the outset, we wanted to define hard and soft tissue reconstruction protocols to standardize the performance of these procedures. This allows for repetition within each technique applied, and thus for continuous improvement of the technique and quality of the postoperative analysis according to the different categories. This is only a classification based on our practice, so must leave room for adaptations specific to each patient.

We have deliberately distinguished between the classification of bone defects and gingival defects even though they are often clinically interconnected.

Bone defects can be classified as follows:

- **GBR 1**: Four-walled bone defect of an immediate implant socket with a buccal wall not exceeding a vertical offset of more than 3 mm with the proximal bone peaks;
- **GBR 2**: Bone defect with vestibular dehiscence exposing less than one-third of the implant volume once the implant is positioned in the socket or vestibular wall, with intact proximal bone peaks;
- **GBR 3**: Bone defect with vestibular dehiscence exposing between one- and two-thirds of the implant volume once the implant is positioned in the socket, with intact proximal bone peaks;
- **GBR 4**: Bone defect with vestibular dehiscence exposing between one- and two-thirds of the implant volume once the implant is positioned in the socket with proximal and/or palatal or lingual involvement.

Gingival defects (GDs) can be classified as follows:

- **GD 1**: Vestibular gingival tissue thickness less than 2 mm;
- **GD 2**: Height of vestibular or lingual keratinized tissue less than 3 mm;
- **GD 3**: Vestibular gingival recession with apical keratinized tissue greater than or equal to 3 mm;
- **GD 4**: Vestibular gingival recession with less than 3 mm apical keratinized tissue.

The treatment protocols that we have standardized against this classification are summarized in Tables 1-1 and 1-2.

Table 1-1 Classification of bone defects.

GBR 1	Tunneling flap	Internal GBR with sticky bone (PRGF + DBBM) + fibrin	Coronal traction of the flap and ASAF suture around the temporary tooth
GBR 2	Full-thickness flap, sulcular incision of + 2 teeth on each side, without discharge	Internal and external GBR with sticky bone profile (PRGF + DBBM) + fibrin. Covered by a collagen membrane scalloped against the temporary tooth	Coronal traction of the flap and ASAF suture around the temporary tooth
GBR 3	Full-thickness flap, sulcular incision of + 2 teeth on each side, with discharge	Internal and external GBR with sticky bone profile (PRGF + DBBM + autogenous chips) + fibrin. Covered by a collagen membrane scalloped against the temporary tooth and stabilized using apical pins	Coronal traction of the flap and ASAF suture around the temporary tooth
GBR 4	Full-thickness flap, sulcular incision of + 2 teeth on each side, with discharge	Internal and external GBR in vestibular, proximal, and/or palatal profile with sticky bone (PRGF + DBBM + autogenous chips) + fibrin. Covered by a collagen membrane transfixed by the temporary tooth and stabilized using apical pins	Coronal traction of the flap and ASAF suture around the temporary tooth

Table 1-2 Classification of gingival defects.

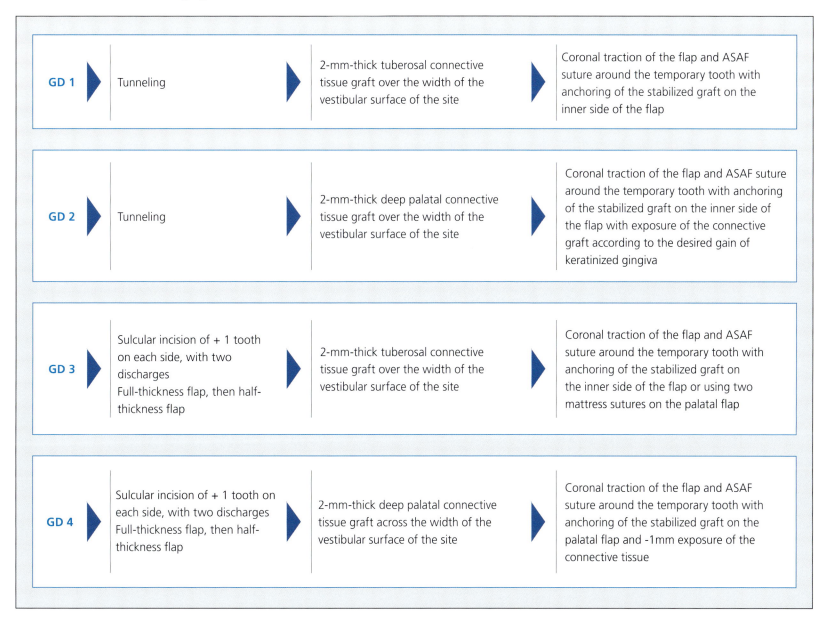

GD 1	Tunneling	2-mm-thick tuberosal connective tissue graft over the width of the vestibular surface of the site	Coronal traction of the flap and ASAF suture around the temporary tooth with anchoring of the stabilized graft on the inner side of the flap
GD 2	Tunneling	2-mm-thick deep palatal connective tissue graft over the width of the vestibular surface of the site	Coronal traction of the flap and ASAF suture around the temporary tooth with anchoring of the stabilized graft on the inner side of the flap with exposure of the connective graft according to the desired gain of keratinized gingiva
GD 3	Sulcular incision of + 1 tooth on each side, with two discharges. Full-thickness flap, then half-thickness flap	2-mm-thick tuberosal connective tissue graft over the width of the vestibular surface of the site	Coronal traction of the flap and ASAF suture around the temporary tooth with anchoring of the stabilized graft on the inner side of the flap or using two mattress sutures on the palatal flap
GD 4	Sulcular incision of + 1 tooth on each side, with two discharges. Full-thickness flap, then half-thickness flap	2-mm-thick deep palatal connective tissue graft across the width of the vestibular surface of the site	Coronal traction of the flap and ASAF suture around the temporary tooth with anchoring of the stabilized graft on the palatal flap and -1mm exposure of the connective tissue

References

1. Araújo MG, Lindhe J. Dimensional ridge alterations following tooth extraction. An experimental study in the dog. J Clin Periodontol. 2005;32(2):212-8.

2. Chen ST, Buser D, Wismeijer D, Belser U. International Team for Oral Implantology, ITI Consensus Conference. *In ITI treatment guide. Treatment options*, Vol. 3. Berlin, London : Quintessence International, 2008.

3. Buser D, Chappuis V, Belser UC, Chen S. Implant placement post extraction in esthetic single tooth sites: when immediate, when early, when late? Periodontol 2000. 2017;73(1):84-102.

4. Prati C, Zamparini F, Pirani C, Gatto MR, Piattelli A, Gandolfi MG. Immediate early and delayed implants: A 2-year prospective cohort study of 131 transmucosal flapless implants placed in sites with different pre-extractive endodontic infections. Implant Dent. 2017;26(5):654-63.

5. Khzam N, Arora H, Kim P, Fisher A, Mattheos N, Ivanovski S. Systematic review of soft tissue alterations and esthetic outcomes following immediate implant placement and restoration of single implants in the anterior maxilla. J Periodontol. 2015;86(12):1321-30.

6. Berglundh T, Lindhe J, Ericsson I, Marinello CP, Liljenberg B, Thomsen P. The soft tissue barrier at implants and teeth. Clin Oral Implants Res. 1991;2(2):81-90.

7. Belser UC, Mericske-Stern R, Bernard JP, Taylor TD. Prosthetic management of the partially dentate patient with fixed implant restorations. Clin Oral Implants Res. 2000;11 Suppl 1:126-45.

8. Belser U, Martin W, Jung R, Hämmerle CHF, Schmid B, Morton D, Buser D. ITI treatment guide, volume 1: Implant therapy in the esthetic zone. Single-Tooth replacements. Berlin : Quintessence International, 2007.

9. Buatois H, Pollini A. Le positionnement tridimensionnel de l'implant. *In L'implantologie supra crestale*. Paris : Quintessence International, 2016 ; p. 97-120.

10. Qahash M, Susin C, Polimeni G, Hall J, Wikesjö UME. Bone healing dynamics at buccal peri-implant sites. Clin Oral Implants Res. 2008;19(2):166-72.

11. Spray JR, Black CG, Morris HF, Ochi S. The influence of bone thickness on facial marginal bone response: stage 1 placement through stage 2 uncovering. Ann Periodontol. 2000;5(1):119-28.

12. Araújo MG, Lindhe J. Dimensional ridge alterations following tooth extraction. An experimental study in the dog. J Clin Periodontol. 2005;32(2):212-8.

13. Hermann JS, Buser D, Schenk RK, Schoolfield JD, Cochran DL. Biologic Width around one- and two-piece titanium implants. Clin Oral Implants Res. 2001;12(6):559-71.

14. Levine RA, Huynh-Ba G, Cochran DL. Soft tissue augmentation procedures for mucogingival defects in esthetic sites. Int J Oral Maxillofac Implants. 2014;29 Suppl:155-85.

15. Cochran DL, Hermann JS, Schenk RK, Higginbottom FL, Buser D. Biologic width around titanium implants. A histometric analysis of the implanto-gingival junction around unloaded and loaded nonsubmerged implants in the canine mandible. J Periodontol. 1997;68(2):186-98.

16. Schropp L, Wenzel A, Kostopoulos L, Karring T. Bone healing and soft tissue contour changes following single-tooth extraction: a clinical and radiographic 12-month prospective study. Int J Periodontics Restorative Dent. 2003;23(4):313-23.

17. Huynh-Ba G, Pjetursson BE, Sanz M, Cecchinato D, Ferrus J, Lindhe J, et coll. Analysis of the socket bone wall dimensions in the upper maxilla in relation to immediate implant placement. Clin Oral Implants Res. 2010;21(1):37-42.

18. Chen ST, Darby I. The relationship between facial bone wall defects and dimensional alterations of the ridge following flapless tooth extraction in the anterior maxilla. Clin Oral Implants Res. 2017;28(8):931-7.

19. Kan JYK, Rungcharassaeng K, Deflorian M, Weinstein T, Wang HL, Testori T. Immediate implant placement and provisionalization of maxillary anterior single implants. Periodontol 2000. 2018;77(1):197-212.

20. Mastrangelo F, Gastaldi G, Vinci R, Troiano G, Tettamanti L, Gherlone E, et coll. Immediate postextractive implants with and without bone graft: 3-year follow-up results from a multicenter controlled randomized trial. Implant Dent. 2018;27(6):638-45.

21. Kois JC, Kan JY. Predictable peri-implant gingival esthetics: surgical and prosthodontic rationales. Pract Proced Esthet Dent. 2001;13(9):691-8; quiz 700, 721-2.

22. Lazzara RJ. Immediate implant placement into extraction sites: surgical and restorative advantages. Int J Periodontics Restorative Dent. 1989;9(5):332-43.

23. Zhou W, Gallucci GO, Chen S, Buser D, Hamilton A. Placement and loading protocols for single implants in different locations: A systematic review. Int J Oral Maxillofac Implants. 2021;36(4):e72-e89.

24. Garcia-Sanchez R, Dopico J, Kalemaj Z, Buti J, Pardo Zamora G, Mardas N. Comparison of clinical outcomes of immediate versus delayed placement of dental implants: A systematic review and meta-analysis. Clin Oral Implants Res. 2022;33(3):231-77.

25. Schropp L, Isidor F. Timing of implant placement relative to tooth extraction. J Oral Rehabil. 2008;35 Suppl 1:33-43.

26. Chen ST, Wilson TG, Hämmerle CHF. Immediate or early placement of implants following tooth extraction: review of biologic basis, clinical procedures, and outcomes. Int J Oral Maxillofac Implants. 2004;19 Suppl:12-25.

27. Chen ST, Buser D. Esthetic outcomes following immediate and early implant placement in the anterior maxilla--a systematic review. Int J Oral Maxillofac Implants. 2014;29 Suppl:186-215.

28. Martin WC, Morton D, Buser D. Pre-operative analysis and prosthetic treatment planning in esthetic implant dentistry. *In Implant therapy in the esthetic zone for single-tooth replacements ITI Treatment Guide* Series Vol. 1. Berlin : Quintessence International, 2006 ; p. 9-24.

29. Kan JY, Roe P, Rungcharassaeng K, Patel RD, Waki T, Lozada JL et coll. Classification of sagittal root position in relation to the anterior maxillary osseous housing for immediate implant placement: a cone beam computed tomography study. Int J Oral Maxillofac Implants. 2011;26(4):873-6.

30. Jung RE, Philipp A, Annen BM, Signorelli L, Thoma DS, Hämmerle CHF et coll. Radiographic evaluation of different techniques for ridge preservation after tooth extraction: a randomized controlled clinical trial. J Clin Periodontol. 2013;40(1):90-8.

31. Chrcanovic BR, Martins MD, Wennerberg A. Immediate placement of implants into infected sites: a systematic review. Clin Implant Dent Relat Res. 2015;17 Suppl 1:e1-e16.

32. Lee J, Park D, Koo KT, Seol YJ, Lee YM. Comparison of immediate implant placement in infected and non-infected extraction sockets: a systematic review and meta-analysis. Acta Odontol Scand. 2018;76(5):338-45.

33. Saijeva A, Juodzbalys G. Immediate implant placement in non-infected sockets versus infected sockets: A systematic review and meta-analysis. J Oral Maxillofac Res. 2020;11(2):e1.

34. Chen ST, Darby IB, Reynolds EC. A prospective clinical study of non-submerged immediate implants: clinical outcomes and esthetic results. Clin Oral Implants Res. 2007;18(5):552-62.

35. Araújo MG, Wennström JL, Lindhe J. Modeling of the buccal and lingual bone walls of fresh extraction sites following implant installation. Clin Oral Implants Res. 2006;17(6):606-14.

36. Fürhauser R, Florescu D, Benesch T, Haas R, Mailath G, Watzek G. Evaluation of soft tissue around single-tooth implant crowns: the pink esthetic score. Clin Oral Implants Res. 2005;16(6):639-44.

37. Kan JY, Rungcharassaeng K, Lozada J. Immediate placement and provisionalization of maxillary anterior single implants: 1-year prospective study. Int J Oral Maxillofac Implants. 2003;18(1):31-9.

38. Evans CD, Chen ST. Esthetic outcomes of immediate implant placements. Clin Oral Implants Res. 2008;19(1):73-80.

39. Cordaro L, Torsello F, Roccuzzo M. Clinical outcome of submerged vs. non-submerged implants placed in fresh extraction sockets. Clin Oral Implants Res. 2009;20(12):1307-13.

40. Girlanda FF, Feng HS, Corrêa MG, Casati MZ, Pimentel SP, Ribeiro FV et coll. Deproteinized bovine bone derived with collagen improves soft and bone tissue outcomes in flapless immediate implant approach and immediate provisionalization: a randomized clinical trial. Clin Oral Investig. 2019;23(10):3885-93.

41. Zaki J, Yusuf N, El-Khadem A, Scholten RJPM, Jenniskens K. Efficacy of bone-substitute materials use in immediate dental implant placement: A systematic review and meta-analysis. Clin Implant Dent Relat Res. 2021;23(4):506-19.

42. Seyssens L, De Lat L, Cosyn J. Immediate implant placement with or without connective tissue graft: A systematic review and meta-analysis. J Clin Periodontol. 2021;48(2):284-301.

43. Tatum CL, Saltz AE, Prihoda TJ, DeGroot BS, Mealey BL, Mills MP, et al. Management of Thick and Thin Periodontal Phenotypes for Immediate Dental Implants in the Esthetic Zone: A Controlled Clinical Trial. Int J Periodontics Restorative Dent. févr 2020;40(1):51-9.

44. Aldhohrah T, Qin G, Liang D, Song W, Ge L, Mashrah MA et coll. Does simultaneous soft tissue augmentation around immediate or delayed dental implant placement using sub-epithelial connective tissue graft provide better outcomes compared to other treatment options? A systematic review and meta-analysis. PloS One. 2022;17(2):e0261513.

45. Atieh MA, Alsabeeha NHM. Soft tissue changes after connective tissue grafts around immediately placed and restored dental implants in the esthetic zone: A systematic review and meta-analysis. J Esthet Restor Dent. 2020;32(3):280-90.

46. Sanz-Martín I, Rojo E, Maldonado E, Stroppa G, Nart J, Sanz M. Structural and histological differences between connective tissue grafts harvested from the lateral palatal mucosa or from the tuberosity area. Clin Oral Investig. 2019;23(2):957-64.

47. Işık G, Özden Yüce M, Koçak-Topbaş N, Günbay T. Guided bone regeneration simultaneous with implant placement using bovine-derived xenograft with and without liquid platelet-rich fibrin: a randomized controlled clinical trial. Clin Oral Investig. 2021;25(9):5563-75.

48. ArRejaie A, Al-Harbi F, Alagl AS, Hassan KS. Platelet-Rich plasma gel combined with bovine-derived xenograft for the treatment of dehiscence around immediately placed conventionally loaded dental implants in humans: Cone beam computed tomography and three-dimensional image evaluation. Int J Oral Maxillofac Implants. 2016;31(2):431-8.

49. Anitua E, Andia I, Ardanza B, Nurden P, Nurden AT. Autologous platelets as a source of proteins for healing and tissue regeneration. Thromb Haemost. 2004;91(1):4-15.

50. Anitua E, Sánchez M, Prado R, Orive G. Plasma rich in growth factors: the pioneering autologous technology for tissue regeneration. J Biomed Mater Res A. 2011;97(4):536.

51. Anitua E, Tejero R, Zalduendo MM, Orive G. Plasma rich in growth factors promotes bone tissue regeneration by stimulating proliferation, migration, and autocrine secretion in primary human osteoblasts. J Periodontol. 2013;84(8):1180-90.

52. Rojo E, Stroppa G, Sanz-Martin I, Gonzalez-Martín O, Alemany AS, Nart J. Soft tissue volume gain around dental implants using autogenous subepithelial connective tissue grafts harvested from the lateral palate or tuberosity area. A randomized controlled clinical study. J Clin Periodontol. 2018;45(4):495-503.

53. Chapple ILC, Mealey BL, Van Dyke TE, Bartold PM, Dommisch H, Eickholz P, et coll. Periodontal health and gingival diseases and conditions on an intact and a reduced periodontium: Consensus report of workgroup 1 of the 2017 World Workshop on the Classification of Periodontal and Peri-Implant Diseases and Conditions. J Clin Periodontol. 2018;45 Suppl 20:S68-S77.

54. Palacci P, Ericsson I. Esthétique et implantologie. Gestion des tissus osseux et péri-implantaires. Quintessence International, 2001.

55. Tavelli L, Barootchi S, Ravidà A, Suárez-López Del Amo F, Rasperini G, Wang HL. Influence of suturing technique on marginal flap stability following coronally advanced flap: a cadaver study. Clin Oral Investig. 2019;23(4):1641-51.

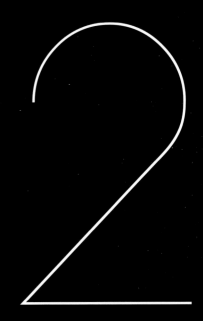

Restoration and immediate loading

Interest 19

Conditions for success 21

Emergence profile, the essential guide 27

The Quokka protocol

Interest

In the mid-1990s, immediate loading became a potential treatment concept for use with osseointegrated implants, which contradicts one of the pillars of Brånemark's osseointegration[1,2]. The aim is to avoid patients experiencing dissatisfaction and discomfort with the removable temporary solution; however, feedback has proven that these transitional removable prostheses:
- cause discomfort for patients due to their instability, functional deficiencies, and limited esthetic result;
- require numerous adjustments by the practitioner that prove time-consuming;
- can be responsible for transmucosal loads if they are too unstable or not sufficiently discharged at the intrados.

The notion of being able to restore comfort to patients as quickly as possible is a real advancement in treatment that plays a significant role in the acceptance of treatment plans. The consideration of the patient's social and professional life during the osseointegration period is more in line with a medical treatment that is about comfort above all (replacement of missing teeth), placing the patient's well-being at the heart of the therapy[3].

In the chapter that presents the Quokka protocol, we will discuss the real clinical benefit of placing the patient in an esthetic and functional situation as soon as possible to optimize the final prosthetic phase. It is desirable and indeed productive (as office time can be optimized) to use this option as a true prosthetic step, in the same way as the fitting of the model and the wearing of a temporary fixed/removable partial denture in tooth-supported restorations. With more than 40 years of clinical experience in this field and having written various scientific publications on the topic, our aim is to bring the management of implant-prosthetic treatment to a level very similar to that of esthetic and/or functional prostheses on natural teeth[4], i.e., to achieve functional continuity, psychological comfort, and improved esthetics.

Immediate loading is subject to a somewhat broad temporal interpretation. If we refer to the ITI classification discussed earlier in this book, it involves delivery of an implant-supported prosthesis within a time frame ranging from 1 to 72 hours postoperatively[5]. It is indisputable that, if considering the social, psychological, and functional factors affecting patients, loading within 1 hour is the option that should be favored. We then speak of **immediate loading** when loading is carried out during the surgical procedure. This is the basis on which we developed our concept of "Smile in 1 hour by Quokka". Our patients must be

The Quokka protocol

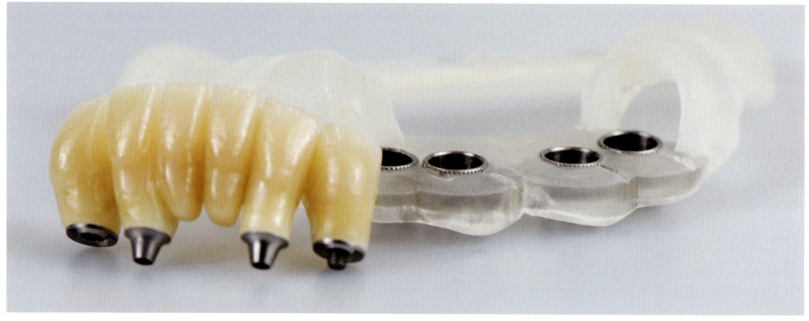

Fig 2-1 A six-tooth partial denture, connected before surgery using four Variobase kits (Straumann, Basel, Switzerland), two for tissue-level (TL) implants in 33 and 43 and two for bone-level (BL) implants in 32 and 42.

able to smile at the end of their surgery. This is an ambitious but realistic goal that will be illustrated in the second part of this book.

With immediate loading, we have gone to the very end of the reasoning with a prosthesis connected to titanium bases in direct implants to reduce the duration of surgery as much as possible, always considering patient comfort, and noted two advantages to doing so. First, it saves time during surgery, making it possible to concentrate on the real added value of implantology, namely the management of hard and soft tissues. Second, it limits the use of resin monomers in the scar area, in the same way as during relining in the mouth. In this context, we speak of **connected immediate loading (Fig 2-1)**. This has a significant impact on the organization of the practice during immediate loading sessions, especially for full arches, in the following ways:

- everything is managed during the surgical appointment;
- patient comfort is increased as they can rest during the postoperative phase without having to undergo another intervention (insertion of the prosthesis) or experience another source of pain and inflammation;
- there is no requirement for additional appointments after surgery for fitting of the temporary prosthesis;
- there is no need to block out a prosthetist for a given period or to have one in the office to insert the temporary prosthesis, as its insertion can be integrated into the standard laboratory schedule.

Following this logic of immediacy, we have increased the number of cases of immediate implantation associated with immediate loading in cases of single or multiple missing teeth or complete edentulism, with success rates quite similar to those provided in the literature; these results make this approach the first choice[6,7].

Having the finalized provisional prosthesis available as soon as the implants are placed is a major benefit. The prosthetic volume in place on the implants can be used with the emergence profiles to guide the 3D periodontal reconstruction. This will apply when performing guided bone regeneration (GBR) in the postextraction socket, and in the periphery if necessary. There will also be a positioning guide for a possible connective graft. This prosthetic volume will constitute a guiding volume for the repositioning of the flap and its stabilization using adapted sutures. **Immediate implantation and instant connected loading therefore introduce the notion of periodontal reconstruction and suturing guided by the prosthesis.** This approach was introduced 6 years ago in our practice and has clearly optimized esthetic results.

Conditions for success

Of course, the evolution towards new clinical protocols must be based on mechanical and biological fundamentals, the pillars of osseointegration[2]. It is not a question here of inventing a new form of implantology, but rather of making it continue to evolve in the years to come as it has done over the previous 50 years. Any therapy is above all a dynamic process. We will review the essential factors that condition the success of immediate loading and that prove truly decisive when they are adhered to in association with immediate implantation.

Patient selection

It is important to identify all the factors that contraindicate implant-prosthetic rehabilitation. As with any dental treatment, but especially periodontal and implant treatment, the patient's healing potential is a key success factor that is based closely on the density and quality of vascularization of the tissues[8]. The establishment of a stable blood clot, capacity for cellular differentiation, and stability of the healing site are well-established notions in reference to the regeneration triad set out by Lynch et al[9].
Candidates for immediate implantation combined with immediate loading or restoration must meet this full potential. In our practice, we apply the same selection criteria as for patients who are candidates for bone or gingival grafts, also including cooperation and compliance with the proposed treatment:
- smoker (fewer than 10 cigarettes per day)[10];
- diabetes compatible with efficient wound healing (HbA1c less than 8%)[11];
- vitamin D deficiency[12];
- absence of active periodontitis (Bleeding Index < 20% and pocket depth < 4 mm)[13];
- ability to understand the functional, physical, and hygiene constraints related to this type of treatment;
- psychological motivation to have a fixed temporary prosthesis and acceptance of the additional financial cost.

Primary implant stability

Of all the pillars of osseointegration outlined by Brånemark in the early 1980s, primary implant stability remains the only one that is essential to achieve bone ankylosis and not fibrous encapsulation; however, bone biology has shown that there is no need for a complete absence of micromovements, but that a threshold exists around 150 mm. Above this threshold, the risk of failure is clearly identified[14]. Primary implant stability in an extraction site is therefore the primary goal of the procedure. Three factors contribute towards achieving this goal:
- bone density;
- implant length;
- implant macrogeometry.

Bone density

As a reminder, the classification outlined by Misch[15] in 1990 is based on the macroscopic structure of the bone with:
- D1: dense cortical bone;
- D2: porous cortical bone with dense cancellous bone inside;
- D3: thin, porous cortical bone with low-density cancellous bone;
- D4: low-density cancellous bone.

Clinically, D2 and D3 bone are most conducive to rapid bone healing because they have the optimal ratio of mechanical stability to vascularization density and therefore cellularity. Mechanically speaking, D1 bone is certainly the most suitable for implant placement, but its capacity for reorganization is time limited in the face of mechanical constraints that will generate remodeling. D4 is the biologic ideal but has no mechanical quality for immediate loading. Modern imaging tools have become extremely helpful for reading bone density, especially CBCT. They allow a reading of the density in Hounsfield units (HUs) and thus make it possible to evaluate the bone classes crossed by the implant subject to immediate implantation and immediate loading. They range from 700 HU for cancellous bone to 3,000 HU for dense cortical bone. This information is frequently found in planning software (Tables 2-1 and 2-2). To level out these differences in density as much as possible, the clinician can capitalize on the under-drilling, tapping in addition to drilling, and implant macrogeometry to achieve optimal primary stability for a given site. According to the literature, the goal is to obtain a theoretical threshold of 35 Ncm[16]; however, some studies show that this can be reduced to 20 Ncm[17]. The threshold is variable and will differ if approaching immediate implantation with single, multiple, or full loading.

Implant length

The second parameter that influences primary implant stability is, of course, the length of the implant receiving the load. There is a general consensus in the literature that the minimum length should be 10 mm[18]. According to a literature review by Tettamanti et al, the most commonly used lengths are between 13 and 15 mm[19]. With regard to long implants, the angled implants introduced by Maló et al have made it possible to increase the length of implants in areas where the anatomy

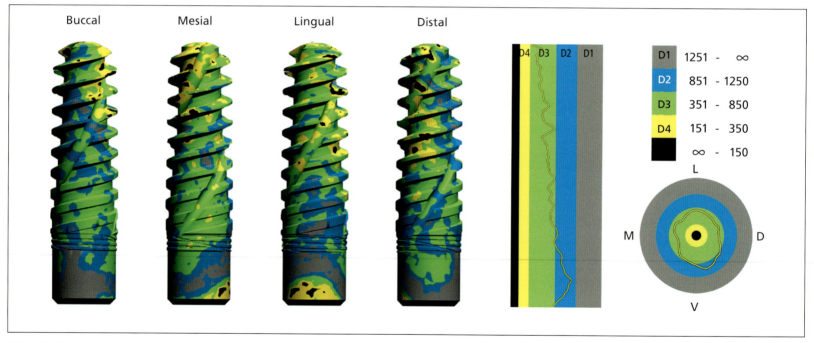

Bone class (Lekholm and Zarb)	Bone density (Norton and Gamble)	Region of interest
Class 1	> +850	Anterior mandible
Class 2/3	+500 to +850	Posterior mandible / Anterior maxilla
Class 4	0 to +500	Posterior maxilla
Class 4*	< 0	Tuberosity region

Table 2-1 In 2001, Norton et al defined a correlation between Lekholm and Zarb's classification of bone class and density expressed in Hounsfield units (HU).

Table 2-2 The updating of density intervals in HU linked to CBCT technologies and the emergence of planning software offer relevant information on the implant's bone environment that is important for both the drilling protocol and the expected primary implant stability.

limits them (sinus, emergence of the inferior dental nerve [IDN])[20,21]. This is therefore an option that has its place in complete rehabilitations, especially in the antesinus, or in cases of rehabilitations with four implants for ten teeth in the mandible, depending on the location of the chin hole. In our practice, we work with 10- or 12-mm implants for cases involving single- or multiple-tooth rehabilitation. For complete rehabilitations, we can use 8-mm implants provided that they are mostly in combination with 12-mm implants.

Implant macrogeometry

The third parameter that impacts primary implant stability is implant macrogeometry. Different design approaches have been developed over the last 40 years, including coils, microspires, macrospires, non–self-tapping implants, self-tapping implants, impacted implants, conical implants, and hollow implants. All these designs had a common goal: to achieve primary stability during the osseointegration period. The coils of Straumann Tissue Level (STL) implant are widely spaced and their design is guided by a strength correlation between the interspiral bone volume and the width of the titanium coil. The implant is not self-tapping. This allows for a combination of under-drilling, no tapping, and tapping to compensate for different bone densities and thus optimize primary stability (Fig 2-2). Currently, the trend is towards a consensus design with aggressive turns such as fins, whose depth accentuates bone anchorage, but also the surface area offered for a given diameter. The new generation of Straumann implants with the tapered tissue-level (TLX) and tapered bone-level (BLX) series has much more aggressive, self-tapping coils that allow for even greater under-drilling to level out primary stability in bone of varying density (Fig 2-3).

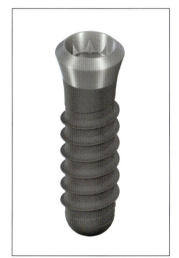

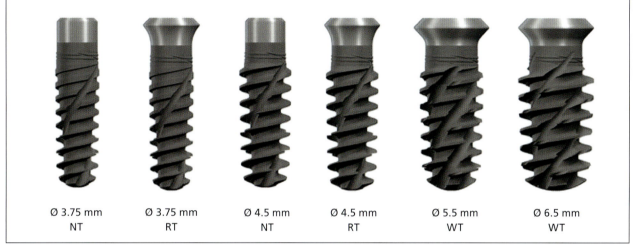

Ø 3.75 mm NT   Ø 3.75 mm RT   Ø 4.5 mm NT   Ø 4.5 mm RT   Ø 5.5 mm WT   Ø 6.5 mm WT

Fig 2-2 The STL range (Straumann). The classic coil design has been used for more than 25 years.

Fig 2-3 The TLX range (Straumann). Note the more aggressive coils. The variety of diameters of the implant necks and bodies makes it possible to choose the implant that is best suited to the bone conditions and prosthetic objectives.

Implant surface condition

In the osseointegration process, not everything is mechanical; indeed, the biologic dimension is the key factor in bone regeneration in contact with the implant body. Stability and the surface of the blood clot between the implant and the drilled bone are the primary factors involved in this healing process. The more the surface allows diffusion of the biologic flows responsible for the process of bone differentiation due to its wettability, the faster this bone apposition will occur and the more important the bone contact surface will be. As the precursor molecules are hydrophilic macromolecules, the higher the surface wettability, the more bioactive it will be in the bone regeneration process around the implant. The SLActive surface by Straumann, a development of the sandblasted, large grit, acid-etched (SLA) implant surface, is one of these high-performance surfaces[22-27].

The combination of deep thread microgeometry and a surface with high hydrophilicity is most relevant and efficient for immediate implantation and immediate loading, according to the current literature[28,29]. Indeed, implant stability must be maintained at a high level throughout the entire osseointegration phase. The transition phase between this primary stability at bone contact during the insertion phase and secondary stability, which is the product of bone remodeling, must be as short as possible in order not to result in too long a mechanical transition period, which is critical during immediate loading (Figs 2-4 and 2-5).

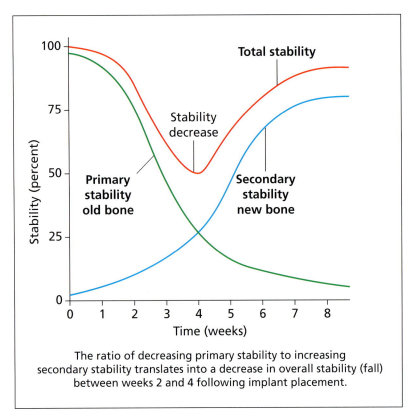

Fig 2-4 Relationship between primary and secondary stability during the osseointegration process.

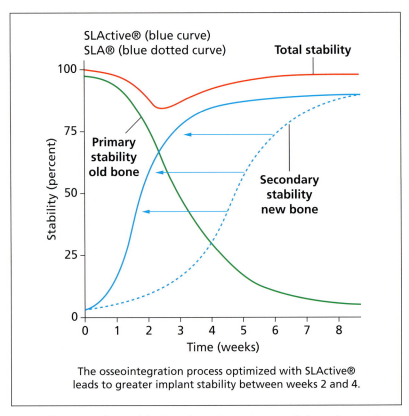

Fig 2-5 Illustration of a principle of accelerated secondary growth due to increased surface wettability (Straumann commercial document).

Number of implants, distribution, and notion of micromovements

For semantic purposes, we will refer to immediate loading for complete restorations since the fixed provisional prosthesis is necessarily loaded. We will also speak of immediate loading for other types of plural or single-unit restorations since the fixed provisional prosthesis is out of occlusal contact, both in centric contact and in eccentric excursion during mastication. In addition to its esthetic, social, and psychological impact, the objective of the prosthesis design is to allow control of the loads transmitted to the implants. In a literature review published in 1998, Szmukler-Moncler et al summarized a theoretical threshold of micromovements transmitted to implants below which osseointegration is possible[14]. This threshold is below 150 mm and will also depend on the shape of the implant (primary stability), the bioactive surface condition, and the load induced by the prosthesis architecture. As such, it is not the lack of early loading that is critical for implant osseointegration, but the absence of excessive micromovements at the bone–implant interface[14].

In this context, TLX and BLX implants offer a clear advantage in providing optimal primary stability. Their SLActive surface is another significant advantage, as is the control of the mechanical load. The current surfaces and designs provide a higher level of tolerance to parasitic loads (tongue, cheek, etc.), making it possible to consider immediate single or multiple restorations provided that there is a total absence of occlusal load in centric contact, as well as in eccentric excursion. Several clinical situations can be distinguished in the management of restorations with immediate loading.

Single restoration

Immediate loading, also known as an immediate esthetic loading, can be done. This can involve any tooth in the arch but will generally be reserved for those whose temporary absence could result in esthetic prejudice. The interarch relationship must allow the tooth to be excluded from any occlusal function and in particular from anterior guidance, without having to vestibulate it too much to ensure an esthetic result for the patient. Class II division 2 dentoskeletal relationships remain the most frequent contraindication for immediate single-tooth esthetics. The implant length must be at least 10 mm, and preferably 12 mm. The insertion torque must be at least 35 Ncm; however, the patient should be careful to follow a semi-solid diet for the first 3 weeks and avoid applying any tearing force in the area during the osseointegration phase (e.g., biting into a sandwich).

Plural restauration

Immediate loading can also be a solution, implying an absence of contact in centric occlusion and during eccentric excursions. In the case of anterior multi-unit restorations, the interarch relationships must be such that the fixed/removable partial denture is not involved in the anterior guidance. In the posterior areas, underbite is easier to achieve. The different possible configurations are:

a/ The anterior edentulous segment does not pass through the median sagittal plane

The classic configuration is two implants for three teeth (5-3, 4-2, 3-1) with implant lengths of 12 mm and a minimum insertion torque of 35 Ncm. If implant lengths of less than 10 mm are used, they should either be combined with 12-mm implants or changed to a configuration of one implant per tooth, i.e., three implants for three teeth, to eliminate the potential axis of rotation defined by the straight line joining the two implants.

b/ The anterior edentulous segment passes through the median sagittal plane

The classic configurations based on the degree of edentulism are:
- two implants for three teeth (12-21 or 22-11);
- three implants for four teeth (13-21 or 23-11);
- two implants for four teeth (12-22);
- four implants for six teeth (13 to 23).

The absence of two teeth engaging a lateral incisor can also be treated with a two-tooth implant (3-2 or 1-2) with a screw-retained prosthesis supporting the extended lateral incisor, provided there is no need for a diastema between the teeth. The implant length must be at least 12 mm.

c/ The edentulous segment is posterior

The presence of the sinus cavity and the IDN often limits the implant length to less than 12 mm. The classic configuration involves planning one implant per tooth. In our practice, we opt for short arches in both full and partial restorations. The classic scheme then involves:
- three implants for three teeth (4, 5 and 6);
- two implants for two teeth (4, 5 or 5, 6).

There is now a history on the combination of sinus grafts during immediate implantation and immediate loading to increase implant length, and the results have been somewhat satisfactory. The configuration does not change and remains, in these cases, one implant per tooth. The decision is always based on the primary implant stability correlated to the residual bone volume and the alveolar volume.

Complete edentulism

In cases of complete edentulism, the implants are brought into function immediately. Micromovements cannot be controlled by moderating the loads transmitted to the implants since they will be subjected to the patient's masticatory load, which we know to be variable. It is done by balancing the forces transmitted to the implants via the prosthesis. To achieve this, there are several factors to validate with the temporary fixed/removable partial denture:

- the rigidity of the resin in its mass and at the level of the prosthetic connections to ensure the principle of contention, called "cross-arch stabilization", to counter the lateral forces applied on one side with a counterforce on the opposite side;
- homogeneous distribution of the implants to support the temporary fixed/removable partial denture evenly. In the maxilla, we find a 6-4-2-2-4-6 configuration with angled or unangled "6s" in the antesinus. In the mandible, the configuration is 6-4-3-4-6 for a 12-tooth fixed/removable partial denture. With four-implant restorations, the configuration becomes 5-2-2-5 for a 10-tooth provisional fixed/removable partial denture, with the possibility of angulation anterior to the emergence of the IDN (Fig 2-6);
- a precise and **balanced occlusion** to counteract the working excursion forces with non-working contacts. This requires precision in the transfer of the occlusion when placing the provisional fixed/removable partial denture, and it is sometimes necessary to make occlusal tracks on the antagonist arch to perfect the functional curves.

The literature advocates the use of six implants, although Maló et al have shown that four give very good results, provided that they are in an extended 5-2-2-5 distribution. With a more limited extension of 4-2-2-4, the results are more uncertain than with six implants[20,21,31,32]. A distinction must be made between a provisional fixed/removable partial denture, which should not have any extension, and a definitive fixed/removable partial denture, which can be designed with distal extensions to complete the arches according to the patient's wishes. The implant length should ideally be 12 mm. For this purpose, placement of implants along an angled axis is a relevant option; however, both in the literature and in our clinical experience, 8-mm

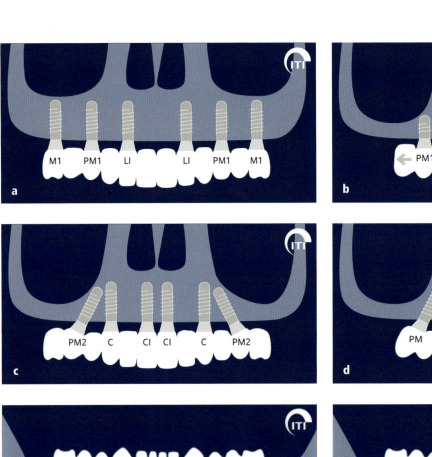

Fig 2-6 a to g The different possible combinations for implant placement depending on the number of teeth that is desired or possible. Note that for configuration (g), a distal angulation is now preferred in the IDN area to extend the bridge connection to the second premolar area.

implants combined with 12-mm implants have been found to work very well[33,34]. As for torque, the theoretical limit is 35 Ncm, but lower torque, such as 20 Ncm, is possible thanks to prosthetic restraint, which allows lower torque resistance[34]; however, the objective is to achieve the highest insertion torque by means of the implant design and drilling protocol. With the latest generation of Straumann implants, TLX or BLX, the drilling protocol is based on bone density. This protocol, combined with the more aggressive design of the self-tapping coils, enables the highest primary stability allowed by the bone site.

Emergence profile, the essential guide

The objective of immediate restoration associated with immediate loading is to accompany the patient during the transition phase in the best esthetic, social, and psychological conditions, as previously discussed. From a clinical perspective, it is also a question of inducing gingival healing in such a way as to ensure that the gingival architecture is optimal at the end of the healing process to receive the final prosthesis. This is done at the end of osseointegration in a provisionalization phase that is recommended according to the consensus in the esthetic zone to develop the soft tissues peripheral to the implant neck that constitute the emergence profile. This same provisional tooth will guide the process of bone reconstruction using GBR and the eventual gingival graft. As such, it plays the role of a true anatomic pilot to ensure the relevance of the peri-implant periodontal reconstruction. In our practice, we have developed the concept of prosthesis-guided sutures with a suture, named the anchored and suspended advanced flap (ASAF) suture, that allow both the necessary sealing of the underlying reconstruction and optimal plating around the provisional tooth to induce optimal healing (Fig 2-7).

In this context, the provisional tooth must of course conform to an ideal coronal morphology according to the recognized macro- and microesthetic criteria, like any provisional prosthesis. There are various tooth libraries in the digital workflow, which makes it possible to quickly build up an esthetic and functional project using digital retouching and morphing tools, and occlusal adjustment. The provisional tooth must also be very elaborate regarding its emergence profile design to reproduce an amelocentric junction line (AJL), which is referred to as prosthetic, in accordance with the tooth to be replaced. Finally, it must have a progressive concave morphology in the transition zone between the implant neck and the strategic zone of the prosthetic AJL to create a space for the development of soft tissue with an optimal thickness. This thickness, which is greater than that around the emergence profile of natural teeth, is intended to compensate for the fragility of the epithelioconjunctive complex that lacks collagen fibers anchored perpendicular to the implant surface; this is a major difference between implants and natural teeth[35]. The histologic arrangement around the implant is limited to connective tissue with peripheral collagen fibers that are closer to scar tissue than a periodontal attachment.

The contribution of CAD/CAM will make it possible to produce these anatomic profiles in a simpler and faster way, because they will be generated without a physical model and thus without specific preparation of a physical model that must anticipate the extraction of the tooth to be replaced and sculpt the emergence profile. We have a digital laboratory in our dental office so we can make the single or multiple small temporary teeth ourselves. This allows us to work in detail on the design of the prosthetic AJL and the junction profile between the implant neck and the AJL. For larger areas, and particularly for complete rehabilitations, these designs are validated remotely with the prosthetist using TeamViewer (TeamViewer, Goppingen, Germany) or other software. Particular attention is paid to the design of the pontics, which follow the morphologic principles of the implant emergence profiles to produce, during gingival healing, a morphologic bed with the presence of pseudopapillae. We draw inspiration from root morphologies that are typical to the teeth to design the horizontal section under the AJL and the vestibular, palatal/lingual, and proximal design of the AJL.

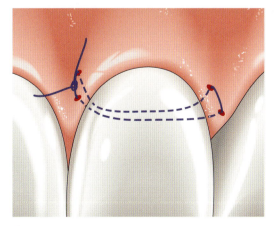

Fig 2-7 Suture ASAF.

References

1. Brånemark PI, Hansson BO, Adell R, Breine U, Lindström J, Hallén O et coll. Osseointegrated implants in the treatment of the edentulous jaw. Experience from a 10-year period. Scand J Plast Reconstr Surg Suppl. 1977;16:1-132.

2. Brånemark PI. Osseointegration and its experimental background. J Prosthet Dent. 1983;50(3):399-410.

3. Dierens M, Collaert B, Deschepper E, Browaeys H, Klinge B, De Bruyn H. Patient-centered outcome of immediately loaded implants in the rehabilitation of fully edentulous jaws. Clin Oral Implants Res. 2009;20(10):1070-7.

4. Gallucci GO, Benic GI, Eckert SE, Papaspyridakos P, Schimmel M, Schrott A et coll. Consensus statements and clinical recommendations for implant loading protocols. Int J Oral Maxillofac Implants. 2014;29 Suppl:287-90.

5. Chen ST, Buser D, Wismeijer D, Belser U. International Team for Oral Implantology, ITI Consensus Conference. In ITI treatment guide. Treatment options, Vol. 3. Berlin, London : Quintessence International, 2008.

6. Eini E, Yousefimanesh H, Ashtiani AH, Saki-Malehi A, Olapour A, Rahim F. Comparing success of immediate versus delay loading of implants in fresh sockets: a systematic review and meta-analysis. Oral Maxillofac Surg. 2022;26(2):185-94.

7. Gamborena I, Sasaki Y, Blatz MB. Predictable immediate implant placement and restoration in the esthetic zone. J Esthet Restor Dent. 2021;33(1):158-72.

8. Zuhr O, Hürzeler M. Chirurgie plastique et esthétique en parodontie et implantologie : une approche microchirurgicale. Quintessence International, 2013;858 p.

9. Lynch SE, Genco RJ, Marx RE. Tissue engineering: Applications in maxillofacial surgery and periodontics. Chicago : Quintessence International, 1999.

10. Mustapha AD, Salame Z, Chrcanovic BR. Smoking and dental implants: A systematic review and meta-analysis. Medicina Kaunas. 2021;58(1):39.

11. Oates TW, Dowell S, Robinson M, McMahan CA. Glycemic control and implant stabilization in type 2 diabetes mellitus. J Dent Res. 2009;88(4):367-71.

12. Werny JG, Sagheb K, Diaz L, Kämmerer PW, Al-Nawas B, Schiegnitz E. Does vitamin D have an effect on osseointegration of dental implants? A systematic review. Int J Implant Dent. 2022;8(1):16.

13. Bouchard P. Parodontologie & Dentisterie implantaire. Volume 2 : Thérapeutiques chirurgicales. Coll. Dentaire. Lavoisier, 2015;491 p.

14. Szmukler-Moncler S, Salama H, Reingewirtz Y, Dubruille JH. Timing of loading and effect of micromotion on bone-dental implant interface: review of experimental literature. J Biomed Mater Res. 1998;43(2):192-203.

15. Misch CE. Divisions of available bone in implant dentistry. Int J Oral Implantol Implantol. 1990;7(1):9-17.

16. Gallucci GO, Hamilton A, Zhou W, Buser D, Chen S. Implant placement and loading protocols in partially edentulous patients: A systematic review. Clin Oral Implants Res. 2018;29(S16):106-34.

17. Benic Gi B, Mir-Mari J, Hämmerle CH. Loading protocols for single-implant crowns: a systematic review and meta-analysis. Int J Oral Maxillofac Implants. 2014;29 Suppl:222-38.

18. Weber HP, Morton D, Gallucci GO, Roccuzzo M, Cordaro L, Grutter L. Consensus statements and recommended clinical procedures regarding loading protocols. Int J Oral Maxillofac Implants. 2009;24 Suppl:180-3.

19. Tettamanti L, Andrisani C, Bassi MA, Vinci R, Silvestre-Rangil J, Tagliabue A. Immediate loading implants: review of the critical aspects. Oral Implantol. 2017;10(2):129-39.

20. Maló P, Rangert B, Nobre M. « All-on-Four » immediate-function concept with Brånemark System implants for completely edentulous mandibles: a retrospective clinical study. Clin Implant Dent Relat Res. 2003;5 Suppl 1:2-9.

21. Maló P, Rangert B, Nobre M. All-on-4 immediate-function concept with Brånemark System implants for completely edentulous maxillae: a 1-year retrospective clinical study. Clin Implant Dent Relat Res. 2005;7 Suppl 1:S88-94.

22. Buser D, Schenk RK, Steinemann S, Fiorellini JP, Fox CH, Stich H. Influence of surface characteristics on bone integration of titanium implants. A histomorphometric study in miniature pigs. J Biomed Mater Res. 1991;25(7):889-902.

23. Bowers KT, Keller JC, Randolph BA, Wick DG, Michaels CM. Optimization of surface micromorphology for enhanced osteoblast responses in vitro. Int J Oral Maxillofac Implants. 1992;7(3):302-10.

24. Raghavendra S, Wood MC, Taylor TD. Early wound healing around endosseous implants: a review of the literature. Int J Oral Maxillofac Implants. 2005;20(3):425-31.

25. Le Guéhennec L, Soueidan A, Layrolle P, Amouriq Y. Surface treatments of titanium dental implants for rapid osseointegration. Dent Mater. 2007;23(7):844-54.

26. Schwarz F, Ferrari D, Herten M, Mihatovic I, Wieland M, Sager M et coll. Effects of surface hydrophilicity and microtopography on early stages of soft and hard tissue integration at non-submerged titanium implants: an immunohistochemical study in dogs. J Periodontol. 2007;78(11):2171-84.

27. Lamers E, Walboomers XF, Domanski M, te Riet J, van Delft FCMJM, Luttge R et coll. The influence of nanoscale grooved substrates on osteoblast behavior and extracellular matrix deposition. Biomaterials. 2010;31(12):3307-16.

28. Steigenga JT, al-Shammari KF, Nociti FH, Misch CE, Wang HL. Dental implant design and its relationship to long-term implant success. Implant Dent. 2003;12(4):306-17.

29. Almassri HNS, Ma Y, Dan Z, Ting Z, Cheng Y, Wu X. Implant stability and survival rates of a hydrophilic versus a conventional sandblasted, acid-etched implant surface: Systematic review and meta-analysis. J Am Dent Assoc. 2020;151(6):444-53.

30. Buser D, Chen S, Wismeijer D. Implant therapy in the esthetic zone: Current treatment modalities and materials for single-tooth replacements. Berlin : Quintessence International, 2019;727 p.

31. Silva GC, Mendonça JA, Lopes LR, Landre J. Stress patterns on implants in prostheses supported by four or six implants: a three-dimensional finite element analysis. Int J Oral Maxillofac Implants. 2010;25(2):239-46.

32. Malo P, de Araújo Nobre M, Lopes A, Moss SM, Molina GJ. A longitudinal study of the survival of All-on-4 implants in the mandible with up to 10 years of follow-up. J Am Dent Assoc 1939. 2011;142(3):310-20.

33. Peñarrocha-Oltra D, Covani U, Peñarrocha-Diago M, Peñarrocha-Diago M. Immediate loading with fixed full-arch prostheses in the maxilla: review of the literature. Med Oral Patol Oral Cirugia Bucal. 2014;19(5):e512-517.

34. Tettamanti L, Andrisani C, Bassi MA, Vinci R, Silvestre-Rangil J, Tagliabue A. Immediate loading implants: review of the critical aspects. Oral Implantol. 2017;10(2):129-39.

35. Sculean A, Gruber R, Bosshardt DD. Soft tissue wound healing around teeth and dental implants. J Clin Periodontol. 2014;41 Suppl 15:S6-22.

3

Presentation of the Quokka protocol

Introduction	33
The prosthetic project	34
Implant-prosthetic planning	49
The surgical guide	52
Guided surgery and immediate loading	55
Transfer of the project to the final prosthesis	62

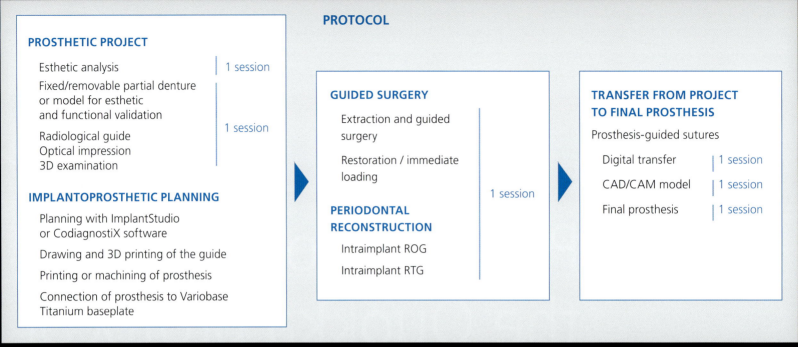

Fig 3-1 Schematic of the Quokka clinical protocol combining the academic principles of preimplant prosthetic study, 3D implant planning guided by the prosthetic project, the introduction of digital guided surgery in the concept of immediate implantation and instant loading via the digital workflow, prosthesis-guided periodontal reconstruction, prosthesis-guided suturing, and finally the transfer to the final prosthesis of the implant-prosthetic project at the end of the periodontal consolidation period.

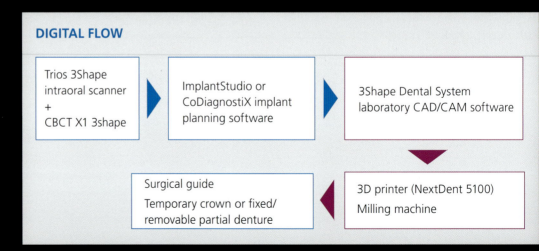

Fig 3-2 Digital flow diagram used in our daily practice for the past 6 years. Initially, in the first 2 years of development of our concept, we attached the provisional abutments to the fixed/removable partial denture in the mouth during surgery, with the relining polished before suturing, before connecting the titanium bases to the fixed/removable partial denture before surgery

Introduction

The Quokka concept, also known as "Smile in 1 hour by Quokka", is a disruptive concept for implant-prosthetic treatment developed in the present authors' practice. Its evolution began in 2016 with the integration of a digital workflow for immediate loading. This immersion in the possibilities offered led us to describe a successful clinical protocol that is now used daily in our practice to manage single, multiple, and complete implants. It is based on four key ideas:
- the central position of the prosthetic project in any major implant treatment, involving a significant modification of the patient's function and/or esthetics;
- the removal of any transitional removable prosthesis while administering patient care;
- a reduction in the overall duration of implant treatment;
- placement during implant surgery of the provisional prosthesis **connected** to the titanium bases **before** surgery, allowing a faster implant placement procedure and especially the development of the concepts of guided bone regeneration (GBR) and sutures guided by the prosthesis.

The strength of this protocol is that it systematizes the meeting of these four axes of reflection within a **standardized, rapid, and reproducible** approach that can be adapted to the different types of edentulism. The digital workflow is an ergonomic tool that then makes it possible to simplify the study procedures, registration procedures and procedures for carrying out our treatments, while improving the quality of the obtained result on a daily basis. We are able to offer treatment for single or multiple missing teeth in four sessions, and for completely edentulous patients in six sessions.

In this chapter, we will present in detail the architecture of this protocol (Fig 3-1). In the second part of this book, we will describe its different clinical applications through cases we have treated in our practice. All these cases, dating from 2016 to 2023, were treated using a digital workflow that has remained unchanged for 7 years, with the exception of regular intrasystem updates. This is the 3Shape workflow (3Shape, Copenhagen, Denmark) performed using a Trios intraoral scanner (versions 3, 4, and 5), Implant Studio planning software and Dental System laboratory software. For the past year, we have been using coDiagnostiX planning software (Dental Wings, Montreal, Canada) for its broader application with the Straumann implant system (Basel, Switzerland), especially in managing the implant abutment library that allows the use of tapered bone-level (BLX) implants and their segmenting possibilities, which represents a real opening to some interesting clinical applications (Fig 3-2).

The prosthetic project

Functional and esthetic analysis

The importance of these analyses will depend on the extent and location of edentulism and the patient's expectations. They may be minor, for example in the case of a single missing tooth, or comprehensive, as with complete rehabilitations to treat multiple missing teeth, terminal tooth migration, and significant esthetic and functional discomfort. The purpose of this chapter is not to go into the details of these analyses, but rather to highlight the protocols used and the digital tools available for analysis. Fundamental knowledge is essential to fuel the reflection. The protocol and digital workflow are only ergonomic tools for reproducibility. We often refer to the concept used in computing of garbage in, garbage out (GIGO), meaning that if incorrect data are entered, the output data (results) will also be incorrect. This is to emphasize how important it is to distinguish clinical and fundamental knowledge from knowledge of technical or digital tools. Knowledge precedes and potentiates the possibilities of tools.

Functional analysis

Functional analysis must precede all other analyses because any prosthetic rehabilitation must be part of a healthy and functional musculoarticular context. Occlusal analysis, like any other analysis, is based on an established protocol that consists of evaluating the musculoarticular system, starting from the temporomandibular joints (TMJs) and muscles, to arrive at the individual dental morphology. The aim is to understand mastication in its entirety, as described in 1920 by Georges S. Monson (Occlusion as applied to crown and bridge-work).

We will discuss occlusal diagnostic strategy as we have been using it in our practice for many years and teaching it at CampusHB. The purpose of this book is not to go into detail on all the elements necessary for functional and esthetic analyses, but to refer to the basic courses that exist in these respective fields; however, we will explain the methodology used in our treatments. There is an opposition between the gnathological school, which is very mechanistic, and the functionalist school, represented by Pedro Planas, but in reality, they are not so different. Everyone is free to use one or the other based on their knowledge and skills. A synthesis of the two approaches dictates clear conditions for functionality (Fig 3-3):

- absence of intracapsular pathology;
- absence of muscular pathology;
- a reproducible and myocentric position of the mandible;
- alternating unilateral mastication.

The occlusal diagnostic strategy starts with the musculoarticular examination and ends with the analysis of the occlusal paths that generate the alternating unilateral mastication, as illustrated in Fig 3-4. In unitary rehabilitations, this complete analysis is questionable if there is no musculoarticular pathology or aberrant functional asymmetry; however, in the context of longer rehabilitation procedures, including those involving the anterior region (which implies reconstruction of the anterior determinant or guide), or that of complete single-arch or maxillomandibular rehabilitation, this analysis becomes essential to ensure symmetrical functional harmony. This is vital to control the forces required for immediate loading. The symmetrical and adapted occlusal load

---

OCCLUSION - FUNCTION

Normality is symmetry and balance,

→ Symmetry of joint amplitudes

→ Symmetry of resting states and states of muscular tension

→ Symmetry of dental volumes

→ Symmetry of functional balance

Pathology is asymmetry and imbalance.

Fig 3-3 Summary of desired functional normality before any immediate loading.

is just as important as the strength of the implant anchors and is a major determining factor in the success of immediate loading. When performing complete rehabilitation, we systematically opt for a balanced occlusion similar as for full removable dentures (FRD) to balance the lateral forces on the implant-supported prosthesis, whatever the material used. In single-arch treatments, it is important to modify the occlusal planes and curves with temporary polymethyl methacrylate (PMMA) resin occlusal tables in the antagonist arch if necessary. The use of nocturnal muscle deprogramming splints is a relevant option that is used during the immediate loading phase and placement of the final prosthesis. It is used systematically in complete treatments, subject to the patient's situation for other rehabilitations (Fig 3-5).

Esthetic analysis

It is difficult to dissociate esthetic analysis from functional analysis because a normal dental morphology is often the result of normal functional coronal volumes; however, smile analysis is a major element in our reconstruction therapies and an esthetic smile remains a major goal for patients that is synonymous with health and anti-aging. It is based on three essential elements:
- facial harmony;
- macroesthetics;
- microesthetics.

The tools currently available for smile design are all based on these elements. We use Smile Design by 3Shape (Copenhagen, Denmark) and have recently also begun using the 3D modeling software RAYFace. For the fundamentals, we recommend the publications by Spear and Kois, Morleys, and Coachman, developer of Digital Smile Design (DSD). Coachman was the first to use the digital tool to standardize the esthetic values described in the fundamental publications. We do not claim to explain the entire esthetic analysis here, but rather to outline some of the basic tools that are sufficient to use in the first instance with smile analysis and design software. Facial harmony through integration of the smile with the face is based on (Figs 3-6 to 3-8):
- three vertical and three horizontal lines (in frontal view);
- a vertical line, an angle, and a vertical length (in profile).

Macroesthetics defines the relationship between tooth volumes and (Figs 3-9 to 3-12):
- the lips;
- the gingiva;
- the adjacent teeth;
- their axis;
- their length/width ratio;
- their intrinsic form.

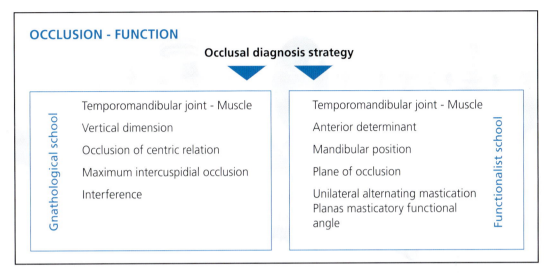

Fig 3-4 The occlusal diagnostic strategy represents the chronology to be followed in the evaluation and correction of occlusal dysfunction.

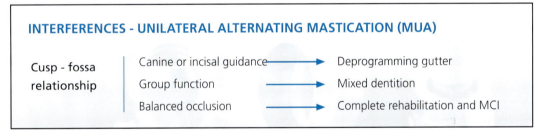

Fig 3-5 Recovery of functional dental relationships according to clinical situations.

Microesthetics is defined by the surface condition of the tooth and its stratification, which determine its visual chromatic rendering based on a priority ratio: brightness, then saturation, then shade. This last element is more concerned with the final prosthetic work carried out by the ceramist. At this stage in producing the provisional models, we limit ourselves to personalized morphological volumes and surface states.

This step enables the creation of a digital model that can be used to produce standard tessellation language (STL) files to:
- create a printed model from which a silicone key can be made to fabricate a mock-up (this option is mainly used for dentoportal restorations with veneers or crowns);
- design a provisional fixed/removable partial denture using CAD/CAM software and then for machining in a PMMA disc (Fig 3-13);
- import an additional file into planning software (an "additional scan" file that can be merged with the patient's STL files) to integrate the future coronal volume into the 3D implant position in accordance with the implant-prosthetic project. This is then referred to as a digital wax-up (Fig 3-14).

The Quokka protocol

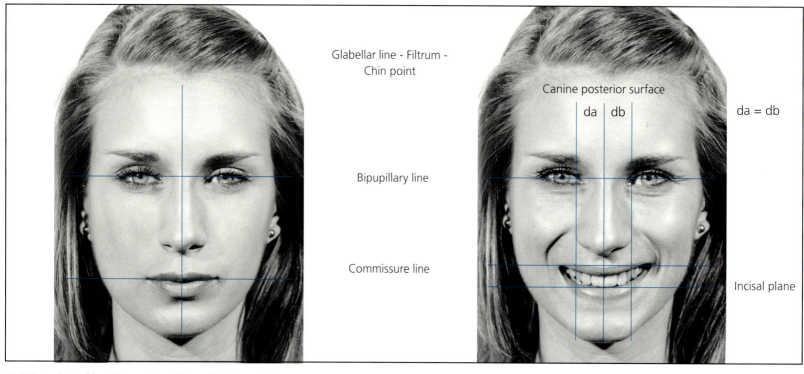

Fig 3-6 Analysis of facial integration of the smile in frontal view.

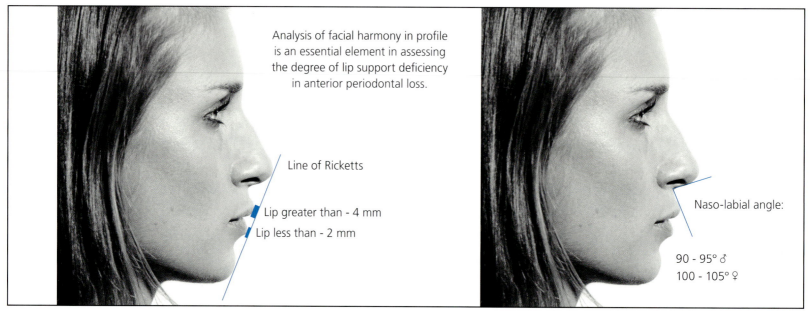

Fig 3-7 Profile analysis of smile integration.

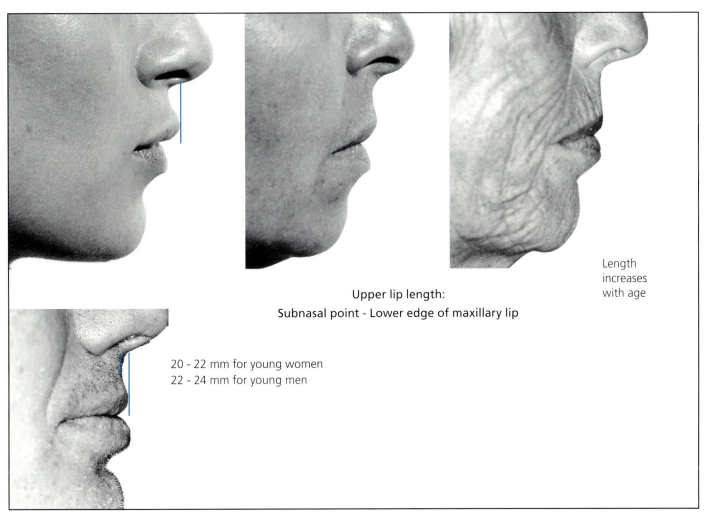

Fig 3-8 Consideration of age and sex criteria in lip support during dental rehabilitations.

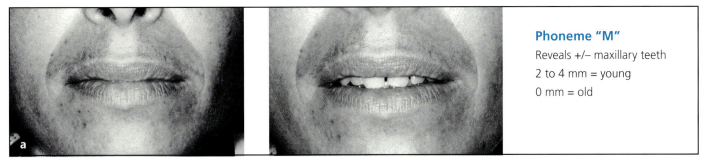

Fig 3-9 a Analysis of length, volume, and tooth–lip axis relationships when articulating the phonemes M.

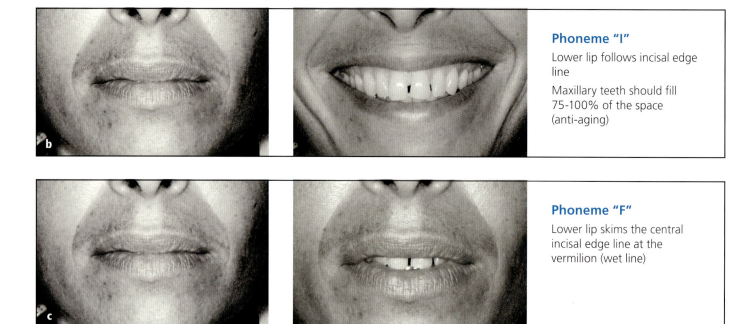

Phoneme "I"

Lower lip follows incisal edge line

Maxillary teeth should fill 75-100% of the space (anti-aging)

Phoneme "F"

Lower lip skims the central incisal edge line at the vermilion (wet line)

Fig 3-9 b and c Analysis of length, volume, and tooth–lip axis relationships when articulating the phonemes I, and F.

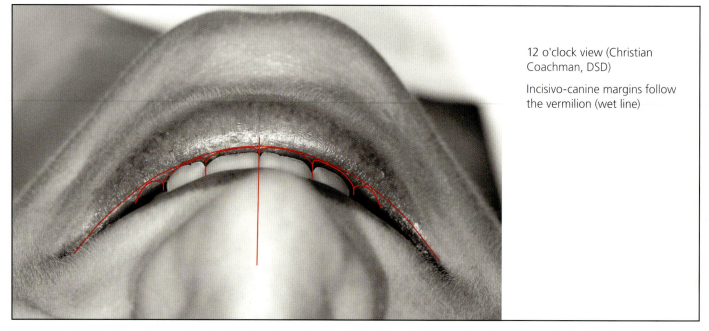

12 o'clock view (Christian Coachman, DSD)

Incisivo-canine margins follow the vermilion (wet line)

Fig 3-10 The 12 o'clock view, introduced by Christian Coachman, allows analysis of the axis of the maxillary incisor group. The incisal edges should follow the vermilion line delimiting the wet lip from the dry lip.

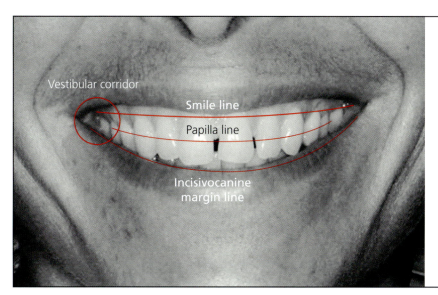

Incisivocanine margin line
The lower lip follows the incisal edge line.
Maxillary teeth should fill 75-100% of the space (anti-aging).

Smile line
Tjian & Miller defined 3 classes: high, medium and low (70% of the population in the medium class). The middle class reveals all maxillary teeth when smiling, following the smile line.

Papilla line
The papilla line follows the papilla points. The height of the papillae is around 40% of the height of the teeth.

Vestibular corridor
The smile line must be filled posteriorly by the dento-gingival volume.

Fig 3-11 Analysis of the relationship of the teeth to the lips, gingival collars, and oral corridors.

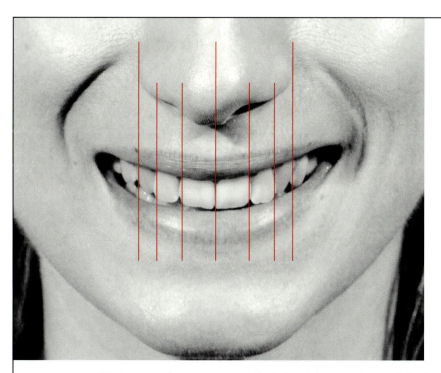
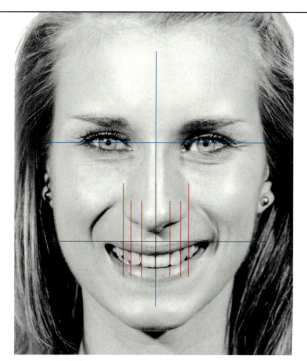

RED proportion: Recurring Esthetic Dental proportion 1 - 0.7 - 0.5. Central incisor proportion: 80% (75 - 85%).

Fig 3-12 The dental proportion to be respected according to the RED ratio by Christian Coachman.

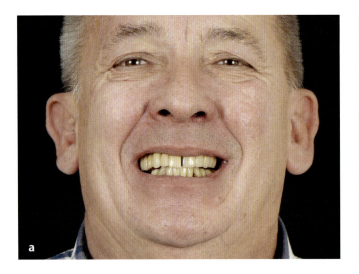
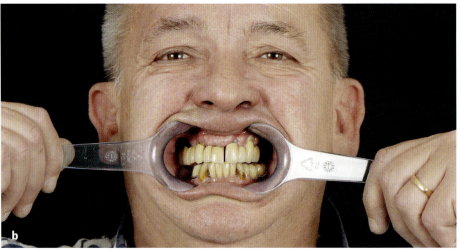
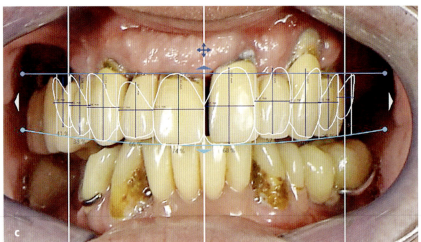
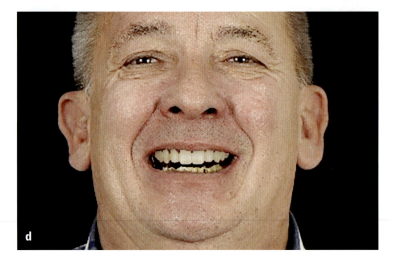
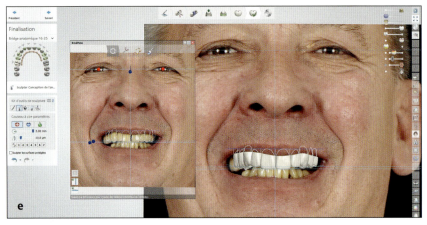

Fig 3-13 a to j *(a and b)* Standardized photos inspired by Digital Smile Design (DSD) by Christian Coachman for esthetic analysis in the 3Shape Trios Smile Design software. *(c)* Elaboration tracing of the new setup integrating the smile line, the RED proportions, and the width and height of each tooth to be reproduced in the CAD/CAM software (Dental System, 3Shape). *(d)* Simulation of the new smile for digital evaluation of the future result. *(e)* Elaboration of the dental assembly in Dental System by Dentitek (Dardilly, France). *(f)* STL file of the bridge elaborated digitally before exporting for machining in a PMMA disk. *(g)* Sizes of the provisionally preserved teeth for the support of the partial denture for validation. *(h)* Partial denture in place with adaptation of the limits with regard to the very provisional function of this partial denture and the future of the teeth. *(i and j)* Frontal and side views of the prosthetic project validated by the patient, both esthetically and functionally.

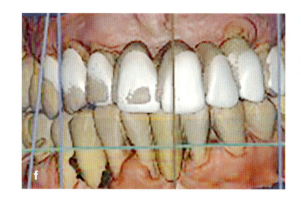
f

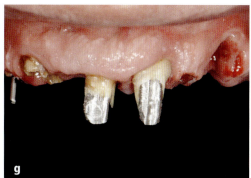
g

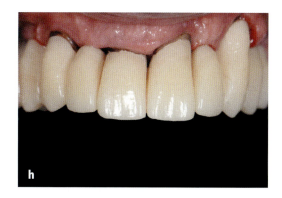
h

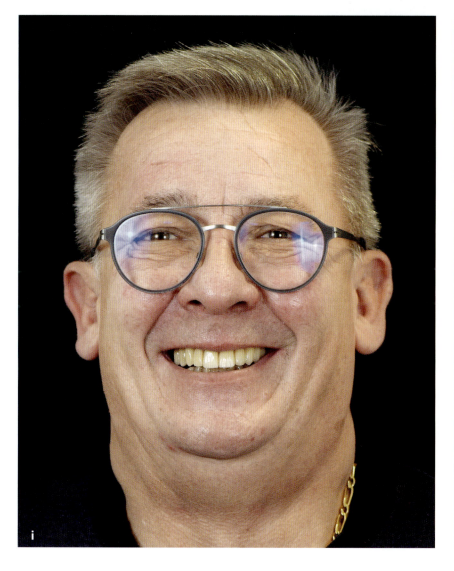
i

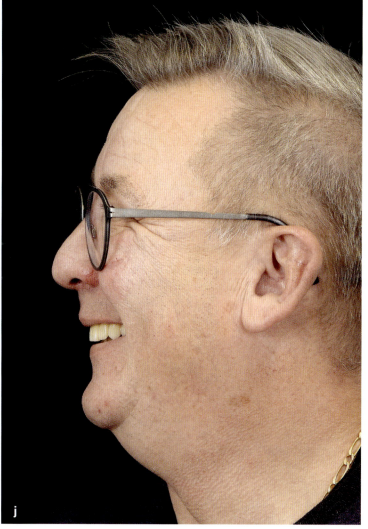
j

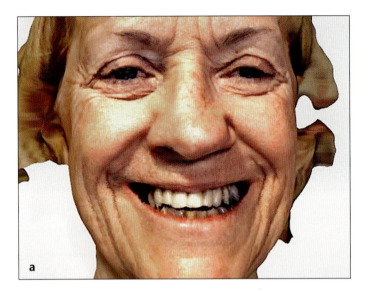
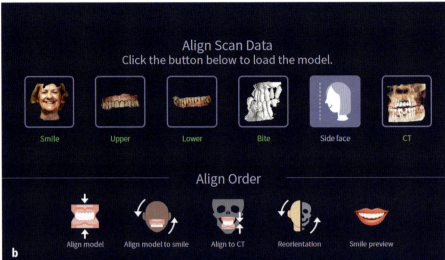
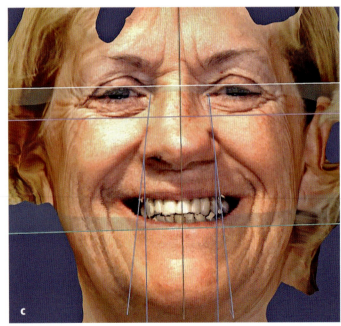
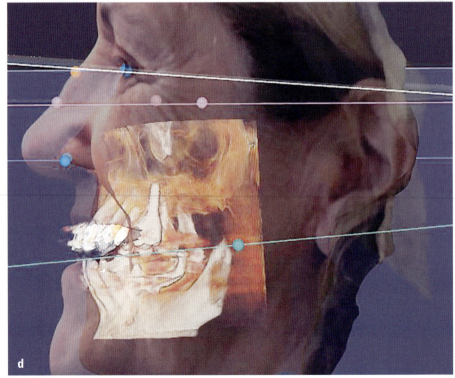

Fig 3-14 a to i *(a)* 3D acquisition of the patient's face using a new modeling tool (RAYFace, Ray Medical). From a near-simultaneous (0.5 seconds) capture of several photos from five angles, the resulting 3D reconstruction provides a model of the patient's face and smile. *(b)* It is then possible to merge the STL files of the dental arches and their bitewings with the DICOM file of the 3D radiological examination through surfacing. *(c)* Once the fusion is complete, reference planes can be drawn, including the Frankfurt, occlusal, sagittal medial, axis-orbital, bipupillary, canine, and other desired planes in order to spatially order the 3D model with respect to these reference reconstruction planes. *(d)* Profile view of the model with the planes and the merged CBCT. *(e)* Elaboration of the smile from a library is then performed in 3D and oriented with the reference planes. *(f)* View of the arch assembly in the STL files without the face layer. *(g)* Profile view with the face layer. *(h)* A useful working window that makes it

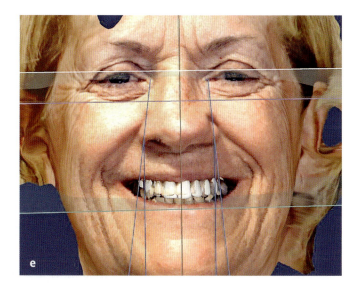
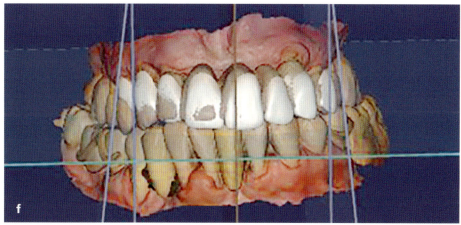
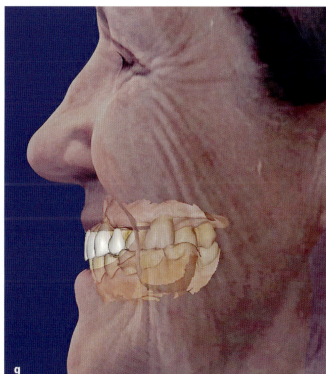
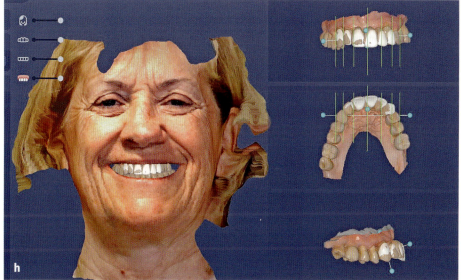
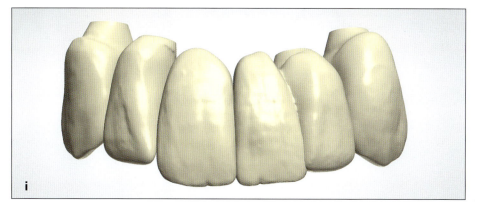

possible to build the virtual wax-up in 3D and check its integration with the patient's face in three dimensions. *(i)* STL file of the instant loading bridge after its elaboration in Dental System after importing the STL file of the assembly made in RAYFace.

Esthetic and functional validation of the removable or fixed partial denture

This is a key element of the Quokka protocol that goes beyond the simple fitting mask, or mock-up, which it can follow or replace. It allows the patient to experience the proposed prosthetic volume and its esthetic and functional result. This concerns pluralistic rehabilitations involving the esthetic zone or complete rehabilitations and relies on roots or teeth to be extracted during implant surgery. The removable/fixed partial denture makes it possible to avoid having to eliminate the removable prosthesis. It is therefore important to study the possible implant options prior to any extraction in order to have a transitional fixed prosthetic solution available even if the patient opts for an implant. We have communicated with dental practitioners in charge of patients in order to avoid extracting any teeth, except in the event of major infection. This has a strong impact on the patient-practitioner relationship: from the second appointment, the patient is in a comfortable situation that is close to the final result. We therefore have a clearly established care contract with the patient and clearly quantified objectives. At the end of this step, we will have identified and corrected the esthetic and occlusal defects. The digital workflow will then allow us to transfer these coronal volumes adapted to the patient's needs throughout the treatment (instant loading fixed/removable partial denture and final partial denture). We will be able to focus on the specific elements of the steps to follow, without questioning the volumes determined initially. This is an intellectual comfort when using a protocol approach. From this point of view, it is of course inappropriate to proceed to implant planning until the project has been validated by the patient. It is also of considerable interest from a medicolegal perspective in that it allows the means used to be justified.

Another advantage of temporary removable/fixed partial denture in esthetically pleasing multiple edentulous teeth and complete restorations is the quality of the radiographs obtained during CBCT. During provisionalization, all metal structures are removed except for any posts that may be useful, in order to prepare the arch for the clearest possible acquisition with the fewest radiographic artifacts (Fig 3-15).

However, there are some situations where a temporary validation removable/fixed partial denture will not be used, namely:

- when the patient wishes to minimize the overall cost in a context with no specific esthetic requirements. The current level of precision of the simulations makes it possible to have a very suitable and often sufficient esthetic result for a patient with no particular demands other than to achieve a balanced standard dental volume (Fig 3-16);
- when it is impossible to place the temporary partial denture due to residual teeth that are too mobile or decayed, especially in cases of multiple missing teeth.

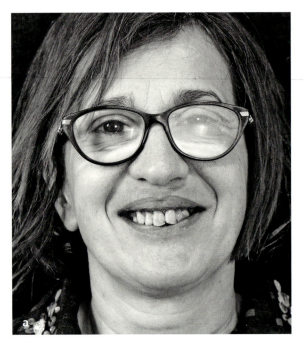
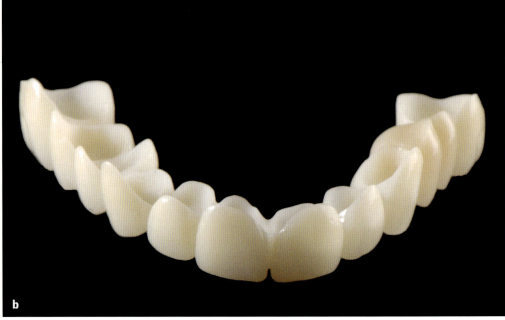

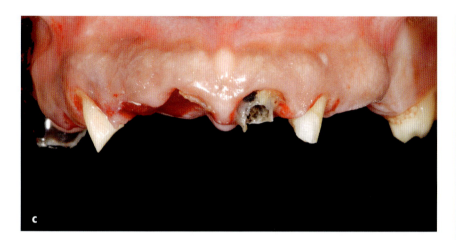

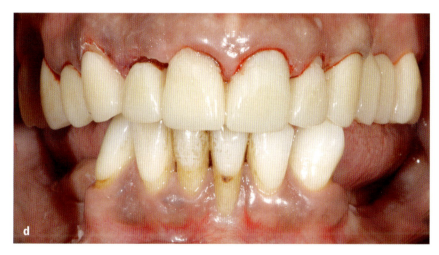

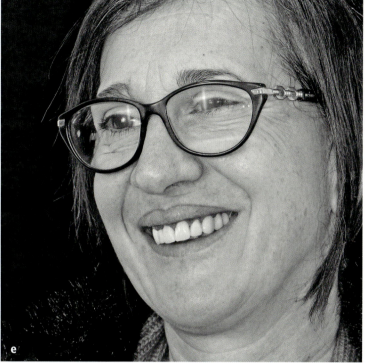

Fig 3-15 a to e *(a)* Situation in the first session during the esthetic analysis. *(b)* Esthetic and functional validation partial denture during the second session. *(c)* Prepared teeth and temporary supports for the validation partial denture. Some teeth that were too decayed were extracted. Most of the metal masses present were removed. *(d)* Partial denture put in place during the second session. *(e)* Situation at the end of the second session validating the prosthetic project and establishing esthetic and functional comfort for the patient.

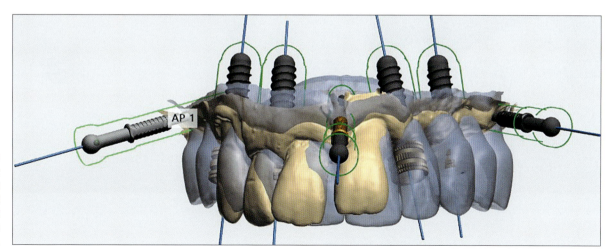

Fig 3-16 Virtual wax-up merged with the STL file of the maxilla for all-on-four planning. As the patient did not make any specific esthetic request, an esthetic and functional validation partial denture was not required. An esthetic analysis, however, was performed to build the virtual wax-up.

Radiographic model

The objective is to transfer the prosthetic project as accurately as possible to the 3D imaging to evaluate the adequacy between the bone volume and prosthetic volume. The STL file of the partial denture for validation, which will be modified or not based on patient feedback, is milled in a radiopaque resin disk. The duplicate of the partial denture thus obtained will be placed in the mouth during an appointment dedicated to recording the information necessary for implant planning. This phase can be combined with placement of the esthetic partial denture for validation to avoid the need for an additional session. The radiopaque partial denture will then need to be rebased in the mouth, as will the partial denture for validation (Fig 3-17). If this step is delayed, extraoral optical impressions of the intrados and extrados will be taken before the partial denture for validation is cemented. This will allow an STL file of the partial denture to be sent and adapted to the natural teeth in the mouth to machine a radiopaque partial denture that will fit with the retained dental supports in an optimal manner, thus avoiding relining (Fig 3-18).

The radiopaque partial denture in place represents the prosthetic project that has been validated by the patient in functional and esthetic terms. This same volume must be recorded in an STL file of the intraoral situation and a DICOM file of the 3D bone situation. It is essential that the position of the partial denture does not change between these two records, as this will allow the files to be merged so the two acquisitions can be superimposed in the planning software. This fusion is facilitated by the absence of coronal metal structures (these were removed during placement of the provisional partial denture) and the replacement of any metal pins with plastic pins when relining the radiopaque partial denture.

This phase may seem tedious, but the ability to connect the partial denture to the titanium bases prior to surgery is linked to a chain of precision from data acquisition to the drilling protocol through the guide. Without this rigor, which we will expand on in the following chapters, it will not be possible to connect the partial denture prior to surgery.

The use of a radiopaque partial denture is essential in certain clinical situations, for example:

- in configurations where the residual teeth have a coronal volume that is too worn to ensure a very accurate overlay of the files. Optimal overlay of STL and DICOM files is key to the workflow;
- in situations where the adequacy between the bone volume and the prosthetic volume is complex due to a reduced bone volume, a challenging prosthetic volume, and high esthetic demand. The presence of a precise 3D radiopaque volume will be a definite qualitative element in the relevance of the planning.

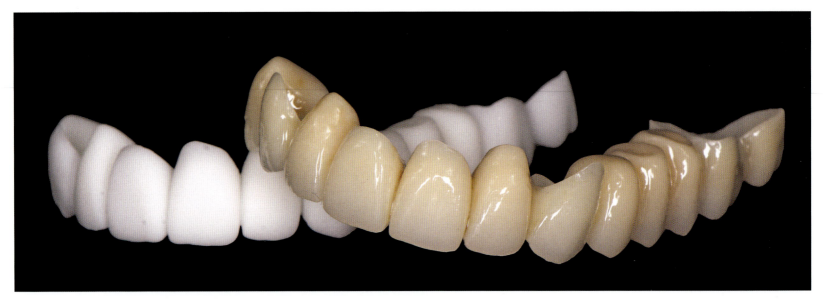

Fig 3-17 The milled esthetic and functional validation partial denture and the milled radiopaque partial denture were delivered to the dental office during the second session. Both partial dentures were relined in the mouth. If a major modification is required to the validation partial denture, both dentures will be modified and milled. An additional session will be necessary. The laboratory cost of the radiopaque partial denture is minimal.

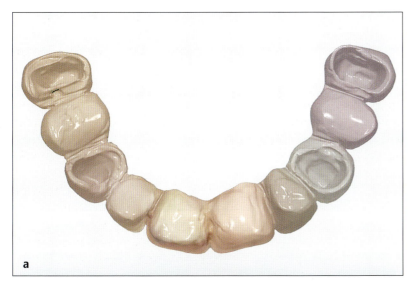
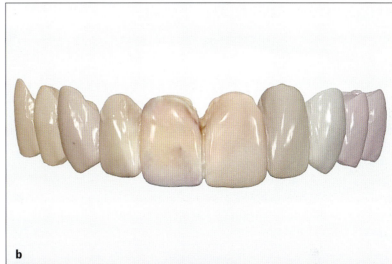
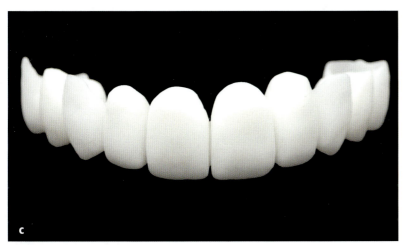
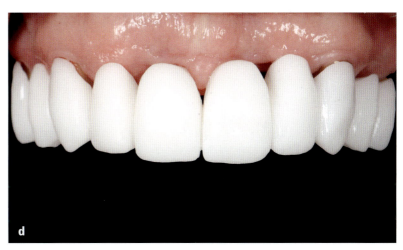

Fig 3-18 a to d *(a and b)* Out-of-mouth acquisitions of the intrados and extrados of the rebased and polished partial denture to generate an STL file that can be directly processed to be sent to the milling machine. *(c)* Receipt of the radiopaque partial denture adapted to the size of the teeth. *(d)* Radiopaque partial denture positioned in the mouth.

However, there are also some clinical situations where a radiopaque partial denture is not essential, for example:

- when only a digital simulation was used to define the implant rehabilitation, as mentioned above;
- when the residual teeth, whether they support the partial denture for validation or not, are large enough to allow fusion with their volume on the DICOM file without artifacts. In this situation, the CBCT examination will be done without the temporary partial denture in place in order to obtain the clearest reading possible. The intraoral scanner record will require a "pre-preparation" file with the provisional partial denture for validation in place in addition to the "preparation" file representing the prepared residual teeth (Fig 3-19);
- partial edentulism;
- unitary edentulism.

The overview in Fig 3-20 shows which approach to use.

The Quokka protocol

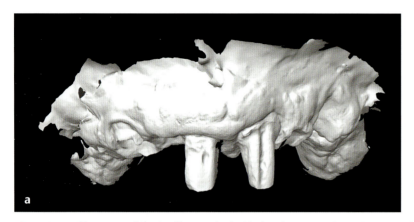
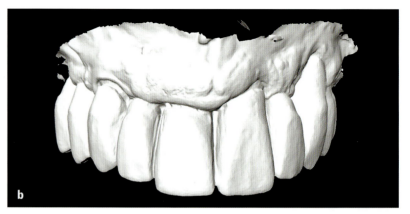

Fig 3-19 a and b Export of the STL files acquired with the Trios scanner in coDiagnostiX: the preparation file (a) on which the planning and surgical guide will be performed in Dental Wings and the so-called "pre-preparation" file (b) that will be merged with the previous file to capture the prosthetic volume during implant planning. This fusion will also take place in the 3Shape ecosystem during the preparation of the instant loading partial denture to reproduce the partial denture validated by the patient. The preparation file will then show the implants.

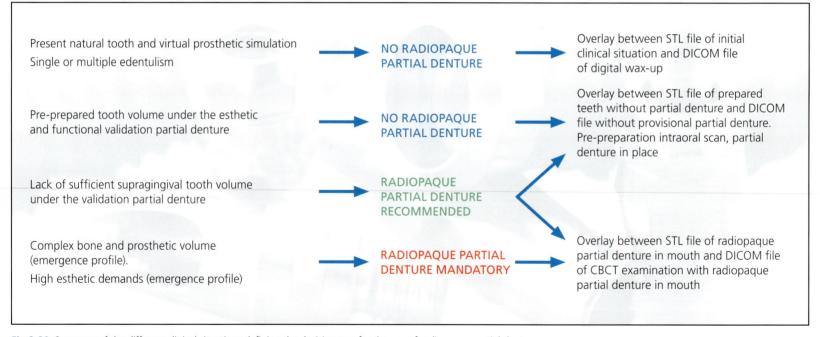

Fig 3-20 Summary of the different clinical situations defining the decision tree for the use of radiopaque partial dentures.

Implant-prosthetic planning

This is the truly innovative step in guided surgery and optical impressions that requires specific training so it can be incorporated into the digital workflow. It involves merging the biologic rules of implant placement with the biomechanical considerations of the prosthesis. It is not about increasing the amount of time spent on a case, as is often claimed by detractors of the digital workflow; it simply involves displacing the time spent thinking about implant positioning during the preoperative period, with greater ease and precision. No time is lost or wasted: on the contrary, there is an overall time saving for a more suitable result. The operating time freed up enables us to focus on what we consider to be the real added value of implant treatment, namely the management of hard and soft tissues. This is another way of approaching implant surgery. In terms of the net amount of time spent on this step, it is by no means time-consuming, but undeniably valuable in terms of implant positioning.

It involves the use of implant planning software that requires the integration of STL files from digital impressions of the maxilla and the occlusal relationship taken using intraoral scanners, as well as DICOM files acquired from 3D radiographic images (CBCT, computed tomography [CT] scans). We use Implant Studio and coDiagnostiX, as mentioned earlier. The principle behind both types of software is the same; it is based on superposition of the two files by surface recognition. This step is essential because it defines the accuracy of the modeling based on the accuracy of the relationship between the two files. We use a colorimetric scale in Implant Studio to adapt the two files to control the level of precision obtained. In this context, it is useful to employ a radiopaque partial denture that will enable optimal merging of the two files. We obtain a 3D model of the patient's bone, gingival, and dental structures (Figs 3-21 and 3-22).

On this model, we can appreciate the relations between the gingiva, mucous membranes, teeth, and bone. We can extract teeth virtually and position implants and virtual teeth based on an adapted prosthetic project and apply the rules of 3D positioning of the implant precisely, in correlation with the optimal prosthetic volume. This makes it possible to identify the prosthetic or bone limits and make the necessary corrections (GBR, guided tissue regeneration [GTR], prosthetic screw axis) (Fig 3-23).

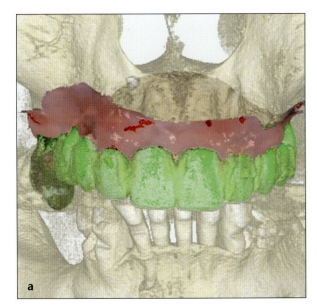
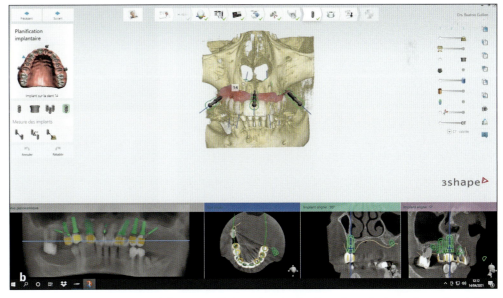

Fig 3-21 a and b Merging the STL file of the arch with the radiopaque partial denture in the mouth and the DICOM file in Implant Studio. The color scale shows the quality of the fusion. The green color represents a deviation of 0 mm. Its uniformity across the whole partial denture shows optimal fusion. Such uniformity of the fusion scale is only possible with the radiopaque partial denture. In the planning phase (b), the gingival and dental bone structures are read together.

The Quokka protocol

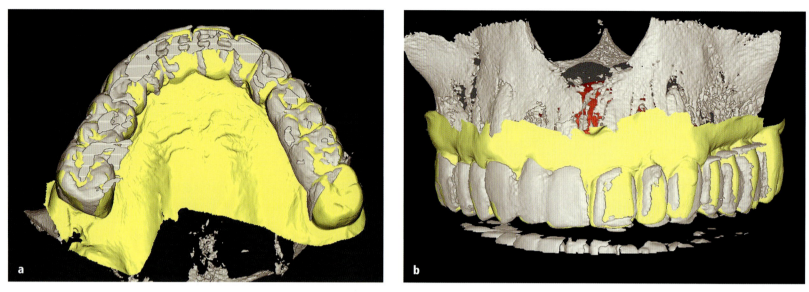

Fig 3-22 a and b   A similar principle shown in coDiagnostiX. There is no colorimetric fusion control scale, but effective manual validation.

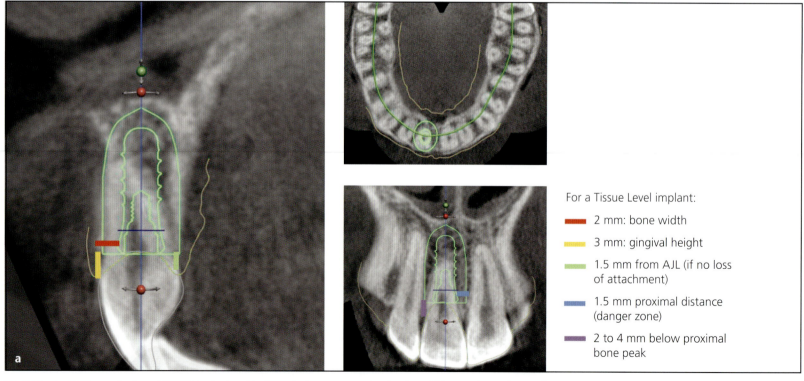

For a Tissue Level implant:

- 2 mm: bone width
- 3 mm: gingival height
- 1.5 mm from AJL (if no loss of attachment)
- 1.5 mm proximal distance (danger zone)
- 2 to 4 mm below proximal bone peak

Fig 3-23 a to d   The application of the 3D implant positioning rules is concrete and makes it possible to evaluate the correlation with the prosthetic and periodontal volume so the need for peri-implant GBR can be established in advance and the type of prosthesis required in terms of connection (cemented or screw-retained) can be defined.

Chapter 3 - Presentation of the Quokka protocol

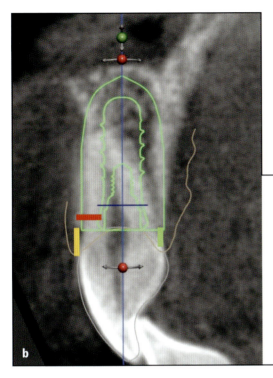

The software we use has various functions and allows us to work with the different files together or separately, and to measure lengths, angles, and interimplant and crown to implant ratio. It is easy to understand that the precision of the measurements is closely linked to the precision of the fusion of the bone and buccal files. After this unitary, plural, or complete planning, we can proceed to fabricate the surgical guide within the same workflow.

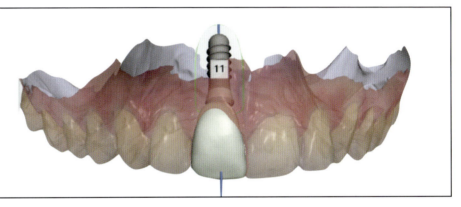

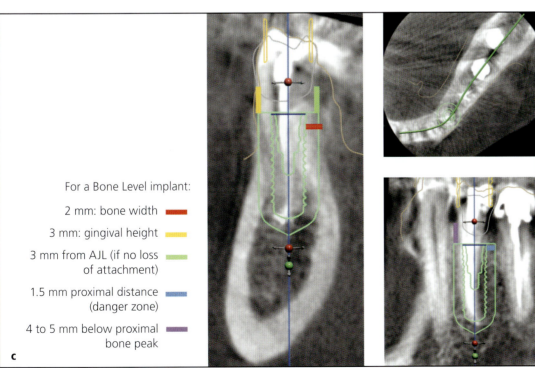

For a Bone Level implant:

- 2 mm: bone width
- 3 mm: gingival height
- 3 mm from AJL (if no loss of attachment)
- 1.5 mm proximal distance (danger zone)
- 4 to 5 mm below proximal bone peak

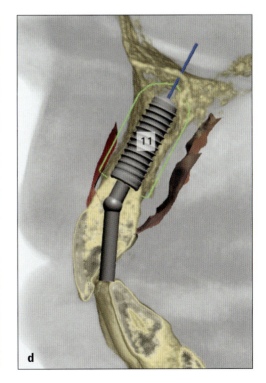

The surgical guide

The surgical guide is the key factor but also the vulnerable variable in the digital workflow. It is the tool used to transfer data from the plan to the surgical site. Any error in the development of the guide or its use will result in an error in the implant positioning and therefore our ability to place the crown or partial denture for immediate loading connected to the abutments before surgery. Thus, a design and development procedure that allows for accurate and consistent transfer of planning data is required. Tooth-supported guides are preferred because they are the most accurate and the literature is clear on this point; however, we have treated completely edentulous arches successfully using the principle of immediate loading. Nevertheless, teeth support is the reference and remains easier to approach than total mucosal support, however it is not always possible. The surgical guide is responsible for allowing the transfer of data to enable immediate loading to occur. At present, the development and accuracy of software and some guided surgery kits are sufficient to standardize immediate loading. As such, everything is based on the transfer of the surgical guide to the mouth. A number of conditions must be adhered to when designing the guide (Figs 3-24 and 3-25), for example:

- the sleeves, linked to the implant system used, are selected while designing the guide in the planning software. They must allow total guidance, i.e., from the start of drilling to implant placement in guided surgery, and should not be substituted for other generic sockets. Their stability in the guide is at stake during drilling.
- When designing the guide, it is crucial to ensure that the sleeves will not interfere with a mucosal support that we have not planned to elevate during surgery;
- the adaptation control windows, at least three (tripod), will make it possible to judge the quality of the adaptation of the guide;
- A cross arch bar ensures the guide resists deformation during drilling;
- Rotational marking on the resin in front of the sleeves is delivered in the planning software. This is essential for single-unit or two-stage multilevel restorations with an intermediate angled abutment;
- transverse stabilizing pins can be added to the guide if the dental supports are insufficient.

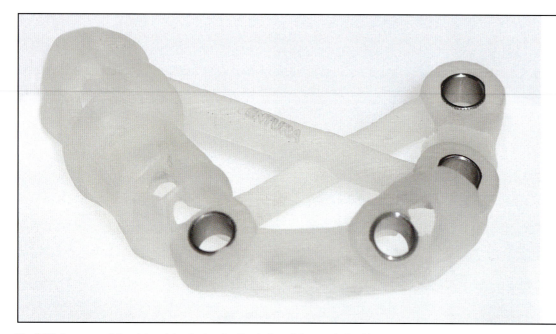

The surgical guide

Precise, consistent transfer of planning data

- Choice of sockets linked to the implant system used
- Sleeve stability
- Fitting control windows
- Through-bars for rigidity
- Tripod dental support
- No interference of sleeves with mucosa
- Rotational marker if MRI/MCI
- 3D printing quality

Fig 3-24 Summary of the determining factors for the design of the surgical guide.

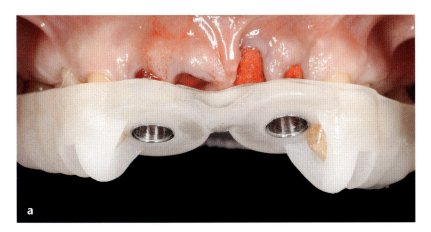
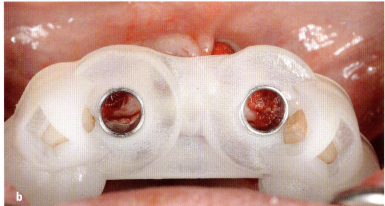
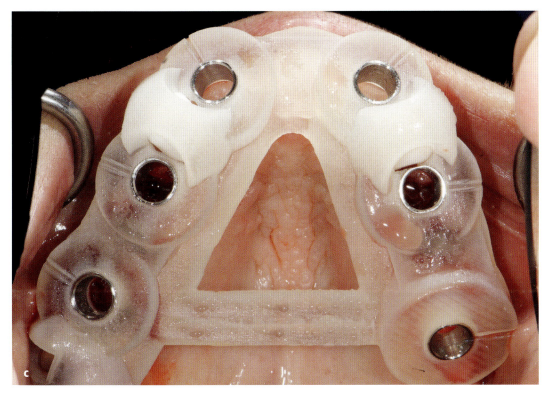

Fig 3-25 a to c Typical drawing of the guide with tripod adaptation control windows and through and side reinforcement to reinforce the rigidity of the guide.

The supports for the guide will depend on the files used to merge with the radiologic images during planning. If a radiopaque partial denture is used, the guide will be supported by the radiopaque teeth of the partial denture, chosen as supports during the planification. If the planning file shows the situation of the present natural teeth or natural stumps, the guide will be made to support these elements.

After validation, the guide is exported as an STL file for printing or machining. Traditionally, resin guides are printed. 3D printing is also a key but variable element of the workflow. The planning software and impressions offer a high level of precision. The accuracy of 3D printers, on the other hand, is heavily dependent on the printer used, the mixing of the resins and the post-treatment of the printed resins. Dental practitioners are very concerned about the reliability of intraoral scanners, but do not pay much attention to the printing procedures used. An analogy can be made with photography. No matter how talented the professional is and how good the camera may be, the quality of the print will be poor if it is printed on an entry-level inkjet machine. The same is true for surgical guide prints. Adjustment of the printing parameters calibrated by targeted tests will help to obtain optimal fit of the guide on the teeth and adequate adaptability of the sleeves for optimal positioning and bonding. In our practice, the printing line for guides and single provisional teeth consists of (Fig 3-26):

- resin stirring rollers;
- a NextDent 5100 printer (Soesterberg, The Netherlands);
- a RAYDENT Studio printer (water-washable resin);
- a post-press isopropyl rinse machine (SpringRay);
- a light-curing unit.

The quality of post-treatment, i.e., cleaning of the resins prior to polymerization, is key to the quality of the adaptation. Suboptimal cleaning will result in polymerization of excess resin from the tray, which may disturb the adaptation of the guide on the teeth or of the sleeve in its housing.

These steps are often carried out in the prosthesis laboratory; however, practitioners must be familiar with them so they can discuss them and control the production line.

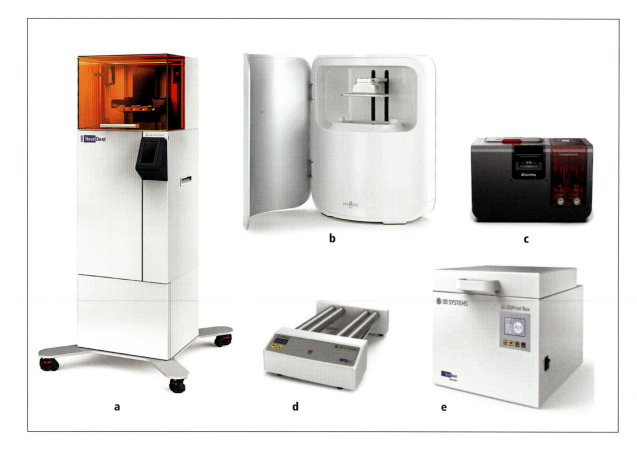

Fig 3-26 a to e *(a)* NextDent 5100 printer in the office for printing surgical guides, single provisional teeth and deprogramming trays. *(b)* In-office integration of Ray Medical's 3D printer with water-washable resins into the chairside chain to facilitate the post-treatment process. *(c)* Automated isopropanol washing of prints simplifies post-processing of resin prints on the NextDent 5100. *(d)* Resin stirring rollers, which are essential before printing to ensure optimal quality. *(e)* Light-curing unit after printing and resin cleaning.

Guided surgery and immediate loading

This is the most disruptive phase of the Quokka protocol. It leads to the insertion of the immediate loading prosthesis during surgery. We distinguish five distinct chronological steps:
- preparation and insertion of the guide;
- drilling and guided implant placement;
- bone preparation and placement of the screwed prosthesis;
- periodontal reconstruction guided by the prosthesis;
- placement of sutures guided by the prosthesis.

Preparation and insertion of the guide

The first step is to extract the teeth involved in the implant placement procedure (immediate implantation) for multiple and single cases, and to check the fit of the guide on the supporting teeth via the selected inspection windows, as well as its stability and fit (Fig 3-27). For full or long multiple-unit cases, the provisional partial denture for validation is removed and, in addition to the extractions performed during its placement, extraction of the teeth involved in the implant sites is performed. Only the guide teeth selected during planning of the guide are retained. If planning was done with a radiopaque partial denture, the radiopaque support teeth, isolated from the partial denture, must be cemented in the mouth (Fig 3-28).

Drilling and guided implant placement

Like implant drilling, guided surgery is brand dependent. There are many different systems, associated with different drilling sequences, settings, and adjustment variables. Not all systems allow for guided drilling over the entire sequence,

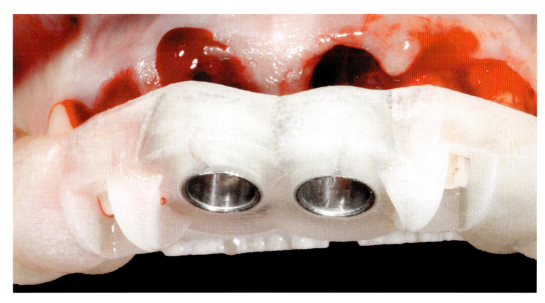

Fig 3-27 Guide placement after extraction of 11 and 21. Note the adaptation control windows at 12 and 22, confirming optimal seating of the guide and the two marks opposite the sockets for rotational positioning of the implant.

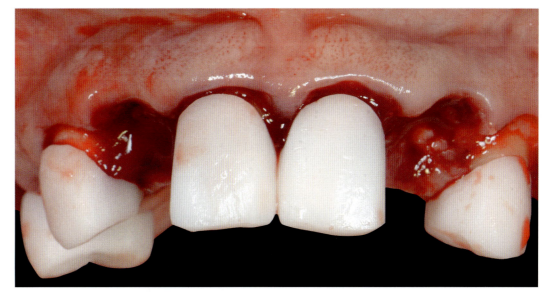

Fig 3-28 Radiopaque teeth supporting the surgical guide, separated from the partial denture and cemented in the mouth after the extractions at the beginning of surgery. They enable seating of the guide according to the configuration in which the guide has been designed.

let alone guided implant placement. It is not possible to obtain the required level of precision without a system that allows guidance over all the drilling and placement stages. Moreover, one may question the need for only partial guidance after precise planning has been carried out using software. The advantage, not to mention the possibility of immediate loading, seems to us to be as partial as the guidance.

We have been using the Straumann guided surgery kit for 6 years, initially with tissue-level (TL) and bone-level (BL) implants, and for the past 18 months with the tapered tissue-level (TLX) and tapered bone-level (BLX) series (Fig 3-29). The guidance is complete, from preparation for the impact of the drill with a flat bur to calibration of the implant bed with a pilot drill and preparation drills, finishing of the site with a profile bur and tap, and finally placement of the implant with precise rotational and vertical registration. No sequence is performed freehand. The guidance is done by means of drill handles, with an inner diameter in accordance with the drill diameter to be used and an outer diameter in accordance with the inner diameter of the guide sleeve present in the guide. This allows the preparation drill to be guided along its entire length. Its design therefore allows for:

- **guided** drilling through the sockets **throughout the** protocol;
- **guided** implant placement;
- management of the precise **vertical positioning** of the implant;
- management of the precise **rotational positioning** of the implant;
- use of a combination of drill lengths to enable placement of implants of different lengths.

We will refer to the **guided length of the drill** as the key principle of guided surgery. This is the distance between the drill stop on the upper part of the sleeve and the tip of the drill. The lower limit represents the apical limit of the future implant.

Four parameters are used to define the guided length of the drill:
- length of the chosen implant: variable from 4 to 16 mm;
- distance between the socket and the bone crest: variable, adaptable in three positions (2, 4, 6 mm);
- height of the sleeve: variable, 5 mm;
- reduction height of the drilling handle (−1 or −3 mm).

The choice of guided drilling length (GDL) is made using the following formula:
GDL = Implant length + Sleeve position + Sleeve height (5 mm) − Drill handle height (Fig 3-30).
Implant Studio and coDiagnostiX software define the drills and handle to be used based on the position of the sleeve. A drilling protocol is generated, it includes the sequences to be performed for each implant.

Depending on the bone density, implant bed preparation can be refined through flaring, coronal widening, and tapping, which will also be guided in accordance with a clinical protocol delivered by the planning software. As such, everything is organized to free up time during the surgical phase for drilling and implant positioning in order to focus on periodontal reconstruction and prosthesis management. The time dedicated to implant placement, and therefore the duration of surgery for the patient, is greatly reduced, and the quality of positioning is superior.

In this specific context, it is easy to understand that the only variable that can alter the positioning of the implant defined during planning is the reliability of the guide. The manufacturing criteria for the guide (thickness, rigidity, precision and stability of support on the teeth, bonding of the sleeves) were mentioned earlier.

During surgery, the main idea is to keep the guide completely passive during drilling. At no point should any stress be exerted that could modify its seating or deform it. If this happens, the implant positioning will be altered, and therefore the ability to achieve immediate loading will be compromised. For a single case, the consequence will be a modified position of the tooth in relation to the design, and for a multiple or complete case, it will be impossible to screw the partial denture onto the implants. This involves **passive drilling for the guide** through the drill handle placed in the socket. We have identified the key factors to be controlled during the preparation sequences and make the following recommendations:

- do not exert any pressure on the guide during drilling (especially with the drill handle);
- do not force the drill stop to rest on the sleeve;
- use the flat drill for guided flattening of the bone crest to allow the pilot drill to start with its penetration axis in an orthogonal position. This step is essential in immediate implantation to create a flat zone on the palatal or lingual alveolar walls, a source of deviation generated by the cortical bone;
- remove any dense bone edges (often the palatal or lingual wall) that could deflect the drill or implant from its path. There must be a circle with a diameter of 4.5 mm and no deviating slopes;
- perform coronal preparation and flaring of the implant bed regardless of bone density to passivate the implants;
- control the parallelism of the H2, H4, and H6 marks present on the guided implant gripper with the edge of the sleeve. This has become essential with the design of the TLX and BLX ranges, as the aggressive coil design of these implants means they are more likely to modify their insertion trajectory based on bone density;
- ensure the accuracy of the vertical limit on the lower edge of the guided implant gripper line corresponding to the chosen height H. The use of optical aids (magnification and light) helps to secure and reproduce the correct vertical stop position on the edge of the sleeve;

Chapter 3 - Presentation of the Quokka protocol

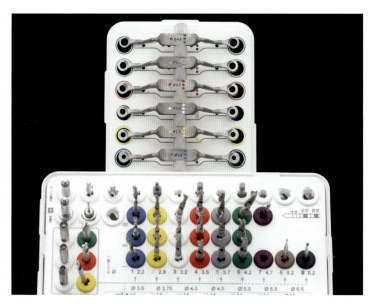

Fig 3-29 Straumann guided surgery kit for TLX and BLX implants, adapted to our daily practice.

Fig 3-30 a to e *(a)* Implant drill from the guided surgery kit in three lengths for each diameter identified by a color code and the presence of a stop that rests on the sleeve. *(b)* Drill handle with the two heights of reduction of the drilling length. *(c)* The three possible vertical positions of the sockets defined during the implant planning stage. *(d)* The combinations of the three determinants of the guided drilling length for implant lengths from 4 to 16 mm. *(e)* Coronal widening protocol according to implant lengths. A complete summary of the drilling sequences, implant by implant, is edited by the software in a detailed drilling protocol.

Drill name	Guided length	Total length	Drill length pictogram
Short	16 mm	34 mm	—
Medium	20 mm	38 mm	=
Long	24 mm	42 mm	≡

a

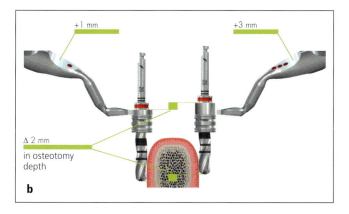

b

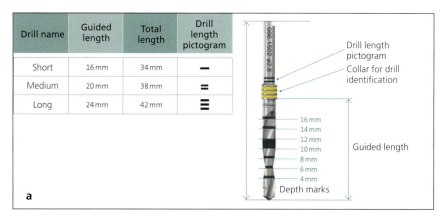

3 PARAMETERS:
- Implant length
- Distance sleeve - bone crest
- Sleeve height

$$L + D + H = \text{guided drilling length}$$

c

Implant length	4 mm	6 mm	8 mm	10 mm	12 mm	14 mm	16 mm
H2, 2 mm		Short drill — + 3 handles •••	Short drill — + 1 handle •	Medium drill = + 3 handles •••	Medium drill = + 1 handle •	Long drill ≡ + 3 handles •••	Long drill ≡ + 1 handle •
H4, 4 mm	Short drill — + 3 handles •••	Short drill — + 1 handle •	Medium drill = + 3 handles •••	Medium drill = + 1 handle •	Long drill ≡ + 3 handles •••	Long drill ≡ + 1 handle •	
H6, 6 mm	Short drill — + 1 handle •	Medium drill = + 3 handles •••	Medium drill = + 1 handle •	Long drill ≡ + 3 handles •••	Long drill ≡ + 1 handle •		

d

Implant length	Coronal widening 6-8 mm	Coronal widening implant 10-18 mm
H2, 2 mm		Short drill — + 3 handles •••
H4, 4 mm	Short drill — + 3 handles •••	Short drill — + 1 handle •
H6, 6 mm	Short drill — + 1 handle •	Medium drill = + 3 handles •••

e

- ensure the accuracy of rotational registration of the guided implant gripper (gripper point opposite the mark on the guide) to the correct vertical position when placing single teeth or using angled abutments (Fig 3-31).

The ease of removal of the implant gripper is a good indicator of passive drilling and positioning of the implant through the guide.

Bone preparation and placement of the screw-retained prosthesis

Once the implant(s) are placed, the guide can be removed and we can proceed to the prosthetic stage of Quokka surgery, i.e., immediate loading.

Implant and pontic emergence profiles were designed in relation to an esthetic and functional objective defined during fitting of the partial denture for validation. The final prosthesis is guiding the project and must be integrated into an adequate periodontal volume during bone and gingival reconstruction. Positioning the prosthesis during surgery therefore offers a real advantage as it becomes a useful guide for reconstruction. The design of the pontics for the removable/fixed partial denture is such that they will deliberately penetrate the soft tissues to generate pseudopapillae for esthetic purposes by the vestibular and proximal height differential. Based on our experience, we have defined subgingival lengths of ovoid pontics whose apex is aligned with the adjacent implant platforms to induce artificially scalloped gingiva. At the same time, 3D positioning in immediate implantation, guided by the architecture of the tooth to be replaced, requires a more apical and palatal position in the extraction sites. This may generate peripheral bone beaks around the connection platform. It is therefore important to check the bone relief around the pontic and implant emergence areas before positioning the crown or removable/fixed partial denture to avoid interference with placement of the prosthesis.

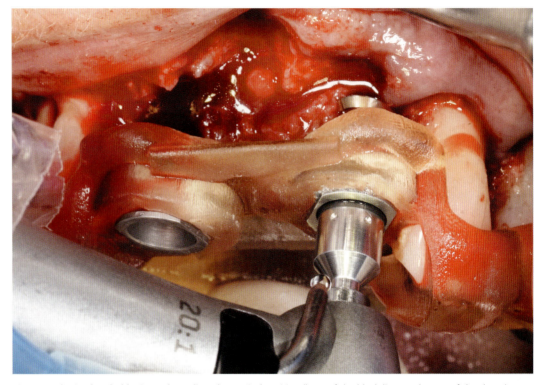

Fig 3-31 The implant holder is used to adjust the vertical position (base of the black line on the top of the sleeve) and the rotational position of the implant (point in front of the mark on the guide resin).

These areas may be either extraction sites or solid bone areas. Attention must be paid to the palatal bone wall and the proximal bone peaks, which may need to be remodeled. The aim is not to flatten the bone, as it is far too precious, but to scallop the bone relief around the implant emergences and pontic volumes to obtain a scalloped gingival contour. For BL and BLX implants, convenient touch-up drills with three flaring diameters can be used (Fig 3-32).

Once this phase has been validated, the crown or partial denture can be inserted for instant loading. For a single tooth, the procedure is very simple and the result highly reliable. For a multiple or full partial denture, the procedure may seem too variable, but our experience has shown it to be reliable. It is based on three factors:

- the viscoelastic properties of the bone. The indispensable passivity of the prosthesis on osseointegrated implants should not be confused with its relative passivity on implants that have just been inserted into alveolar bone, often in immediate implantation;
- the deformation capacity of the PMMA resin even when milled;
- the guided drilling protocol that generates less deviations than the cumulative deformation envelope of the bone and resin.

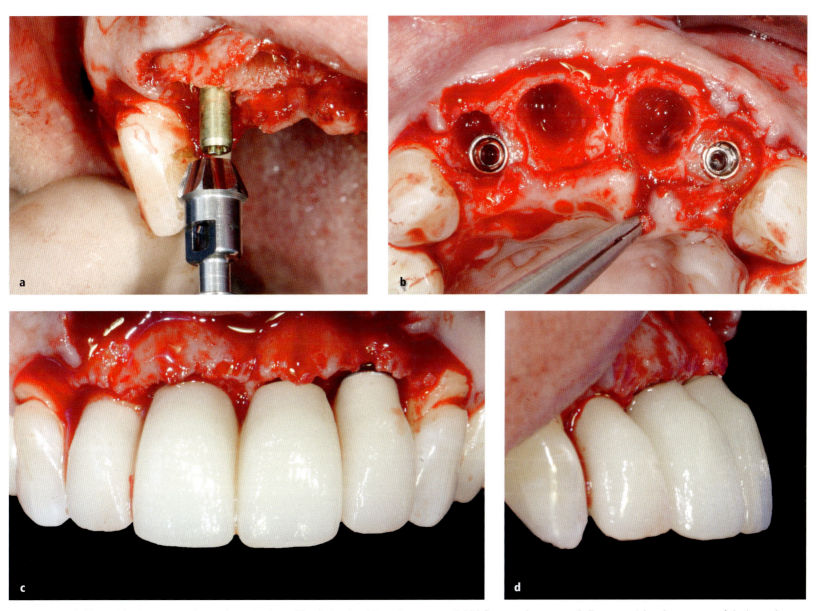

Fig 3-32 a to d *(a)* A guide pin is screwed onto the BL implant. *(b)* A flaring bur (three diameters available) fits onto the stem and allows a peripheral osteotomy of the bone that may interfere with the seating of the titanium baseplate on the implant neck. *(c)* Instant loading partial denture in an optimal position with a pontic design that matches the alveolar bone for an esthetic pontic bed. *(d)* Profile view. Note the matching of the emergence profiles to the bone profiles.

The crowns or partial dentures are then screwed in. The adaptation of the titanium bases on the implants is checked with direct vision, which is made possible by raising flaps. The prosthesis is then blocked at 35 Ncm if the bone density allows it (single tooth) to prevent any loosening during the osseointegration phase.

The objective of this book is to eradicate doubts about the reliability of immediate loading. The main obstacle experienced by dental practitioners is the difficulty of inserting a prosthesis connected to titanium bases before surgery on newly placed implants. The numerous clinical cases to follow largely overcome this obstacle. The second obstacle is the fact that this approach is not 100% successful. We are always surprised by the need to have 100% certainty, or at least reliability, with this protocol in order for it to be included as a treatment option, despite the fact that for all the procedures we use, particularly in implant surgery, 100% reliability does not exist. This is a professional requirement for digital technology. Failures are possible, just as they are with immediate implantation, immediate loading, GBR, bone grafts, or gingival grafts, but what are these failures, and what should be done when they occur? Our clinical experience allows us to list the potential failures that we may face. They may be inherent to immediate implantation or immediate loading.

Immediate implantation

Inherent failures in immediate implantation involve:
- insufficient implant stability to be left in situ or loaded due to an error in the planning protocol, the choice of bone anchorage, or the indication for immediate implantation;
- the impossibility of tightening the prosthesis due to a lack of resistance to the torque of the implant placed, due to an error in the drilling sequence in relation to the available bone site (over-drilling).

Immediate loading

Inherent failures of immediate loading involve too great a deviation of one or more implants from the prosthesis as a result of an error due to a constraint on the guide, suboptimal surfacing in the planning software, or a poor-quality or retouched radiographic image (cleaning of artifacts).

The solutions are as follows:
- for a complete denture: the implant may not be connected to the denture
- for a single tooth: the tooth morphology can be modified by adding or removing resin and polishing as in the more traditional immediate loading procedures;
- for a plural or complete denture: the denture can be sectioned with a resin disk and repaired in a passive position, ideally with a metal reinforcement.

We have treated and followed up around 200 patients, using solutions from single units to complete dentures. With the exception of two patients (complete denture), all of them left with the provisional prosthesis in place following an immediate loading procedure, i.e., having been placed before the flaps were sutured, with or without all the implants loaded. With regard to the two failures, the dentate patient left with his esthetic and functional validation partial denture cemented to the guide teeth and the implants not loaded, and the other patient, who was edentulous, left with his complete removable prosthesis that he had had already and with the implants placed but not loaded.

Prosthesis-guided periodontal reconstruction

Reconstruction techniques and a decision tree were presented in Chapter 1. In the second part of the book, the different reconstruction situations will be illustrated through clinical cases. In this chapter, we seek to emphasize use of the prosthesis as a volumetric guide for GBR and the conjunctive graft in addition to immediate implant placement. The desired final tooth volume is the best possible guide; thus, the extent of the reconstruction must be designed in view of the optimal emergence profile. Although the decision tree for choosing GBR or a connective graft is based on biologic rules, the volume of these reconstructions is based on a precise prosthetic objective. Our specifications are underpinned by several criteria (Fig 3-33):

- the extraction gap must be completely filled around the implants and at the extraction sites where no implants are placed;
- the desired bone volume must be in line with the designed prosthetic emergence profile. GBR should overcorrect this volume by 1 mm. A minimum thickness of 2 mm is required;
- vertically, GBR must be overcorrected in the concave profile of the provisional tooth and stabilized by the horizontal projection of the coronal base of the implant emergence profile;
- the proximal bone festoon must be reconstructed within the limits of the proximal bone peaks;
- the gingival tissue must be at least 2 mm thick in the 4-mm coronal area;
- the presence of 3 mm keratinized gingiva at the neck of the prosthetic reconstruction must be ensured.

Sutures guided by the prosthesis

Sutures are even more essential in this type of surgery than others. It is also vital to protect GBR, which is crucial in immediate implantation, tighten the emergence profiles of the prosthetic teeth that are present, and stabilize the blood clot for rapid and controlled healing. At the same time, to create deep pontic beds, secondary intention healing must be induced around the subgingival prosthetic profile. The prosthesis will therefore help to protect the site. Over the years, we have made progress in developing a suture that is better able to meet all these objectives. We now use a modified version of

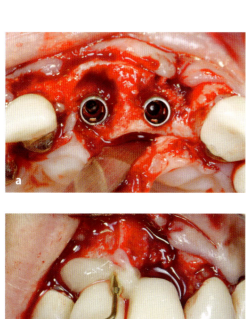
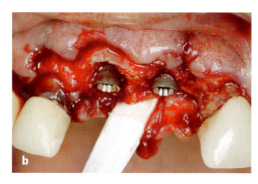
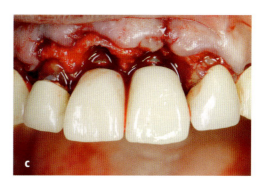
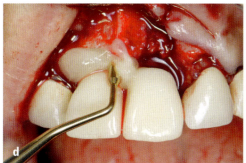
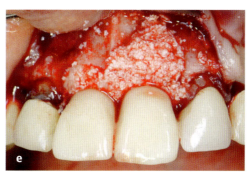
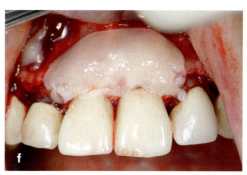
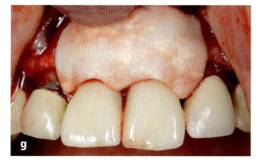
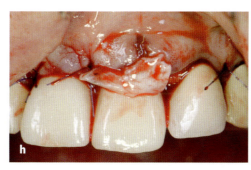
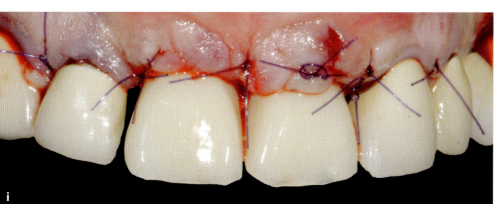

Fig 3-33 a to i *(a)* Two BL immediate loaded implants in the maxillary central incisor sites illustrating the hiatuses of the extraction sites.
(b) Frontal view with buccal and proximal dehiscence present in 21.
(c) The two immediate loaded provisional teeth in place serve as a guide for reconstruction.
(d) Filling of the hiatuses with PRGF and autogenous drill bone at the bottom of the alveolus.
(e) Placement of composite graft, consisting of deproteinized bovine bone mineral (Bio-Oss, Geistlich) incubated in PRGF phase 2. Note the proximal and vestibular overcorrections to follow the subgingival prosthetic contour, guiding the future implant emergence profile.
(f) Covering with fibrin membrane from phase 1 plasma.
(g) Covering with a resorbable collagen membrane (Bio-Gide, Geistlich).
(h) Harvesting of a tuberous connective graft to thicken the vestibular flap at the neck of 21.
(i) ASAF sutures associated with a horizontal mattress suture in 21, stabilizing the connective graft against the vestibular flap.

the SAT ("Sling and Tag") suture by anchoring the first pass palatally around the tooth and suspending around the palatal aspect of the tooth. The entries are distal to the bases of the papillae and the exits mesial to the base of the same papillae. We call this the anchored and suspended advanced flap (ASAF) suture. The mechanical resultant allows the flap to rise toward the center of the collar in a coronal direction, which results in protection of GBR and vestibular and proximal plating of the flap in a coronary direction on the prosthesis emergence profile. The sutures are made from resorbable 6/0 thread. The milled surface of the subgingival resins, the plated sutures, the use of plasma rich in growth fiber (PRGF), and the short duration of the surgery to limit inflammation allow rapid healing to occur, in 8 days.

A minimum of 3 months of osseointegration and gingival maturation are observed. The aim is to obtain bone maturation in the context of immediate implantation, but also, and above all, gingival maturation of the implant and pontic emergence profiles, which is often associated with a connective graft. A period of 6 months would be ideal.

Transfer of the project to the final prosthesis

Following the osseointegration and gingival maturation period (at least 3 months), the implants can be tested. The denture or crown is removed and the implant is tightened with a 35 Ncm healing screw to ensure that it is well integrated into the bone. At this stage, the prosthetic phase can begin to create the final prosthesis adapted to the patient. We exclusively use a digital workflow for impressions in single and multiple cases. We use it increasingly often in full-arch cases, with increasingly precise results accordingly. Given the current state of clinical and technological developments, we believe that optical impressions are the ideal replacement for traditional physical impressions. Practitioners are free to continue taking physical impressions at this stage of the Quokka protocol; we simply aim to share the advantages we benefit from by using a fully digital workflow during this phase. We use a digital approach in the final prosthetic stages with success and with a very satisfactory level of reliability. We are aware that the reliability of digital in implantology, particularly for completely edentulous patients or those with multiple missing teeth, has yet to be established in clinical studies. Here again, the intraoral camera models, acquisition techniques (path and fluidity), and also the 3D printing of the models are all factors that impact the results. Our clinical experience currently allows us to use intraoral cameras on a daily basis. Deviations in results are more common for fully edentulous mandibles. We systematically validate the impressions using a plaster index according to the recognized standards. If the plaster index fractures, we take a conventional impression and splint the transfers with DuraLay resin (Reliance Dental Manufacturing, Alsip, IL, USA). We distinguish three clinical situations related to the type of edentulism:
- single-unit;
- plural-unit;
- complete maxillary or mandibular edentulism.

For such situations, we can define a level of reliability and the number of appointments required for the final prosthesis.

Single-unit

Single-unit impressions are the simplest procedure and are as reliable clinically as conventional impressions. Only two appointments are required to make the final prosthesis. The impression procedure includes taking the antagonist arch impression, implant arch impression, gingival profile impression, and implant situation impression with the scan body in place, followed by registering the lateral bites with the opposite arch (Fig 3-34). In office workflow we use the 3Shape Trios 5, the files are sent to our laboratories either through the 3Shape Communicate portal (Laboratoire Mathias Berger, Lyon, France) or by exporting the files in STL format and sending them via Dropbox (Dental Art Technology laboratory, Richard Demange, Nice, France). The architecture of single-unit restorations is based on a zirconium coping screwed onto a titanium base (Variobase straight or Variobase angulated screw, Straumann) laminated with ceramic.

The unitary Quokka protocol therefore allows for the extraction of a tooth, its replacement with an implant, the management of an anatomic emergence profile and the fabrication of the final prosthesis in four sessions over 3.5 months (Fig 3-35).

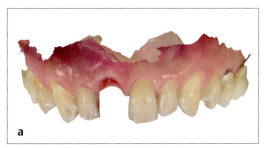
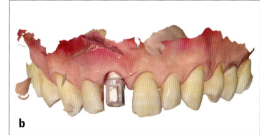
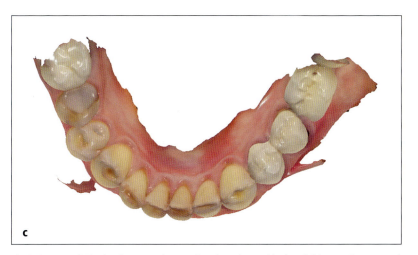
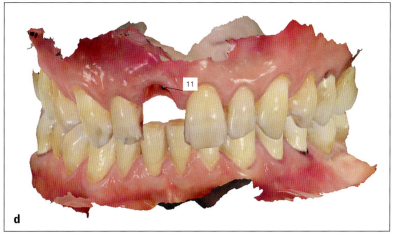

Fig 3-34 a to d The implant-type intraoral registrations with, in addition to the two arches and the occlusion, the registration with the scan body in place to transfer the implant position, a digital version of the transfer of mark-dependent implant impressions in physical impressions.

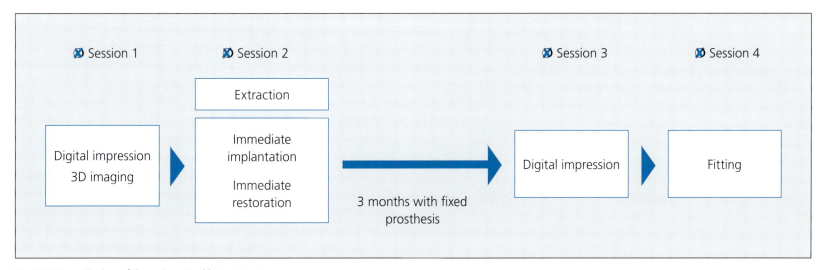

Fig 3-35 Synoptic view of the unitary Quokka treatment.

Plural-unit

For patients with multiple missing teeth, depending on the extent and location of the edentulism, we use two protocols based on whether the edentulism concerns:
- an esthetic area (cf. exposure during speaking or smiling);
- or more than two implants on more than four teeth.

In the esthetic zone, it is necessary to validate the mounting and the esthetic and functional integration of the instant loading partial denture. In addition to the standard scans taken for single implant registration, the digital impression requires an additional file, called a "pre-preparation" file, which will enable the morphology of the partial denture in the mouth to be transferred to the prosthetic laboratory. This file will be superimposed on the gingival scan and will serve as a prosthetic key that is much more precise than the silicone keys, and will remain in a digital workflow via the CAD/CAM software. At this stage, a framework design following the principle of homothetic reduction will be easier to achieve (Fig 3-36).

To complete the design for the pontic supports and implant emergence profiles following gingival healing induced by the provisional prosthesis, it may be necessary to balance the volumes. In this situation, a temporary resin model connected to temporary abutments or titanium bases is fabricated. It is scanned in its entirety to record its 3D volume in the prosthetic laboratory before being sent to the dental office. The model is tried in the mouth so the esthetics and **occlusion** can be assessed. Once validated by the patient, the model is left in the mouth to sculpt the gingiva and allow the patient to integrate the modifications. If significant occlusal or esthetic modifications are made, the model is sent back to the laboratory to be scanned and used as a guide in the CAD/CAM design of the framework and the ceramic. This is especially important in the case of full zirconia prostheses on which occlusal alterations are not recommended, and will allow the dental laboratory to proceed to direct finishing of the ceramic partial denture. In the esthetic zone, three sessions are allocated to finalizing the final prosthesis.

If the partial denture spans fewer than four teeth with two or three implants, it is not necessary to control the impression with a plaster key in our protocol, as our clinical experience has shown. If it spans more than four teeth, we consider it important to use a plaster key. In this case, we group the fitting of the key with the esthetic model, if necessary. We therefore continue to work on a three-session basis. If key fracture occurs, a

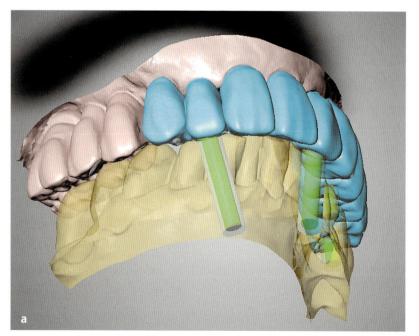
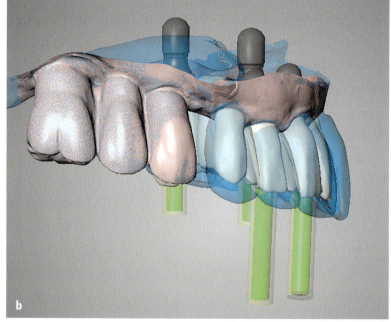

Fig 3-36 a and b (a) Importing the STL files of the impression of a multi-unit implant rehabilitation with the scan of the immediate loading partial denture as an additional layer in Exocad software (Dental Art Technology, Richard Demange, Nice, France). (b) Use of the volume of this partial denture to design the zirconia framework of the partial denture according to reductions in accordance with the support of the future ceramic layering.

physical or digital impression will be made. The validation model, if approved, will be sent back with the physical impression to complete the work in accordance with a traditional workflow, or registered in a pre-preparation scanner if the digital is used again. Classically, the architecture of the multiple-unit prosthesis, as for the single-unit prosthesis, is a partial denture on a milled zirconia base that is laminated in ceramic and screwed directly onto TL or TLX implants or intermediate abutments of the SRA type (multi-unit abutments) on BL or BLX implants. The Quokka protocol, with its fully digital workflow, makes it possible to treat a multi-faceted rehabilitation from conception to the final prosthesis in four sessions, or five sessions in the esthetic zone (Fig 3-37).

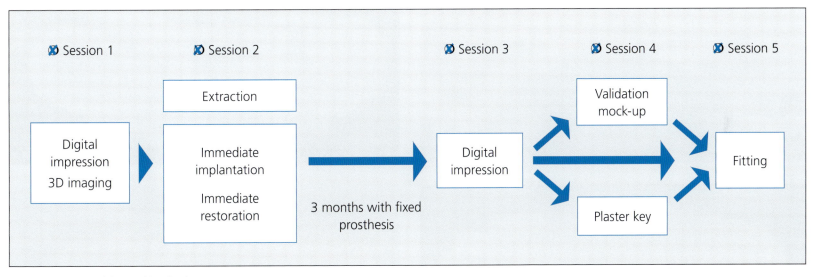

Fig 3-37 Overview of the Quokka plural treatment.

Complete rehabilitation

Complete edentulism requires the use of both a validation model and a plaster key. Physical impressions may be required rather than use of an intraoral camera. In the digital workflow, we can treat cases in three sessions. When using a physical impression, we plan four sessions, with one being spent validating the impression with the plaster index and transferring the occlusion chairside using the temporary instant-load partial denture onto the articulator. The digital workflow is clearly faster, and its use is becoming systematic in the dental office for maxillary treatment. It has not been used to treat many cases in the mandible thus far, so less feedback has been received on this. What is certain is that the greater the level of resorption of the edentulous ridges, the more difficult it is to take a digital, which impacts its potential accuracy. The proximity of the labial mucosa and the narrowness of the mandibular ridges make it difficult for the camera to move forward.

The architecture of prostheses in complete rehabilitations is more varied in terms of the materials used and the prosthetic volumes. Typically, in complete treatments, it is often necessary to compensate for lost periodontal volumes with a "pink" prosthesis. At the same time, mechanical stresses and occlusion have a major impact on the load exerted on the implants and thus on their durability. The use of various evolving materials, enhanced by CAD/CAM, allows us to adapt prosthetic structures to the specific constraints of each patient. Framework designs can be managed in the prosthetic laboratory (Laboratoire Mathias Berger) or by specialist machining companies, such as Createch Medical (Dental Art Technology laboratory).

Currently, in our therapeutic arsenal, we work with three options:
- screw retained full-zirconia partial denture on titanium bases with anterior buccal reductions for ceramic veneering (Fig 3-38);

The Quokka protocol

- a screw-retained zirconia (ZrO$_2$) framework with ceramic veneering with or without a artificial gingiva (Figs 3-39 and 3-40);

- a screw-retained polyetheretherketone (PEEK) framework with composite layering of the teeth and pink artificial gingiva in cases of significant vertical defect (Fig 3-41).

The Quokka protocol, with its complete digital flow, makes it possible to perform complete rehabilitation from conception to placement of the final prosthesis in six sessions (Fig 3-42).

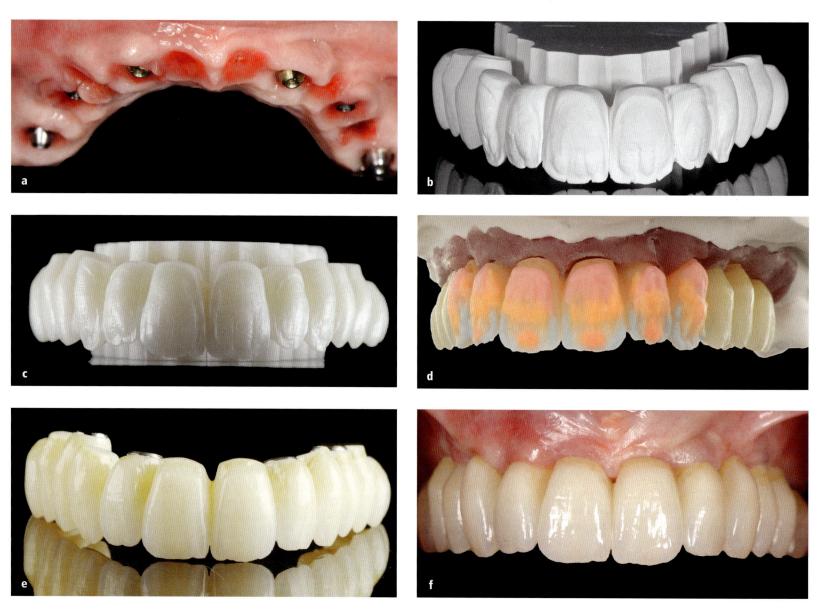

Fig 3-38 a to h Twelve-unit partial denture, screw-retained on six Straumann BL implants with SRA abutments, with a full-volume zirconia design except for the six anterior teeth. A buccal reduction is provided in the partial denture on these six teeth to allow for ceramic veneering. The posterior areas were colored. The occlusion was optimally adjusted on the CAD/CAM model to leave no retouching to be done on the stained, nor on the full volume of zirconia (Laboratoire Vinci, Geneva, Switzerland).

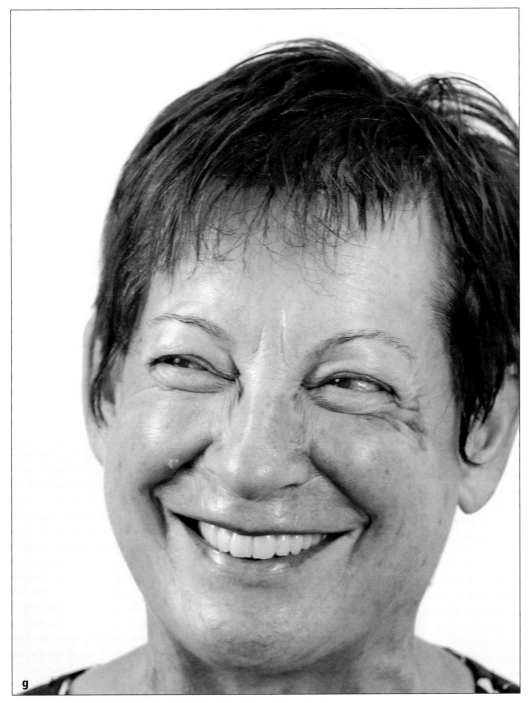
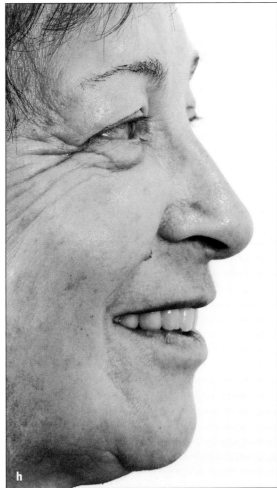

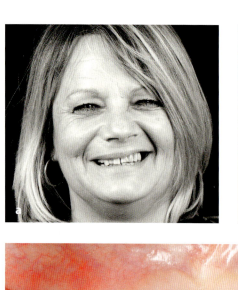
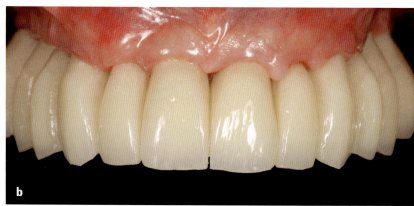
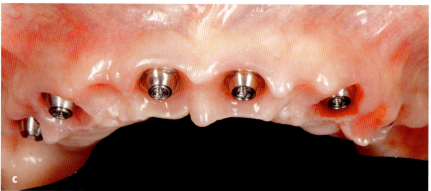
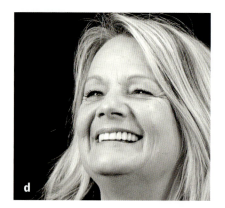
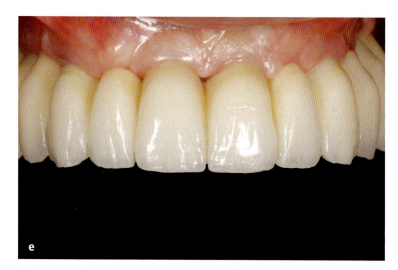
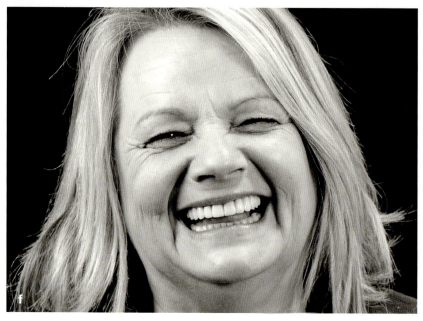

Fig 3-39 a to f Twelve-unit partial denture with ceramic-laminated zirconia framework, screw-retained on SRA abutments on six Straumann BL implants. The three stages are shown at the beginning of treatment, with the instant loading partial denture and finally with the final ceramic bridge (JC Allègre Laboratory, Champagne-au-Mont-d'Or, France).

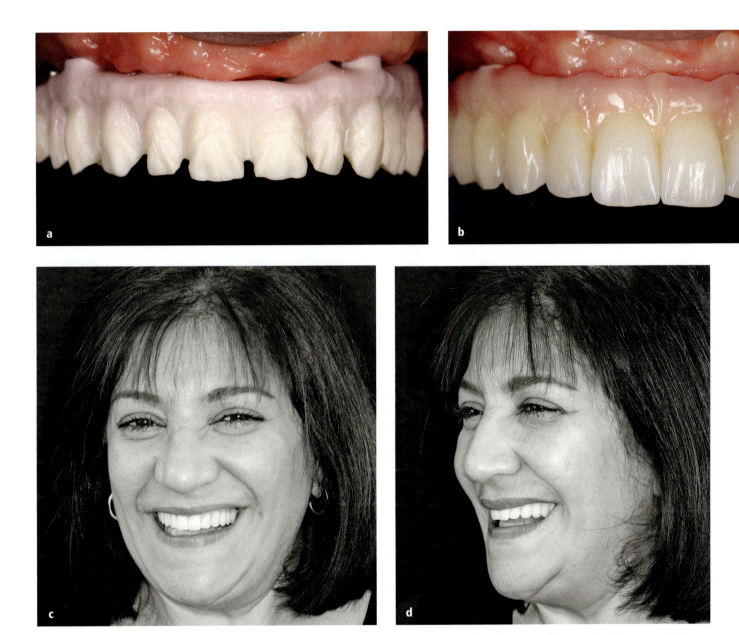

Fig 3-40 a to d Twelve-unit bridge screwed directly onto a Straumann TL implant via titanium sockets. The zirconia framework will support a pink ceramic layering to complement the dental volumes (JC Allègre, Champagne-au-Mont-d'Or, France).

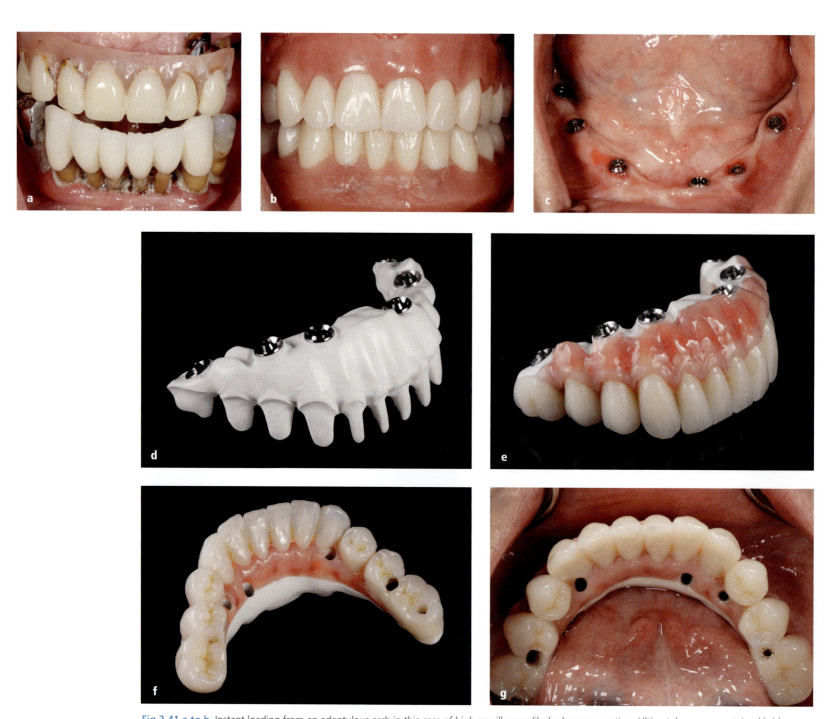

Fig 3-41 a to h Instant loading from an edentulous arch in this case of high maxillomandibular bone resorption. Ultimately, a screw-retained bridge was fabricated on six TLX implants with a Createch-milled PEEK framework and a composite mounting of the false gingiva and teeth. This highly elaborate work was performed by Richard Demange (Dental Art Technology, Nice, France). Note the lingual design and the supports on the PEEK ridge to reduce bacterial biofilm adherence. The embrasures are calibrated at 1.2 mm for interdental brushes.

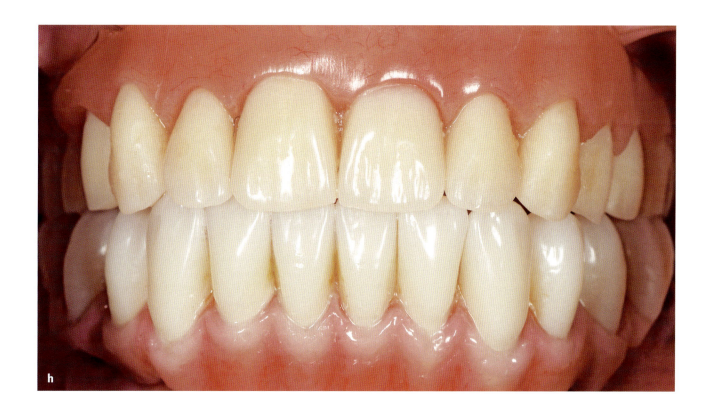

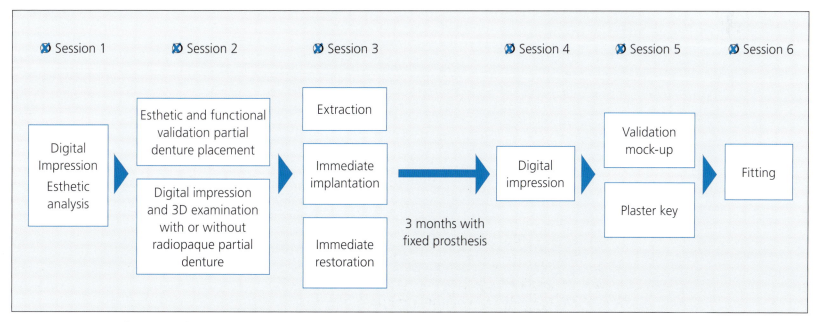

Fig 3-42 Synoptic view of the Quokka full-arch treatment.

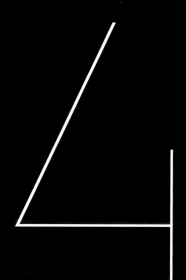

Single-unit clinical applications

Alveolus intact, vestibular bone wall preserved
Single-unit cases 1 to 5 75

Alveolus with narrow vestibular dehiscence
(< 1/3 of root exposure volume)
Single-unit cases 6 to 9 113

Alveolus with medium vestibular dehiscence
(1/3 to 2/3 of root exposure volume)
Single-unit cases 10 and 11 141

Alveolus with large vestibular dehiscence
(> 2/3 of root exposure volume)
Single-unit cases 12 to 15 155

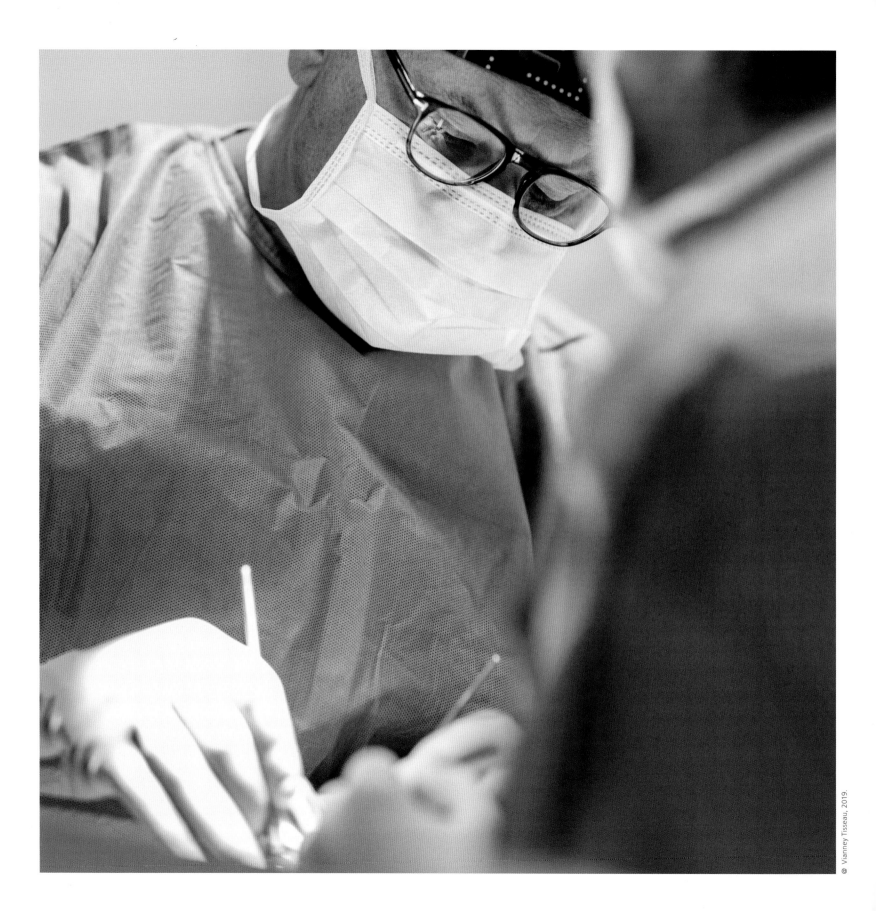

© Vianney Tisseau, 2019

Single-unit clinical case 1

42-year-old man.

Clinical data

- Devitalized and crowned tooth 11 prone to recurrent infections, despite an apical resection performed in 2017 by the treating dentist.
- Case treated in November 2019.
- Vestibular bone wall present.
- Good mucogingival architecture.

Presurgical treatments

- Optical impression taken using Trios 3 (3Shape, Copenhagen, Denmark) and 3D examination performed using Planmeca ProMax (Helsinki, Finland).
- Planning using Implant Studio.
- Straumann RN Standard Plus Roxolid SLActive Implant (3.3 × 12.0 mm) (Basel, Switzerland).
- 3D printing of the guide designed in Implant Studio (Dentitek Laboratory, Dardilly, France).
- First-generation Straumann socket.
- Temporary crown milled in polymethyl methacrylate (PMMA) (Ivotion Dent Multi, Ivoclar Vivadent, Schaan, Liechtenstein) (Dentitek Laboratory).
- Variobase RN used for crowns bonded with Multilink Hybrid Abutment (Ivoclar Vivadent).

Assessment of the intervention

- Case treated in **three appointments at the office** (impression and 3D examination, surgery, control at 3 months).
- Final prosthesis made in the office (JC Allègre Laboratory, Champagne-au-Mont-d'Or, France).

Additional treatments

- In addition to the treatment of 11, we performed internal whitening of 22 and redid the incisal composite in 21.

The Quokka protocol

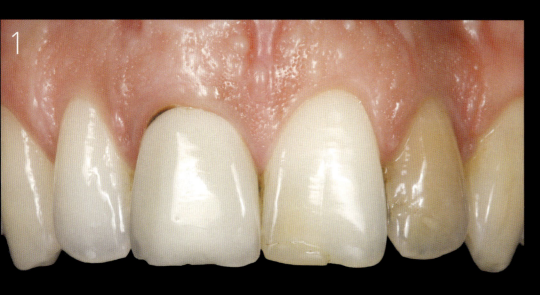

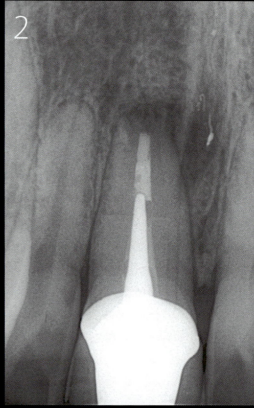

Initial clinical situation with the presence of devitalized and crowned tooth 11, subject to recurrent infections. Note the lack of alignment of the necks between teeth 11 and 21, and that tooth 22 is devitalized and will be treated with internal bleaching.

Preoperative radiograph. Periapical curettage surgery involving apical resection and retrofilling was performed by the referring dentist in 2017, but tooth 11 was still prone to infectious episodes. Tooth extraction was recommended.

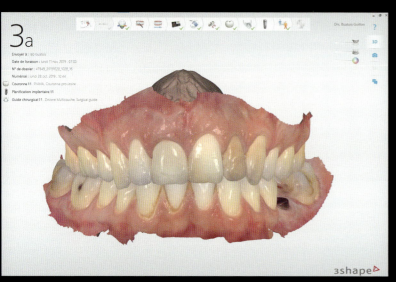

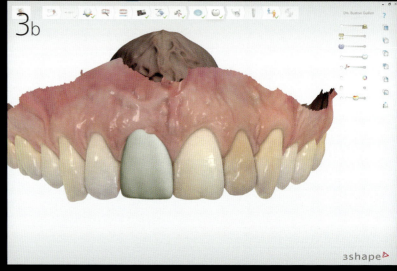

Purchase order made in Implant Studio 3Shape planning software with digital impression taking (Trios 3) and DICOM scanner importation (Planmeca ProMax) for immediate implantation and restoration.

Digital design of the prosthetic project to achieve prosthetically guided implant placement. Note the collar of the prosthetic design in relation to tooth 21. The vertical positioning of the implant will play a major role in this final goal.

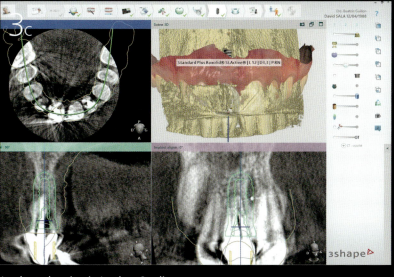

Implant planning in Implant Studio.

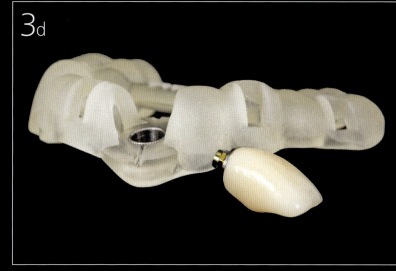

Surgical guide and immediate temporary crown (made by Dentitek Laboratory), cemented with Variobase before surgery.

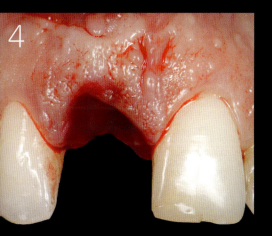

Single avulsion of tooth 11.

Fitting of the surgical guide. Note the good adaptation of the surgical guide thanks to the control windows.

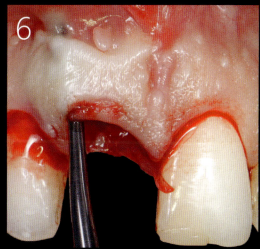

Creation of a superperiosteal flap by tunneling with a Black Series #1 tunneling knife (Hu-Friedy, Chicago, IL, USA).

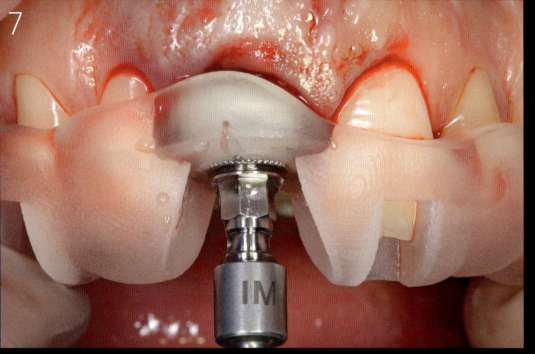

Guided implant placement. Note that for the guided BL and TL first-generation implants, the implant holder was connected to the implant. The depth markings (H2, H4, and H6) are rails that receive a locking key. Alignment was performed on the apical edge of the groove (here H6). For first-generation TL guided implants, rotational positioning is achieved by aligning the surgical guide markings with the edge of the guided implant holder.

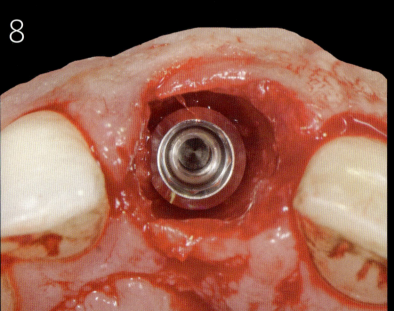

Axial view of the 3D implant positioning.

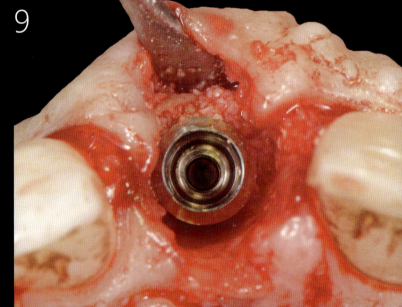

Filling of the gap between the implant body and the vestibular bone wall with a

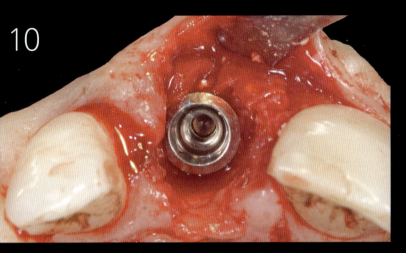

Covering of the vestibular bone cortex and filling with a bi-layer collagen membrane of resorbable porcine origin (Bio-Gide Perio, Geistlich).

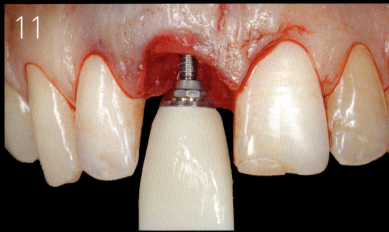

Presentation of the temporary PMMA screw-retained immediate crown. Note the polished surface for gingival maturation.

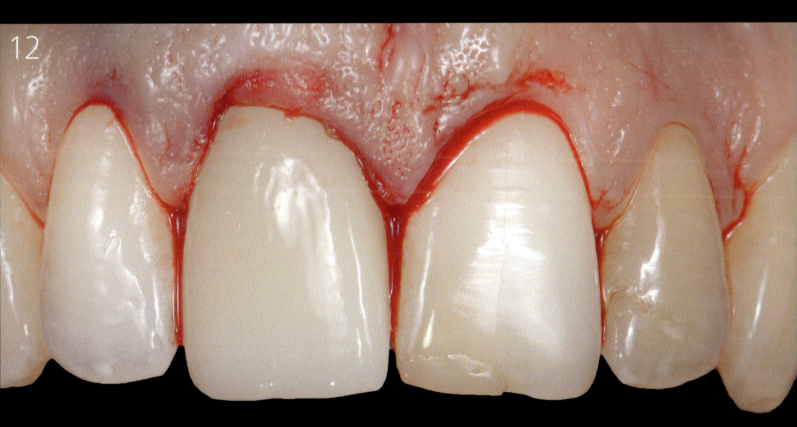

Immediate crown screwed into the implant. Note the adaptation of the temporary crown (free edge, collar).

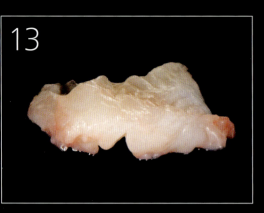

Harvesting of a tuberous epithelioconjunctival graft, which was subsequently de-epithelialized. A connective graft was indicated in this case to support the peri-implant emergence profile.

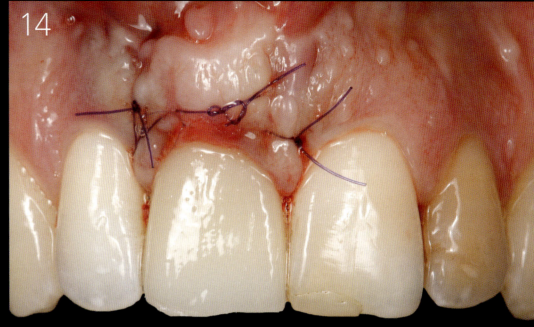

Stabilization of the connective tissue graft with a horizontal mattress suture, and an ASAF suture around the temporary tooth.

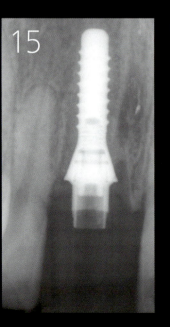

Postoperative radiographic control. Note the adaptation of the implant abutment to the

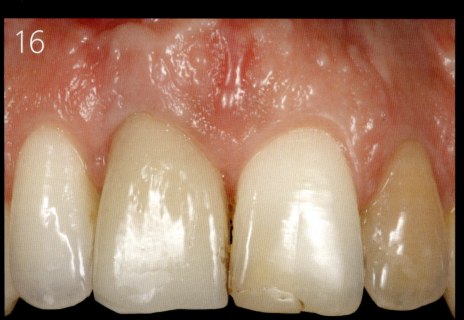

Clinical control of healing and implant osseointegration at 3 months, frontal view.

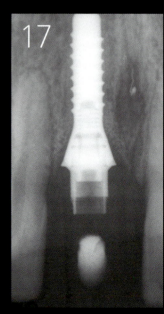

Radiographic control 3 months after implant surgery.

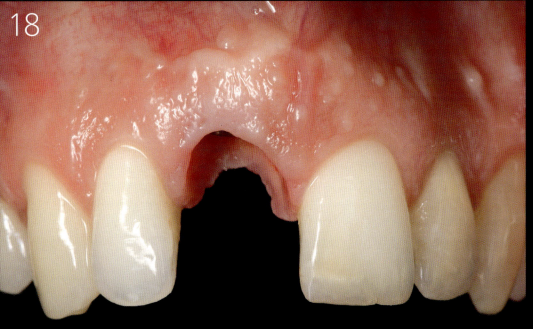

Frontal view of the implant emergence profile after the temporary crown was unscrewed. Gingival maturation was guided by the immediate temporary prosthesis. Note the absence of inflammation of the implant emergence profile due to the lack of relining of the provisional prosthesis.

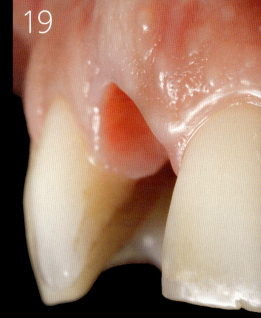

Side view.

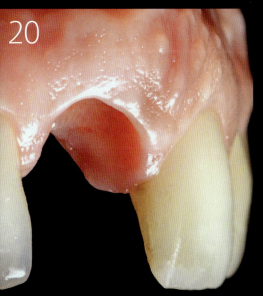

Another side view.

Axial view. Note the good vestibular volume of the peri-implant mucosa, guaranteeing long-term implant stability.

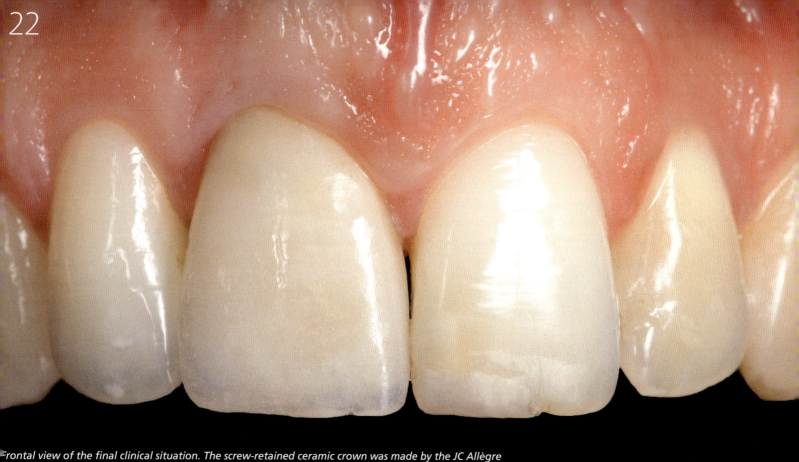

Frontal view of the final clinical situation. The screw-retained ceramic crown was made by the JC Allègre laboratory. Internal bleaching of tooth 22 was performed in the office to harmonize the dental shades. Note the alignment of the collars between teeth 11 and 21 that was managed by implant planning, vertical implant positioning through guided surgery, GBR, and connective tissue grafting.

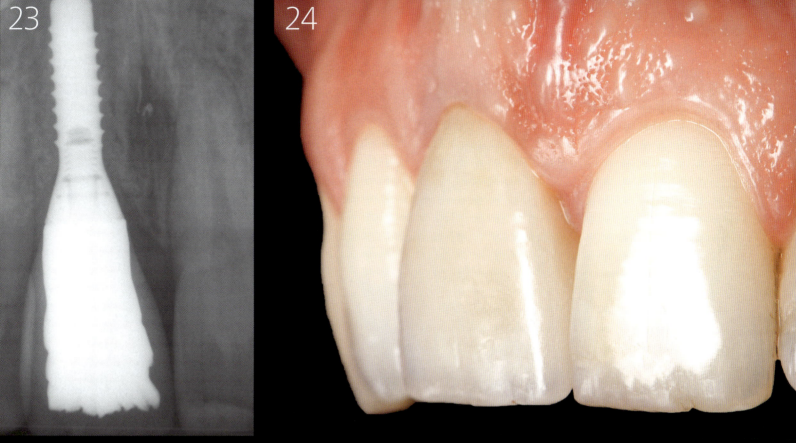

23 Radiograph of the ceramic crown screwed into the implant.

24 Lateral view of the final clinical situation.

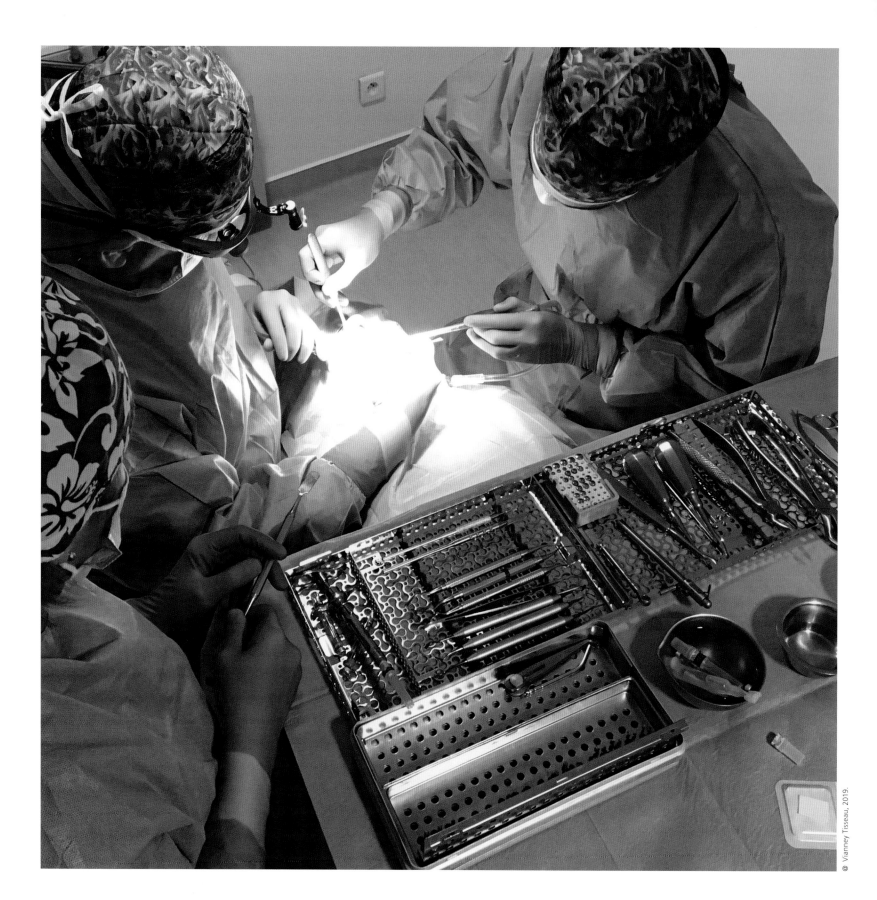

© Vianney Tisseau, 2019.

Single-unit clinical case 2

43-year-old woman.

Clinical data

- Chronic pain in the tooth, especially when chewing. Tooth devitalized many years previously. Suspicion of a crack.
- Case treated in May 2018.
- Vestibular bone wall intact.
- Good mucogingival architecture.

Presurgical treatments

- Trios 3 used to take an optical impression and Planmeca ProMax used to perform the 3D examination.
- Planning using Implant Studio.

- Straumann RC TiZr SLActive implant (4.1 x 12.0 mm).
- Surgical guide designed in Implant Studio and printed in Dentitek Laboratory.
- First-generation Straumann socket.
- **Instant** temporary tooth milled on a PMMA disc (Ivotion Dent Multi, Ivoclar).
- Variobase RC used for crowns bonded with Multilink Hybrid Abutment (Ivoclar).

Assessment of the intervention

- Case treated in **three appointments at the office** (impression and 3D examination, surgery, control at 3 months).
- Final prosthesis made by the referring dentist.

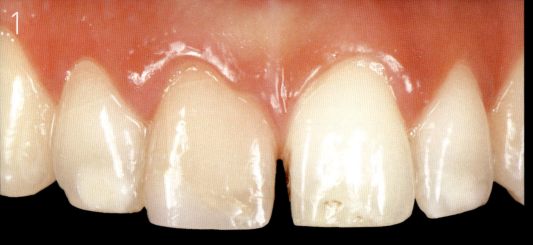

Frontal view of the initial clinical situation.

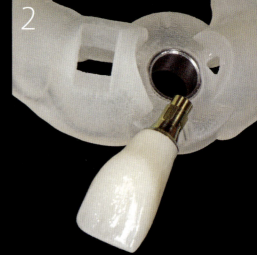

*Surgical guide and **immediate** temporary crown. Note the surface condition of the cervical portion of the milled **immediate** crown.*

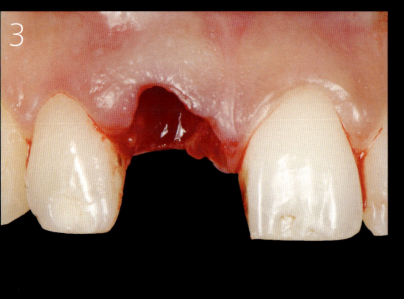

Frontal view after extraction.

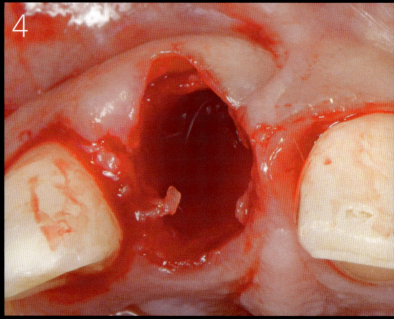

Axial view of the postextraction socket.

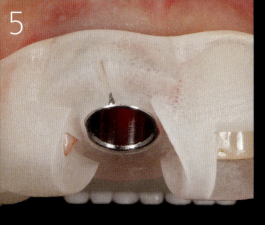

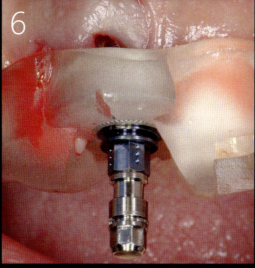

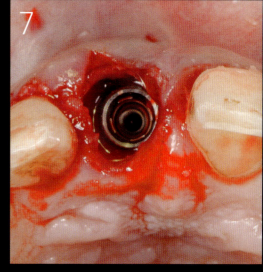

Frontal view of the surgical guide positioned in the mouth. Note the groove for rotational positioning and the inspection windows.

Guided implant placement in 11. Due to a shift of one-sixth of a turn in the implant coordinates between the Implant Studio (implant planning) and Dental System (laboratory CAD/CAM) software, the implant positioning was determined by the flat face of the loxim. Vertical positioning of the implant in H6.

Axial view of the implant position. The vestibular bone cortex remains intact.

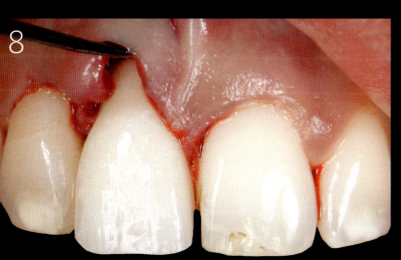

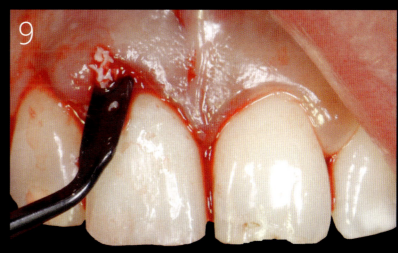

Placement of the **immediate** temporary crown screwed into the implant. The patient's wish to keep her diastema was respected.

Guided bone regeneration with a DBBM slow resorption bone substitute (Bio-Oss, Geistlich) with a fine particle size (0.25 to 1.00 mm) with a Rompen Black Series drill (Hu-Friedy). The filling was inserted between the implant body and vestibular bone cortex. The presence of the vestibular wall and the fact that it was more than 1 mm thick meant that only internal filling of the socket could

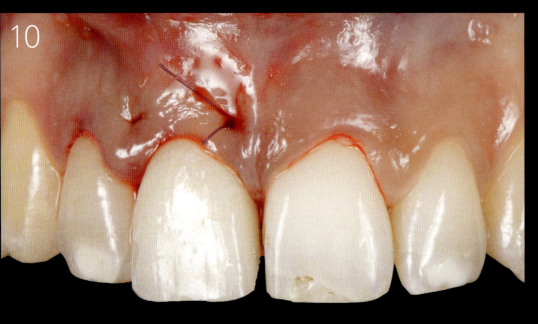

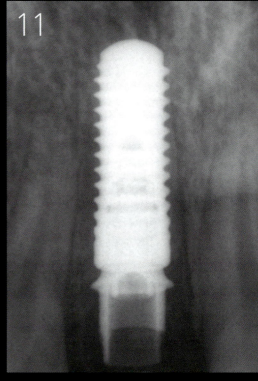

Frontal view of the postoperative situation with an ASAF suture around the **immediate** temporary crown.

Postoperative radiograph.

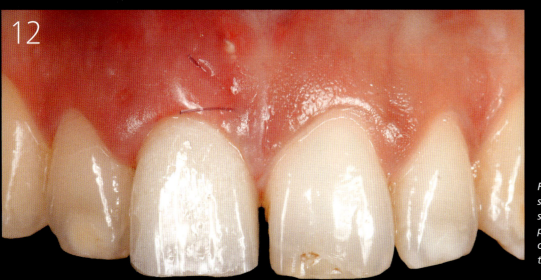

Frontal view of the clinical situation 7 days after surgery. Note the quality of healing around the smooth prosthetic surface. A parasitic Bio-Oss particle, originating from an excess during filling, occluded the alveolar mucosa. It migrated during the filling process.

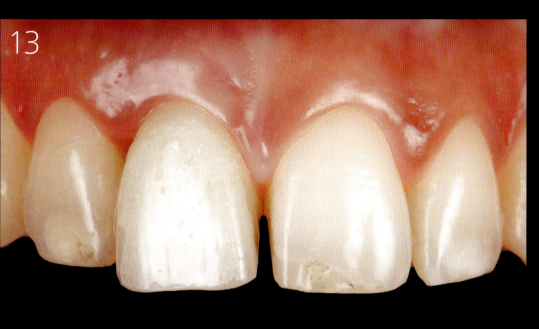
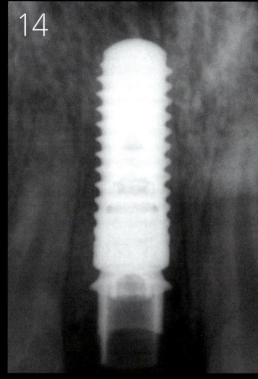

Frontal view after 3 months of healing. Note the quality of the texture and gingival architecture.

*Radiograph at 3 months after surgery. The proximal bone peaks were preserved. The **immediate** crown served as a protection and guide for GBR:*

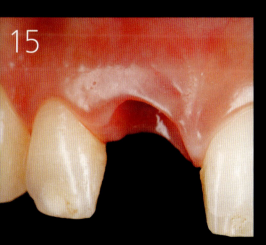
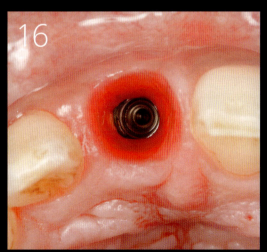
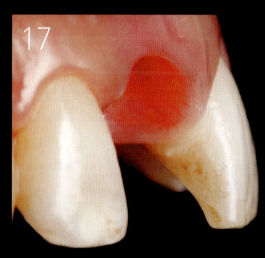

Frontal view of the implant bed and emergence profile.

Axial view. Note the induction of a prosthetic anatomy of the implant bed and the absence of inflammation of the sulcus. At 3 months, all the necessary work had been done to continue with a qualitative implant impression.

Lateral view of peri-implant gingival health. The density of the tissues allowed stable support of the emergence profile that was not dependent on the support of the prosthesis.

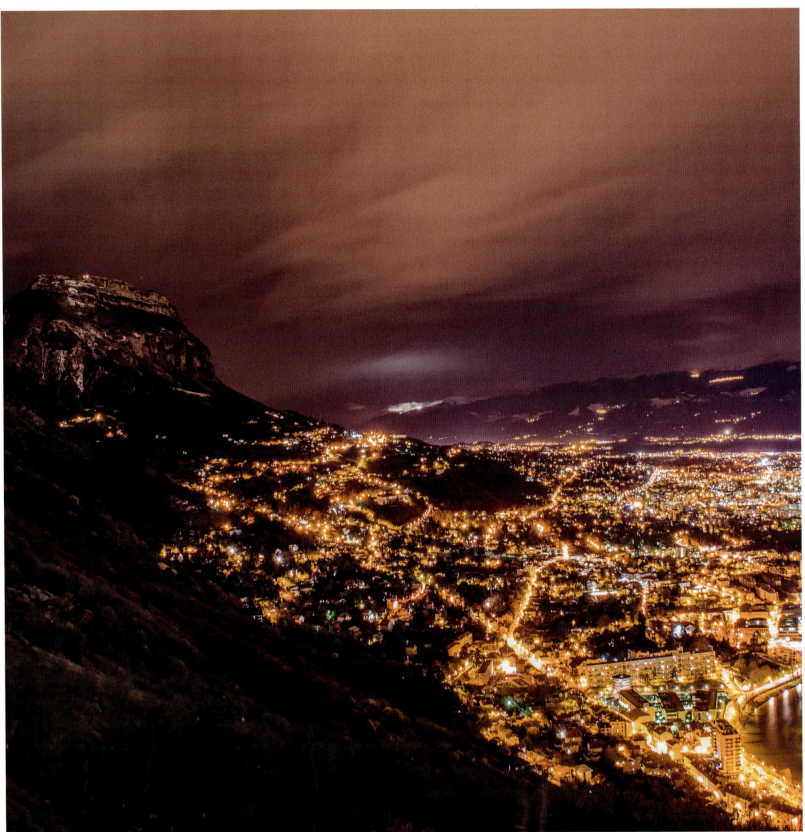
© Martin Boutière, 2016.

Single-unit clinical case

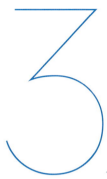

60-year-old man.

Clinical data

- Vestibulopalatal mobility of the crown in 11. Localized 10-mm periodontal pocket opposite the vestibular bone cortex, synonymous with a vertical crack. Suspicion of a crack on retroalveolar radiography, confirmed on 3D examination.
- Case treated in June 2018.
- Vestibular bone wall present.
- Good mucogingival architecture.

Presurgical treatments

- Trios 3 used to take an optical impression and Planmeca ProMax used to perform the 3D examination.
- Planning in Implant Studio.
- Straumann bone-level (BL) RC Roxolid SLActive implant (4.1 x 12.0 mm).
- 3D printing of the guide designed in Implant Studio (Dentitek Laboratory).
- First-generation Straumann socket.
- Temporary crown milled in PMMA (Ivotion Dent Multi, Ivoclar) (Dentitek Laboratory).
- Variobase RC (GH 1 mm) used for crowns bonded with Multilink Hybrid Abutment (Ivoclar).

Assessment of the intervention

- Case treated in **three appointments at the office** (impression and 3D examination, surgery, 3-month control).
- Final prosthesis made by the attending dentist.
- Surgery performed live during a CampusHB session on the Quokka protocol for single-unit edentulism.

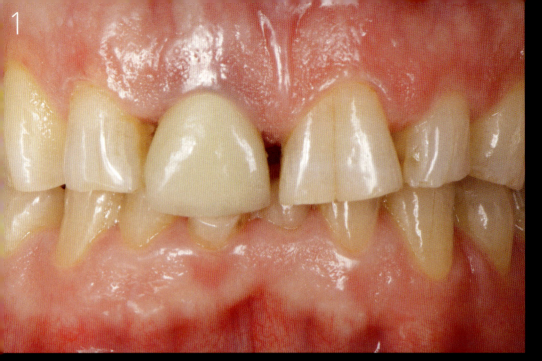

Frontal view of the initial clinical situation.

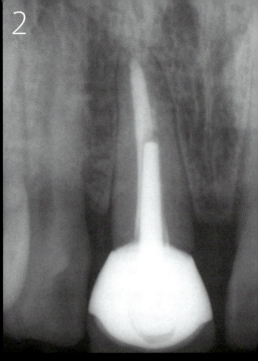

Preoperative radiograph.

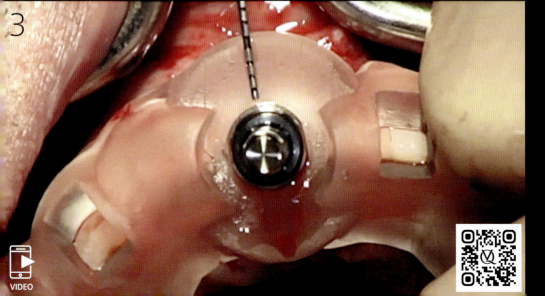

Sequenced video: implant placement, GBR, and ASAF suture. Note the positioning of the implant in the socket, the thin vestibular bone wall requiring bone augmentation (releasing incision in addition to the initial flap). Bio-Oss small and Bio-Gide Perio membrane (Geistlich Pharma France).

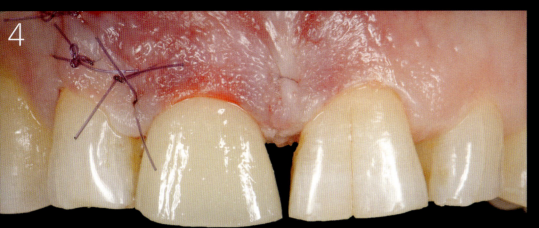

Postoperative clinical situation with the immediate screw-retained temporary crown in 11, ASAF sutures and single sutures of the distal releasing incision.

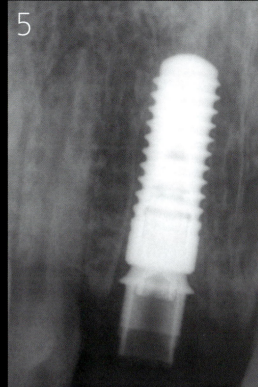

Postoperative radiograph.

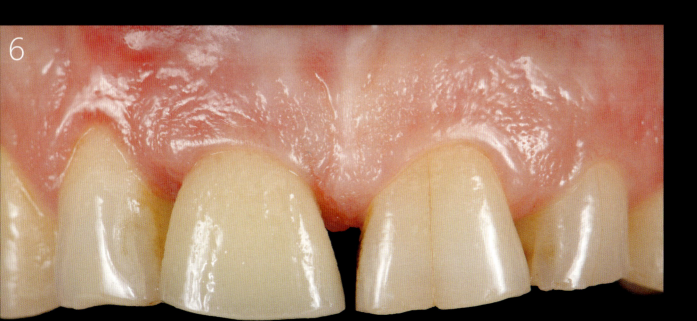

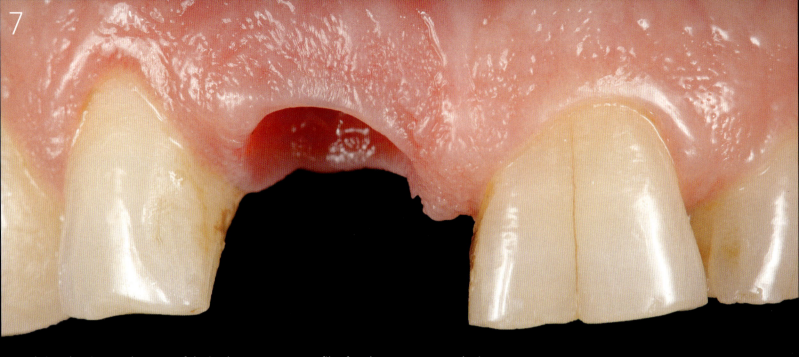

Frontal view showing good support of the implant emergence profile after the temporary prosthesis was unscrewed.

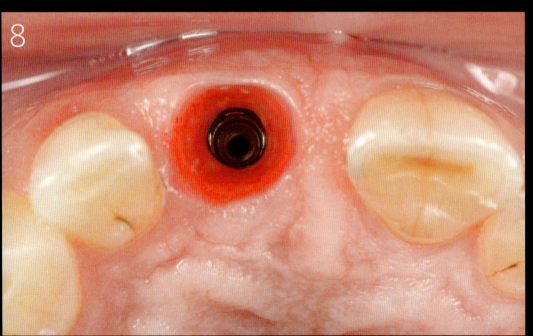

Axial view of the implant bed. Note the absence of inflammation of the gingival bed.

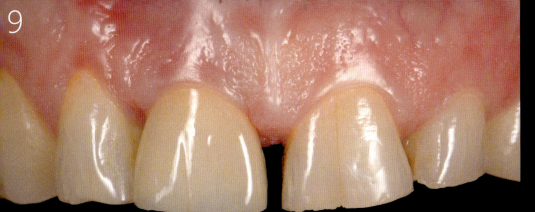

Frontal view of the clinical situation with the screw-retained ceramic crown.

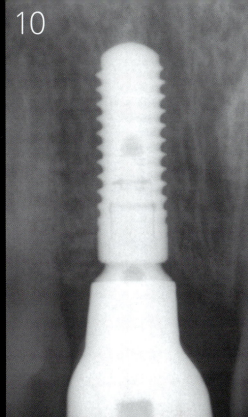

Radiograph showing the screw-retained ceramic crown at 1 year.

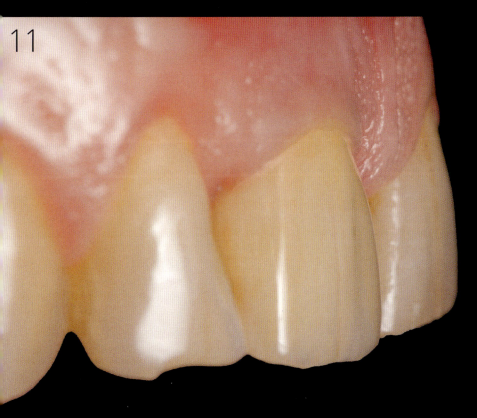

Profile view showing stable 3D support at 1 year.

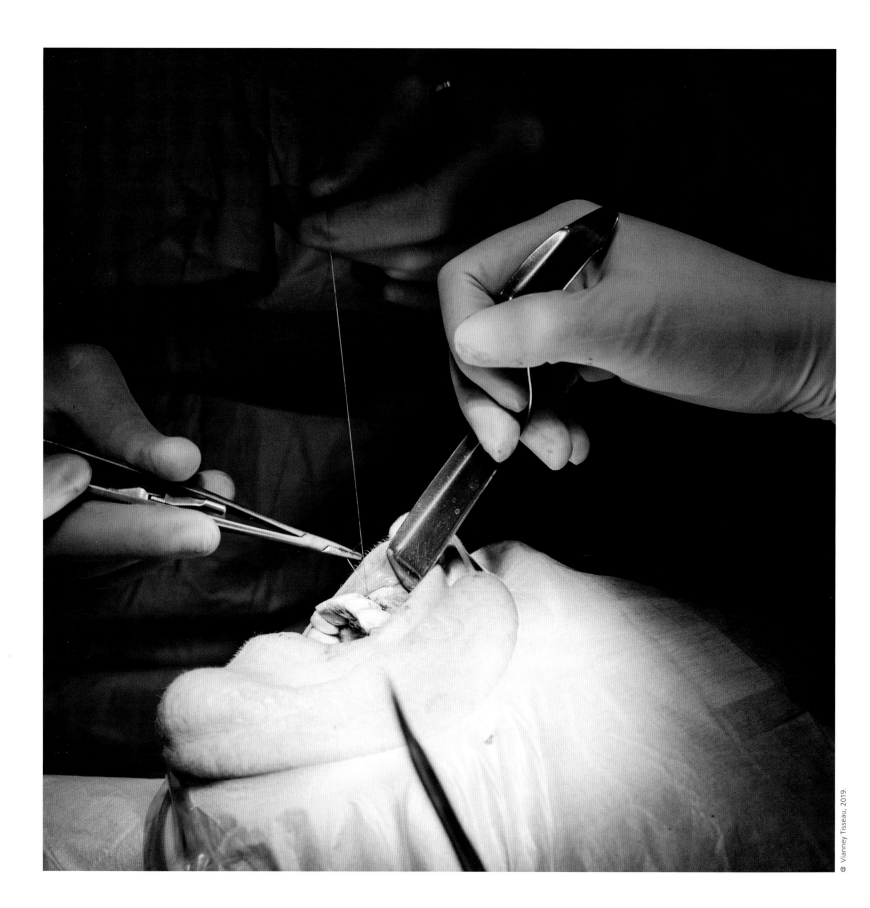

© Vianney Tisseau, 2019.

Single-unit clinical case 4

47-year-old woman.

Clinical data

- Agenesis of teeth 12 and 13, presence of 52 and 53.
- Case treated in February 2019.
- Buccal bone defect in 52 and 53 area requiring a preimplant bone graft. Implantation 6 months after grafting.
- Good mucogingival architecture.

Presurgical treatments

- Trios 3 used to take an optical impression and Planmeca ProMax used to perform the 3D examination.
- Planning in Implant Studio.
- Straumann BL NC TiZr SLActive 12-mm implant to replace tooth 12 with a morphology of 13 in a symmetrical 23 position.
- 3D printing of the guide designed in Implant Studio (Dentitek Laboratory).
- First-generation Straumann sleeve.
- Temporary screw-retained crown, shade A2, milled on a PMMA Ivotion Dent Multi disc on a Roland milling machine (Hamamatsu, Japan) (Dentitek Laboratory).
- Use of Variobase NC for crowns bonded with Multilink Hybrid Abutment.

Assessment of the intervention

- Case treated in **three appointments at the office** (impression and 3D examination, surgery, control at 12 months).
- Final prosthesis made by the referring dentist.
- Patient referred by Dr. Prévé, an orthodontist in Grenoble, France, for management of agenesis in 12 and 13. Immediate implantation and loading were performed in a grafted site at 6 months in 12 in order to achieve, at the end of osseointegration, orthodontic traction of 14 in the site of 13. The morphology of 12 was that of a canine, mirroring 23 according to the patient's wishes.

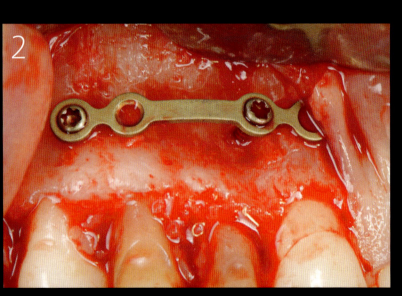

1. Initial clinical situation with the presence of teeth 52 and 53, which were esthetically disturbing to the patient without significant mobility. Due to the agenesis, the bone volume in front of the two milk teeth was horizontally deficient, making it impossible to position the implant in the 12 site in a correct prosthetic axis.

2. A pre-implant bone graft was performed while keeping the two milk teeth to avoid the patient having to wear a transitional removable prosthesis. We use a published technique that was developed in our office. It consists of a formwork made from osteosynthesis plates, filled with a graft composed of cortical bone chips that may or may not be mixed with DBBM, and taken from the external oblique line with a single-use bone chisel (derived from the Merli technique).

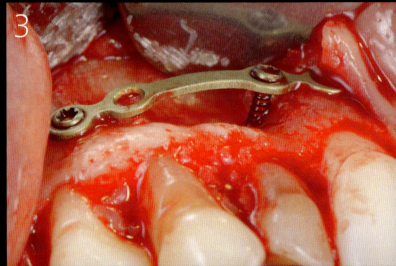

3. Axial view showing the bone undercut, which justified the use of a graft.

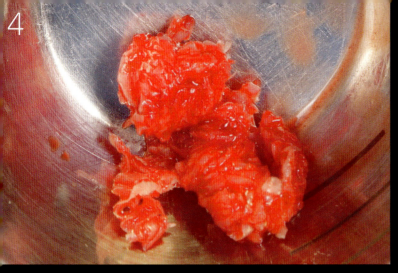

Cortical bone chips removed with a bone chisel (Safescraper Curve META, PP Pharma France).

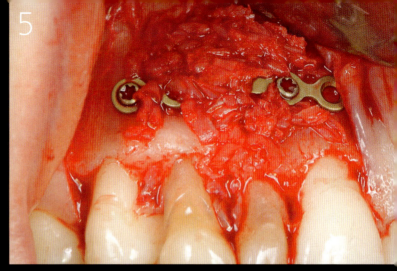

Chips filling the space defined by the vestibular cortex and the osteosynthesis plate.

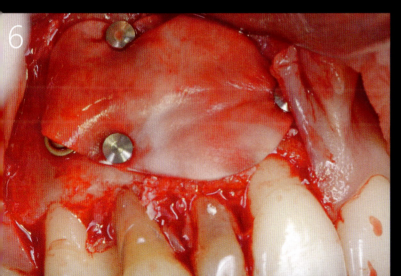

Filling with a bilayer collagen membrane of resorbable porcine origin (Bio-Gide Perio) and stabilization of the membrane with three impacted pins (Geistlich).

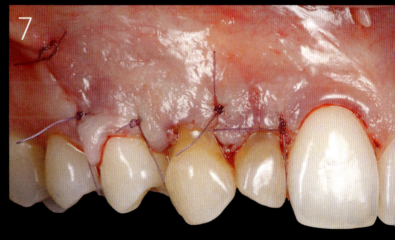

After a half-thickness incision and coronal traction, the flap was sutured with single stitches (discharge and papillae).

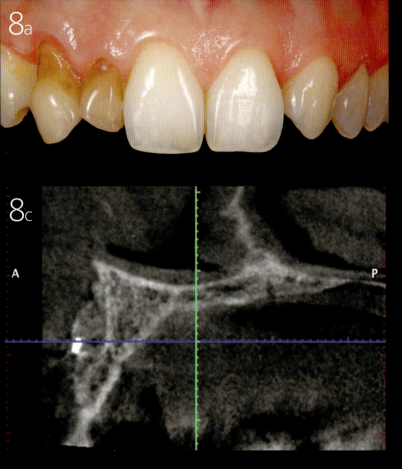

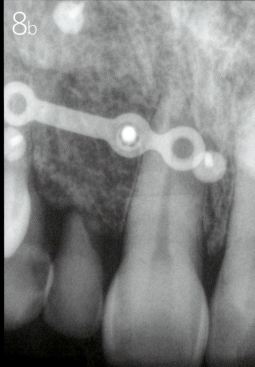

Clinical situation at 6 months. Note the preservation of the milk teeth to increase patient comfort. At this stage, a maxillary and mandibular optical impression (Trios 3) was taken and a 3D radiological examination (Planmeca ProMax) was performed to create the implant plan, the surgical guide, and the screw-retained temporary tooth in 12. Note the bone gain in the vestibular depression.

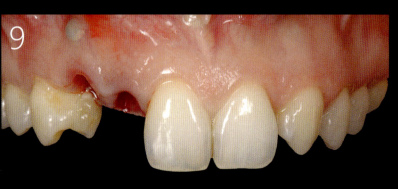

*Second procedure: extraction of the milk teeth and placement of the implant with **immediate** restoration. Note the membrane stabilization pins that were removed with the osteosynthesis bar before guided implant drilling.*

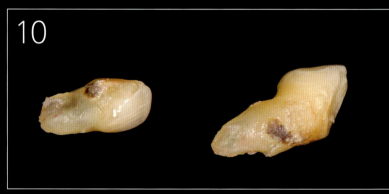

Extracted teeth 52 and 53.

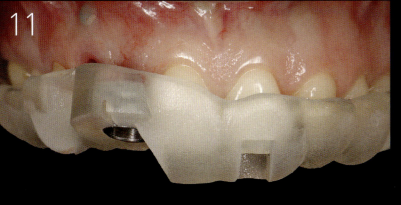

The 3D printed surgical guide (Dentitek Laboratory) was tried in before raising the flaps to check the fit was optimal through the inspection windows. First-generation Straumann sleeve in 12 with rotational registration grooves present on the guide.

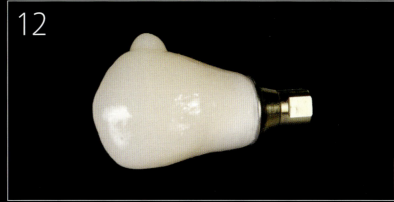

Temporary tooth connected to a Variobase NC for Crown **before** surgery. Milled crown (Dentitek Laboratory), shade A2. Note the resin bead added distally to allow for suture suspension.

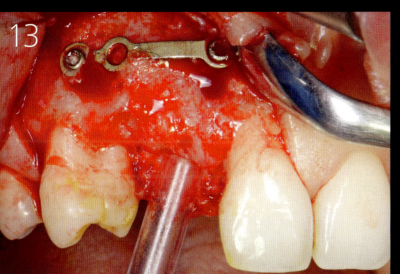

Flap removal exposing the osteosynthesis plate.

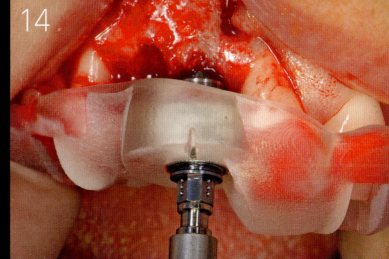

Guided implant placement. For the first-generation guided BL and TL implants, the implant holder was connected to the implant. The depth markings (H2, H4, and H6) are rails that receive a locking key. Alignment was performed on the apical edge of the groove, in this case H6. The points are supposed to align with the rotational registration line, but with the 3Shape Dental System we had a 1/6 turn offset (flat without point in front of the groove). We therefore have guided implant positioning in its axis, depth, and rotation.

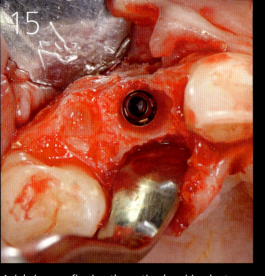

15 Axial view confirming the optimal peri-implant bone environment. A proper implant axis was permitted by the pre-implant bone graft.

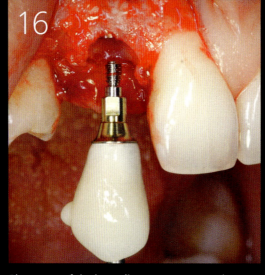

16 Placement of the **immediate** temporary tooth during surgery to serve as a guide for possible bone or gingival reconstruction.

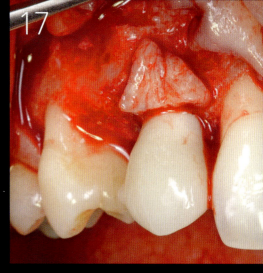

17 Placement of a connective graft from a de-epithelialized tuberosal harvest to better support the emergence profile.

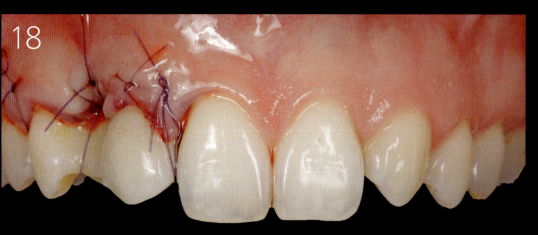

18 ASAF suture combined with a hanging suture distal to 12 and vestibular padding to stabilize the graft against the medial aspect of the vestibular flap, with single sutures on the discharge distal to 14.

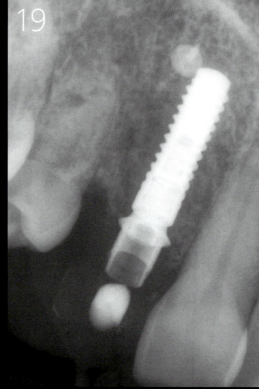

19 Postoperative radiologic check confirming the optimal adaptation of the temporary tooth screwed into the BL NC implant.

Chapter 4 - Single-unit clinical applications

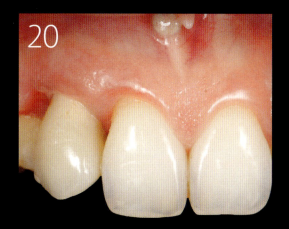

Frontal view of the clinical situation 3 months after surgery when the implant osseointegration was checked.

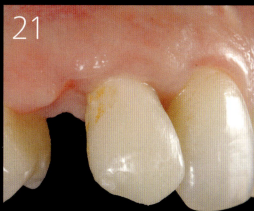

Side view.

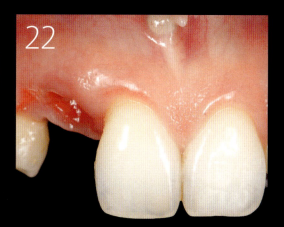

Frontal view of the emergence profile after removal of the provisional tooth for implant control.

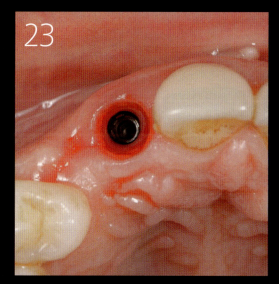

Axial view of the emergence profile. Note the rounding and alignment of the buccal emergence profile and the absence of inflammation of the sulcus due to the smooth surface of the milled resin not relined in the mouth. Orthodontic treatment could be carried out before the final prosthesis was made by the referring dentist.

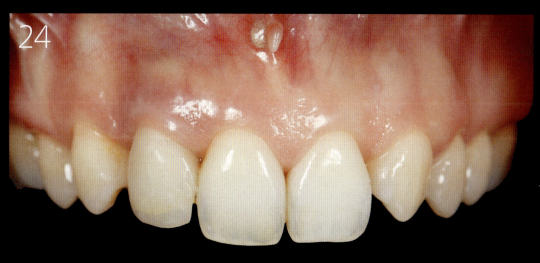

Final situation after 4 years.

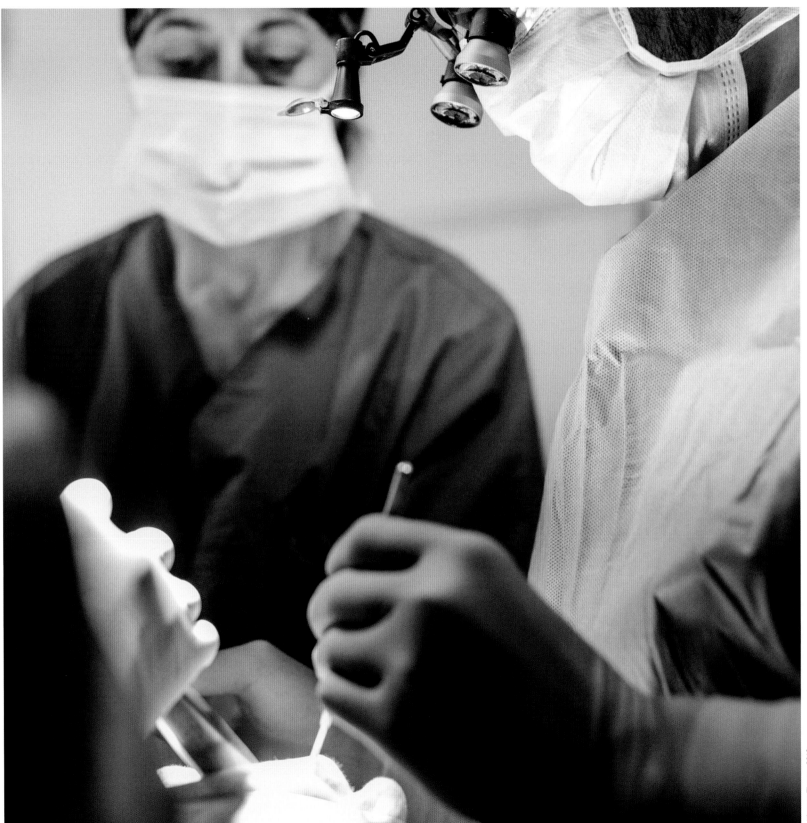
© Vianney Tisseau, 2019.

Single-unit clinical case 5

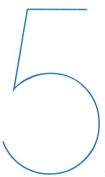

71-year-old woman.

Clinical data

- Periodontal loss of teeth 12 and 22. Type 2 mobility, which made it difficult for the patient to chew as she had lost confidence in the retention of these teeth.
- Case treated in April 2022.
- Apical bone volume integrity (horizontal loss on two-thirds of the roots in 12 and 22).
- Fragile mucogingival architecture to be reinforced by a buried connective tissue graft to stabilize the context locally.

Presurgical treatments

- Trios 4 used to take an optical impression and a 3Shape X1 used to perform the 3D examination.
- Planning in Implant Studio.
- Placement of a Straumann TLX SP NT implant (3.75 x 10.00 mm) to replace tooth #12 and tooth #22.
- 3D printing of the guide designed in Implant Studio, in the office on a NextDent 5100 printer (Utrecht, The Netherlands) with NextDent SG resin and polymerized in an LC-3D 3D polymerization unit.
- Straumann TLX PEEK T-socket, self-locking.
- Interim crowns 12 and 22, shade A3.5, printed in the office on a NextDent 5100 printer with NextDent N1 resin, polymerized in the LC-3D 3D polymerization unit and stained on an A3.5 base with the Optiglaze Color Set (GC Europe, Leuven, Belgium).
- Variobase used for NT crown bonding to Multilink Hybrid Abutment HO.

Assessment of the intervention

- Case treated in **three appointments at the office** (impression and 3D examination, surgery, control at 3 months).
- Final prosthesis made by the referring dentist.
- It was not a question of considering a global periodontal or prosthetic treatment. There was no indication for this in this case, nor any desire from the patient to correct the esthetic appearance of the gingiva or teeth; she simply wanted to regain two reliable lateral incisors.

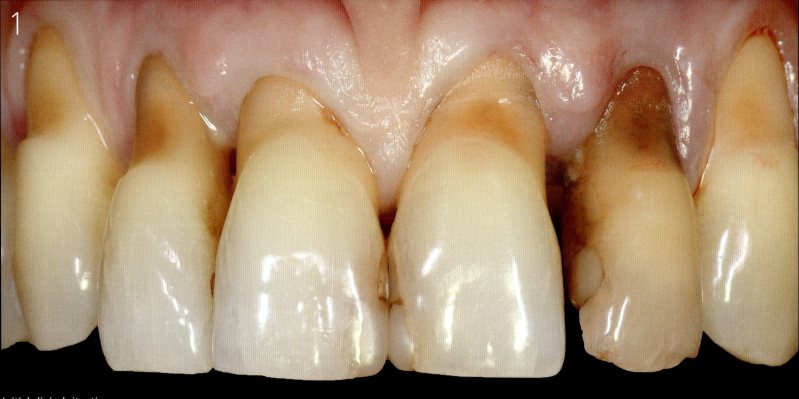

Initial clinical situation.

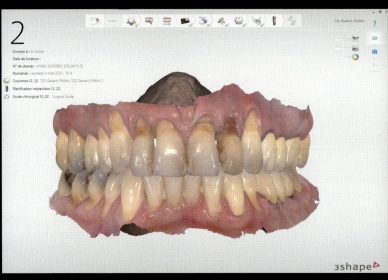

Optical impression taken using Trios 4 in a preparatory session combined with the 3D examination using a 3Shape X1.

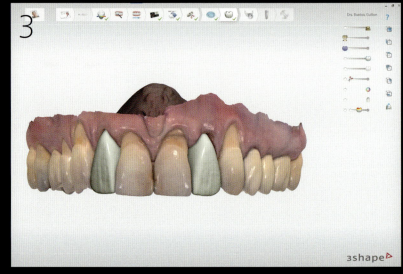

Virtual "avulsions" of teeth 12 and 22 and creation of two prosthetic teeth as a guide for 3D positioning.

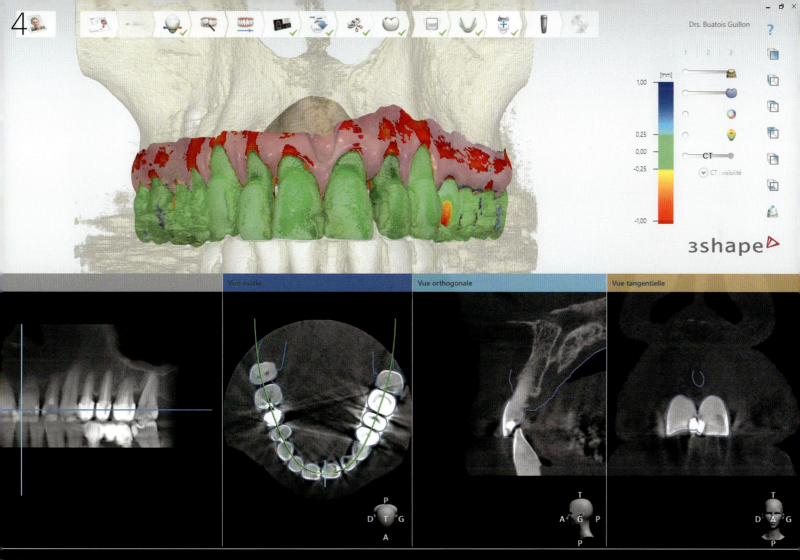

Surfacing of the intraoral STL file and the bone DICOM file. Colorimetric index showing perfect matching between the two files.

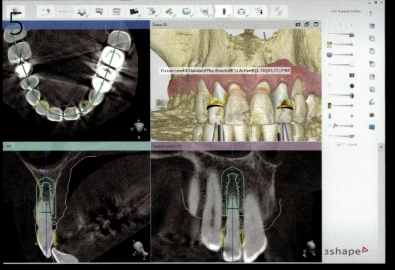

Positioning of the implant in 12.

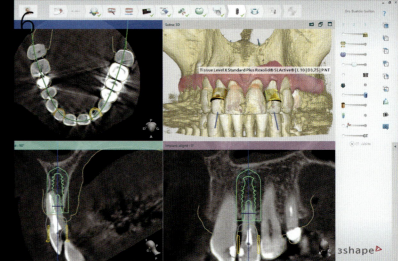

Positioning of the implant in 22.

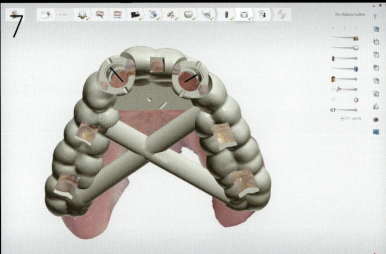

After implant positioning and selecting the height of the sockets (H2, H4, or H6), the surgical guide was designed, with inspection windows, reinforcement bars, sockets, and rotational marking. This was followed by validation of the plan in the workflow to edit the CAD/CAM files required to print the guide and create the prostheses.

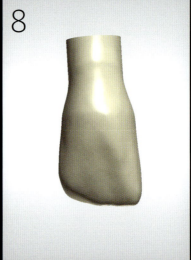

After exporting the planning data to Dental System, the screw-retained prosthesis was fabricated in 12. Note the drawn emergence profile.

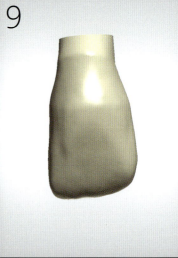

Same for 22.

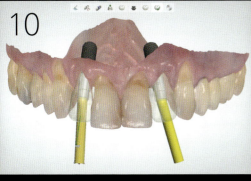

Transparent view of the individual layers showing the screw shaft and the necessary angulation of the screw axis to secure the esthetics and strength of the incisal edge. Variobase SA was required.

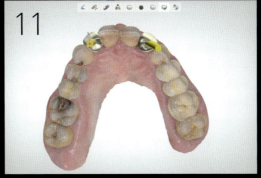

Occlusal view.

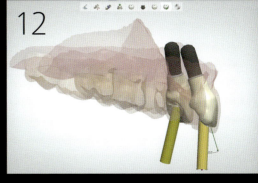

Side view.

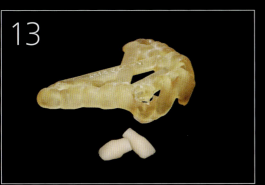

The guide and teeth printed in the office.

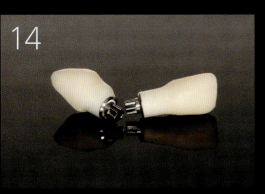

***Immediate** temporary teeth connected to Variobase SA for NT.*

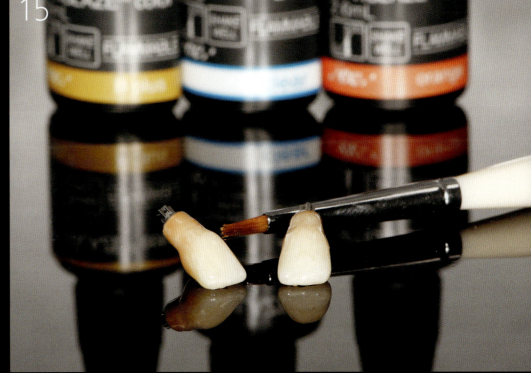

Stained teeth.

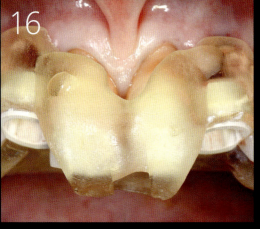

Placement of the surgical guide after avulsion of teeth 12 and 22. Note the control of the fit of the guide via the inspection windows.

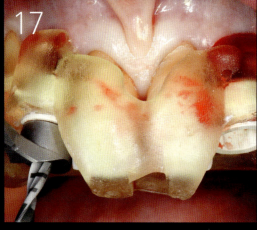

Drilling sequence.

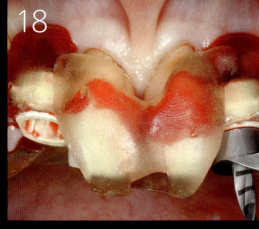

Drilling sequence continued.

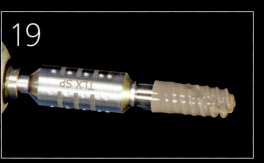

TLX NT 3.75 x 10.00 mm implant on the guided implant gripper for TLX SP.

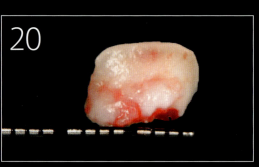

Harvesting of connective tissue grafts from both tuberosities.

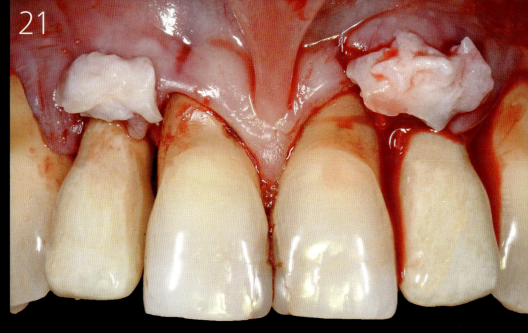

Presentation of the two de-epithelialized and open grafts.

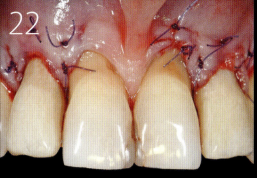

Horizontal mattress suture vestibular to teeth 12 and 22 for the connective graft on the medial side of the vestibular flap, and ASAF suture around 12 and 22.

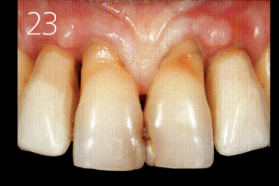

Clinical situation at 3 months with **immediate** provisional teeth in place.

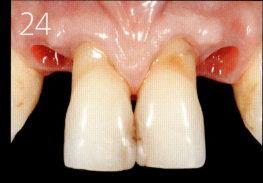

Frontal view of the emergence profile in 12 and 22 with vertical gain in the collar position.

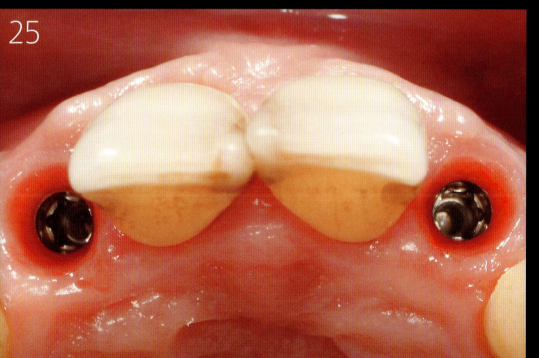

Axial view of the emergence profile and implant beds.

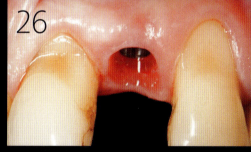

Implant bed in 22. Note the absence of inflammation.

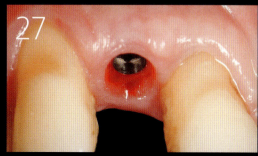

Implant bed in 12. Note the absence of inflammation.

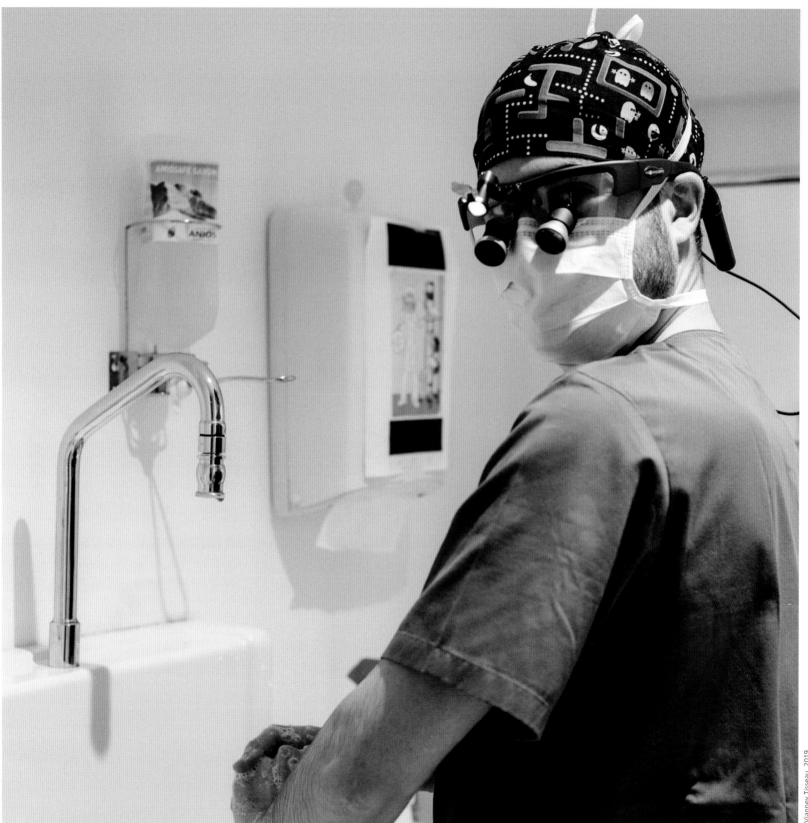
© Vianney Tisseau, 2019.

Single-unit clinical case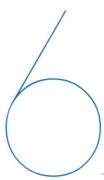

40-year-old woman.

Clinical data

- Loss of 21 due to carious regrowth under the crown, short tapered root and fracture of the coronal root margin.
- Case treated in October 2018.
- Vestibular bone wall had a dehiscence affecting one-third of the alveolus which was to be managed by guided bone regeneration (GBR) under tunneling (Bio-Oss and Bio-Gide, Geistlich, Wolhusen, Switzerland).
- Good mucogingival architecture, but a connective graft would be used to secure the inflammatory gingiva present.

Presurgical treatments

- Trios 3 used to take an optical impression and Planmeca ProMax used for the 3D examination.
- Planning in Implant Studio.
- Straumann BL RC TiZr SLActive 12-mm implant to replace tooth 21.
- 3D printing of the guide designed in Implant Studio (Dentitek Laboratory).
- First-generation Straumann socket.
- Temporary screw-retained crown, A2 shade, milled on a PMMA Ivotion Dent Multi disc on a Roland milling machine (Dentitek Laboratory).
- Dynamic abutment with angled screw hole Medentika RC (Straumann) for crowns bonded to Multilink Hybrid Abutment.

Assessment of the intervention

- Case treated in **three appointments at the office** (impressions and 3D examination, surgery, control at 4 months).
- Final prosthesis made by the referring dentist.

Additional treatments

- The patient was referred for management of a 21 that had become too unstable. She was embarrassed by the low esthetic nature of her smile but could not afford a more extensive esthetic rehabilitation. She wished to regain functional stability for this tooth. Restoration of the composites was not her priority; however, we pointed out the benefit of this to the referring dentist. The patient agreed with the option of immediate loading despite the additional cost. This allowed her to postpone the fabrication of the final prosthesis by the referring dentist for 1 year and therefore delay the financial implications of the prosthetic work.

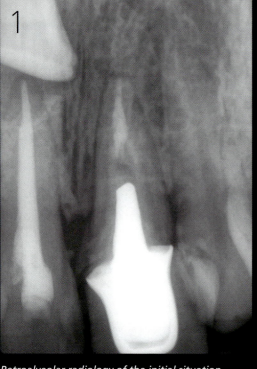

Retroalveolar radiology of the initial situation. Note the impacted tooth 13.

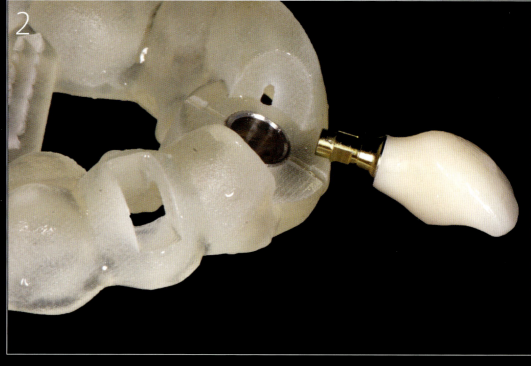

Guide and *immediate* temporary tooth on Variobase BL for Crown (Dentitek Laboratory).

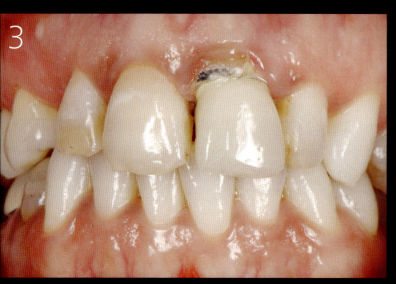

Clinical situation on the day of surgery.

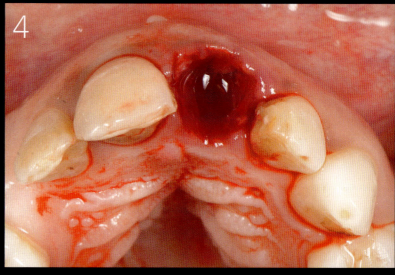

Extraction of 21, curettage of the site, and rinsing with Betadine.

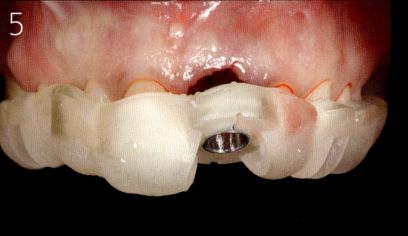

Guide in place with inspection windows to ensure an optimal fit.

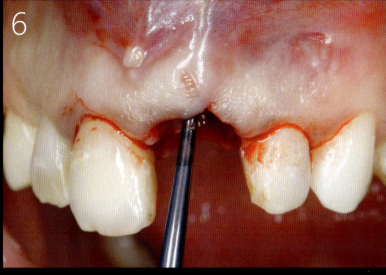

Sulcular incision from 11 to 22 and full-thickness then half-thickness tunneled flap. Good laxity of the flap was thus obtained without exposing the vestibular cortex. The limitation of the vestibular dehiscence of the alveolus allows this type of approach, which is more respectful of the vascularization of the site.

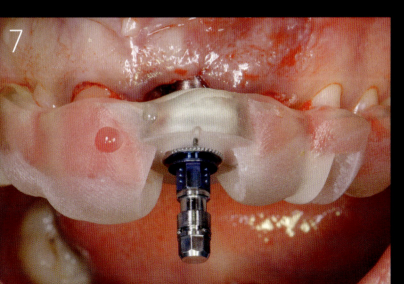

Guided implant placement, still with a one-sixth turn offset for the correct tooth position from the 3Shape implant holder registration.

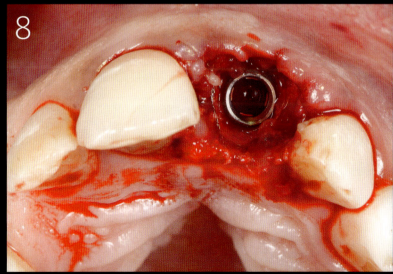

Axial view of the implant in place according to the recognized 3D positioning criteria.

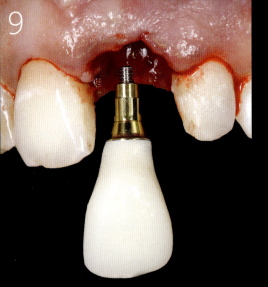

Immediate temporary tooth.

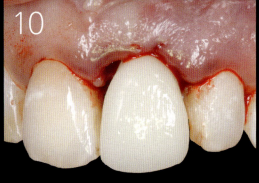

Note the very good positioning of the provisional tooth, confirming the quality of the data transfer by guided surgery.

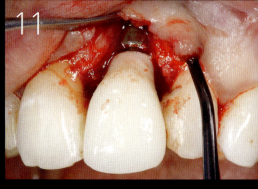

Note the optimal fit of the **immediate** tooth on the implant.

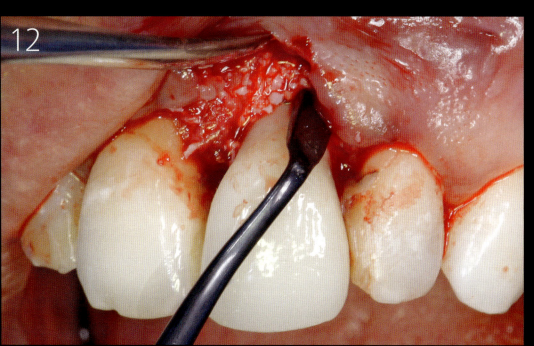

Performance of perimplant GBR guided by the prosthetic volume. Filling of the extraction hiatus and closure of the vestibular dehiscence (Bio-Oss) covered by a resorbable collagen membrane (Bio-Gide).

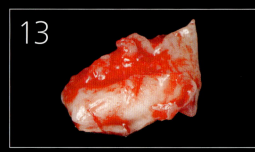

Harvesting of a tuberous connective tissue graft.

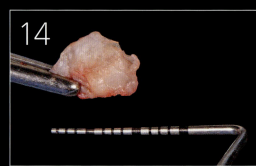

De-epithelialized and opened graft. The tuberosal graft treated in this manner is the optimal half-moon volume for reinforcing the neck of an implant unitary zone.

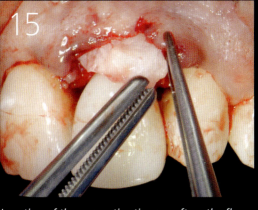
Insertion of the connective tissue graft on the flap.

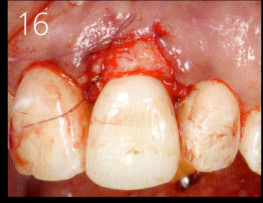
Proximal single-stitch suture of the graft.

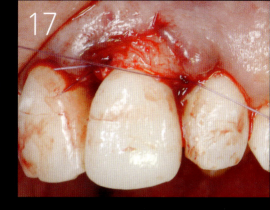

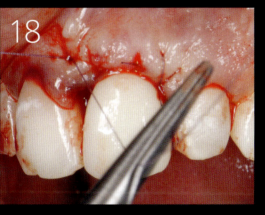
ASAF suture.

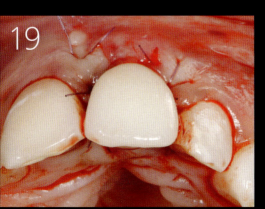
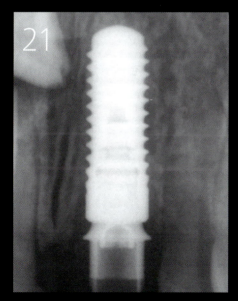

Axial and vestibular views illustrating the benefit of the ASAF suture, which allows the flap to be pulled up in a "roll-neck" fashion around the temporary tooth *instantly*. We thus define the suture guided by the prosthesis.

Postoperative retroalveolar radiograph confirming the very good connection between the implant and the tooth. Note the usefulness of planning and guided surgery in this case for homogeneous bone volume between the adjacent tooth, the impacted canine, and the anterior palatal canal.

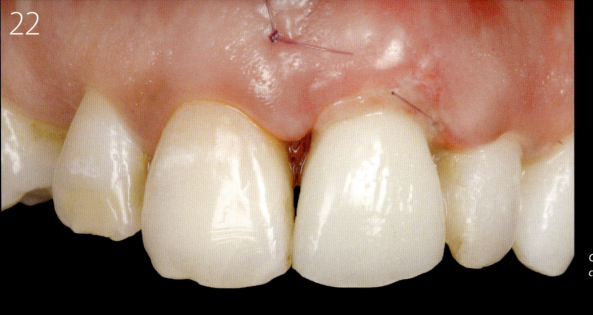

Clinical appearance at 8 days with connective tissue graft revascularization

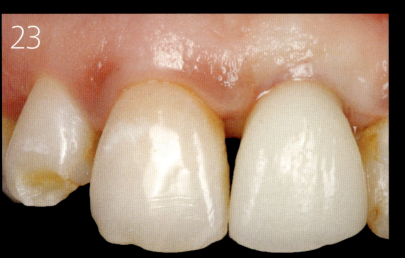

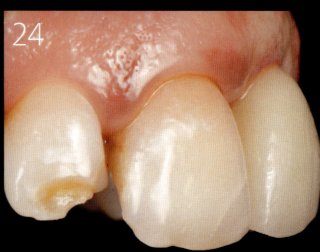

*Clinical appearance at 3 months with the **immediate** denture in place. Note the very good vestibular support of the periodontium and the quality of the emergence profile. This is a consequence of GBR and the connective graft guided by the **immediate** prosthesis.*

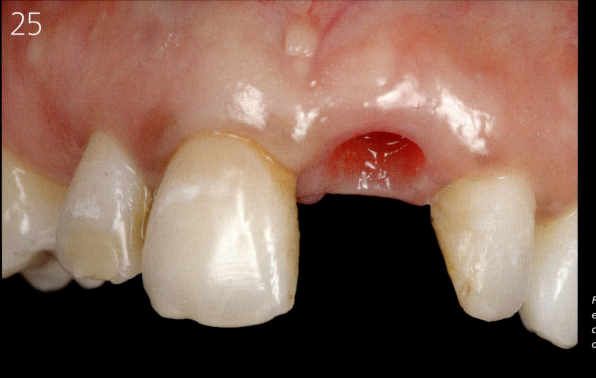

Frontal view of the dense, stable emergence profile with GBR and connective graft after removal of the temporary tooth.

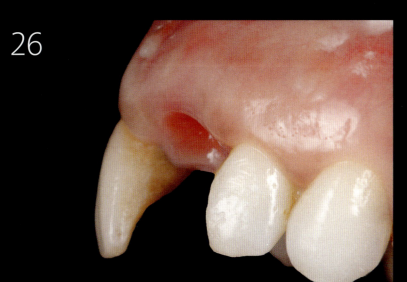

Lateral view of the healthy and stable implant bed.

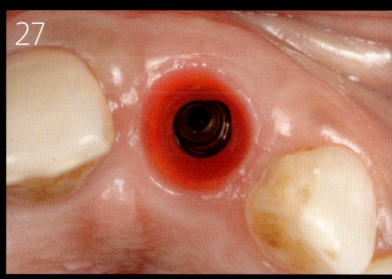

*Occlusal view of the implant bed. Note its anatomy guided by the **immediate** prosthesis and the good vestibular volume.*

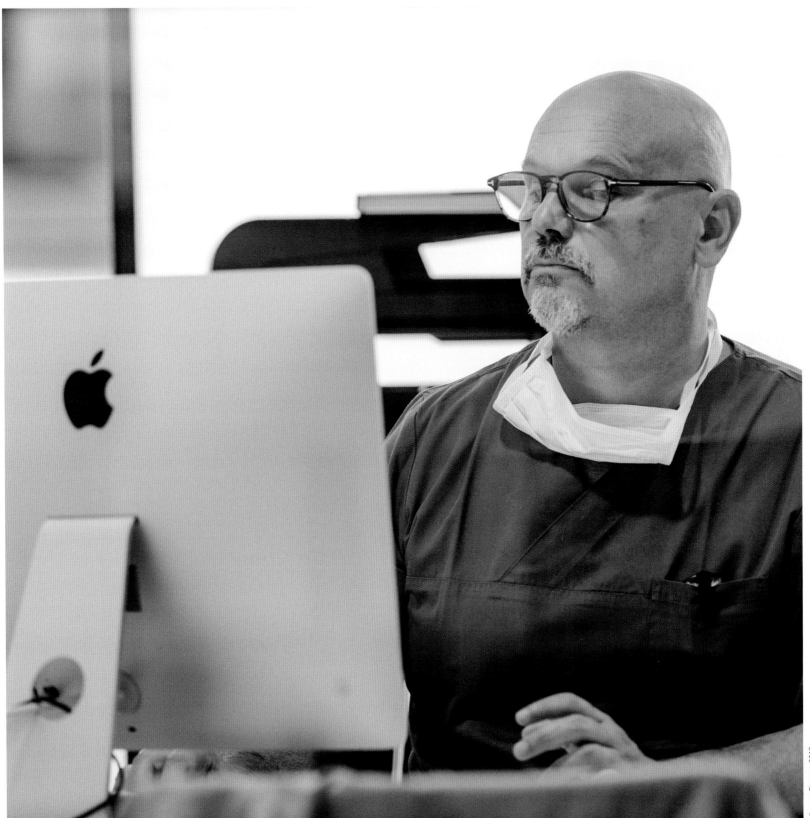

© Vianney Tisseau, 2019.

Single-unit clinical case 7

52-year-old woman.

Clinical data

- Vertical root fracture of 21 involving half the root.
- Case treated in September 2017.
- Vestibular dehiscence not exceeding one-third of the residual root managed by GBR (Bio-Oss and Bio-Gide, Geistlich Pharma France).
- Good mucogingival architecture in a thick periodontium.

Presurgical treatments

- Trios 3 used to take an optical impression and a Planmeca ProMax used to perform the 3D examination.
- Planning in Implant Studio.
- Placement of a Straumann BL RC TiZr SLActive 12-mm implant to replace tooth 21.
- 3D printing of the guide designed in Implant Studio (Dentitek Laboratory).
- First-generation Straumann socket.
- Provisional screw-retained crown, A3 shade, milled on a PMMA Ivotion Dent Multi disc on a Roland milling machine (Dentitek Laboratory).
- Variobase RC used for crowns bonded with Multilink Hybrid Abutment.

Assessment of the intervention

- Case treated in **two appointments at the office** (surgery, control at 3 months).
- Final prosthesis made by the referring dentist (Dr Philippe Aymoz, Varces-Allières-et-Risset, France).
- The patient was seen within 48 hours of her fracture, referred by her dentist, and treated within 8 days of the fracture after information required for planning was gathered on the day of the consultation. This allowed her to avoid the need for a temporary removable prosthesis.

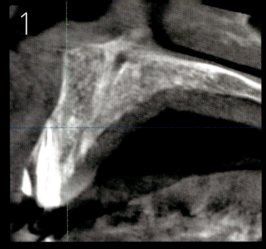

Sagittal view of the 3D examination of the initial clinical situation. The examination was done on the day of the consultation because of the urgency of the situation due to the mobility of the tooth, and the optical impression was taken in the same session. This approach allowed the patient to avoid wearing a temporary removable prosthesis after surgery and restoration took place 8 days later.

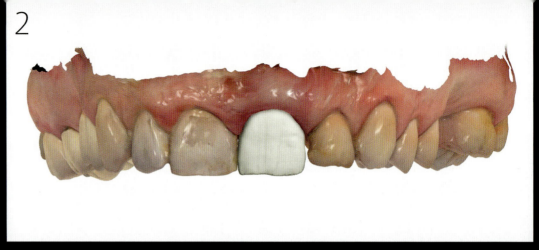

Design of 21 by symmetrical copying of 11 during the planning of guided surgery and the **immediate** restoration. This prosthetic volume allowed 3D implant positioning in adequacy with the prosthetic volume and replaced the radiologic guide.

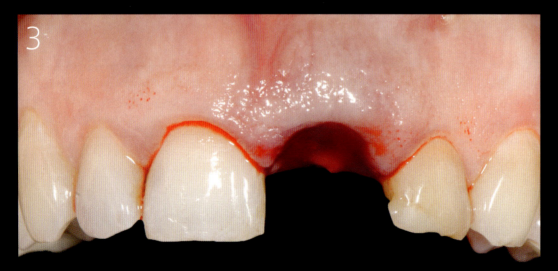

Extraction of 21 at the beginning of surgery.

Longitudinally fractured root of 21.

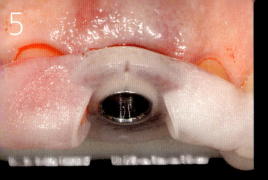

Fitting of the surgical guide with the inspection windows, the rotational registration groove, and the first-generation Straumann sleeve.

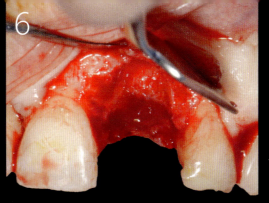

Elevation of a flap from 11 to 22 (sulcular incision without unloading) exposing a dehiscence not exceeding one-third of the root. Note the good integrity of the proximal bone peaks.

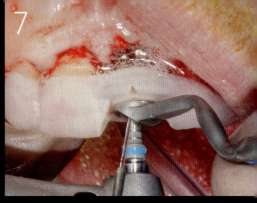

With the guide in place, guided drilling was performed with the drill handles and drills in the guided surgery kit according to the drilling protocol edited in the planning software.

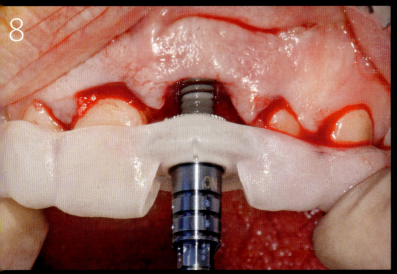

Guided implant placement with vertical and rotational registration.

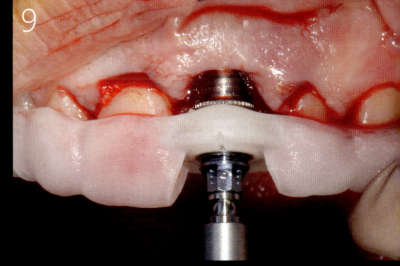

Implant in a vertical position, in the correct rotational position.

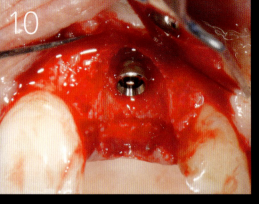

BL implant in place illustrating the vestibular dehiscence. Note the implant platform positioned 3 to 4 mm apically according to the recommendations of 3D positioning.

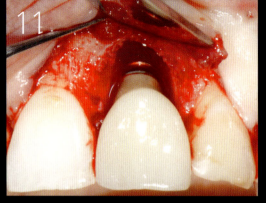

Immediate temporary tooth in an optimal position. Note the management of the emergence profile with the more palatal and apical position of the implant, which is typical in immediate implantation, and the alignment of the prosthetic CEJ in accordance with the contralateral tooth.

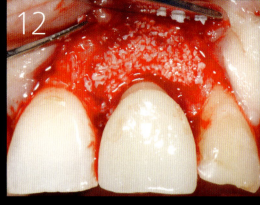

Prosthesis-guided dehiscence closure GBR (Bio-Oss fine-grained, Geistlich). Note the advantage of using a projected emergence profile for the provisional tooth rather than a progressive one to leave as much space as possible for GBR.

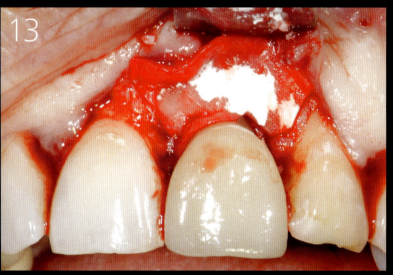

Resorbable collagen membrane (Bio-Gide Perio).

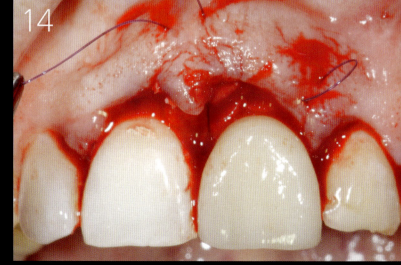

ASAF suture before tightening.

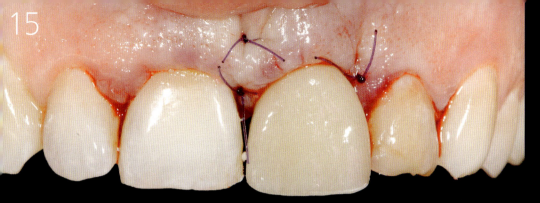

...ight suture with this "roll-neck" movement, guided by the **immediate** prosthesis.

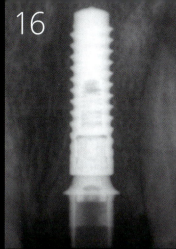

Postoperative radiograph.

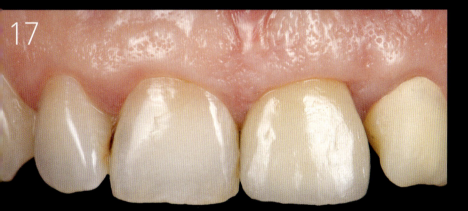

Frontal view at 2 years with the final prosthesis in place. Note the very good gingival level.

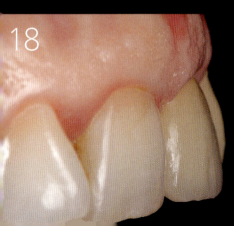

Profile view at 2 years. Note the adapted emergence profile of the implant rehabilitation, the result of 3D positioning and adequate GBR.

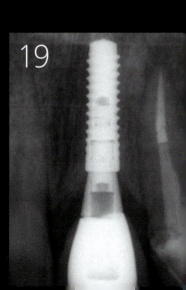

Radiograph taken at 2 years. Note the optimal bone integration of the BL implant at 2 years.

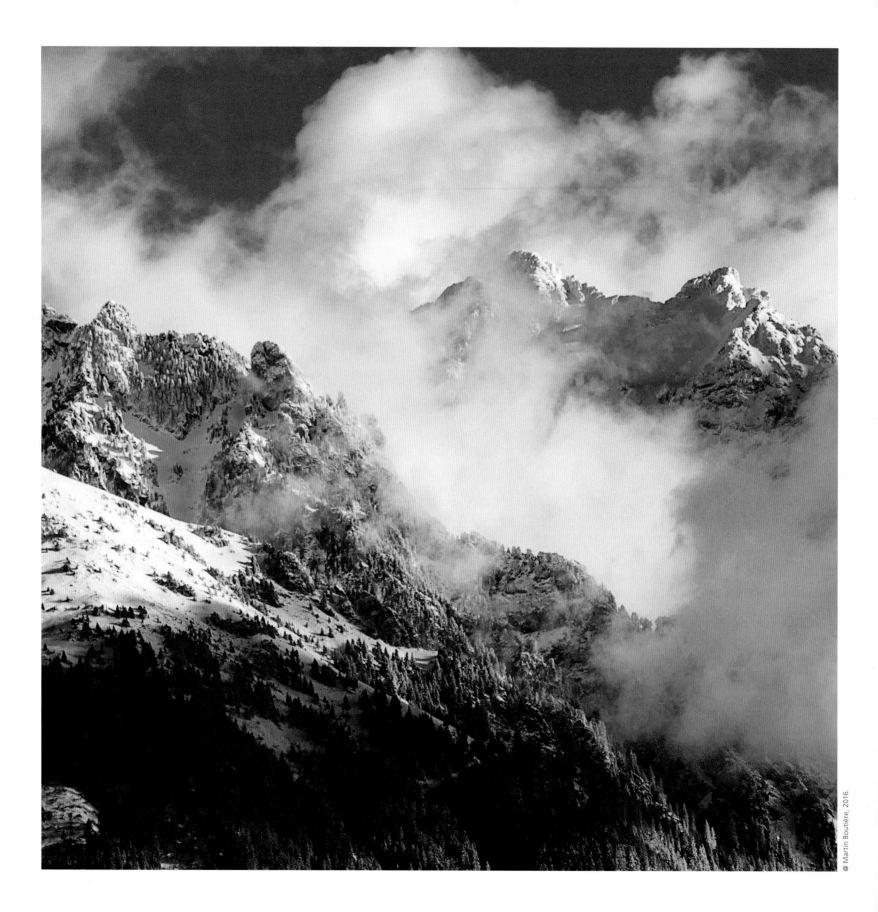

Single-unit clinical case 8

51-year-old woman.

Clinical data

- Loss of the 12 in egression as a result of periodontal disease stabilized by the referring dentist. The tooth was becoming increasingly mobilized due to periodontal bone loss.
- Case treated in April 2022.
- Vestibular dehiscence not exceeding one-third of the residual root managed by GBR (Bio-Oss and Bio-Gide, Geistlich Pharma France) and a plasma rich in growth factors (PRGF; Endoret).
- Good mucogingival architecture, but a buried connective tissue graft would thicken the gingiva and stabilize the flap in this context of periodontal loss.

Presurgical treatments

- Trios 4 used to take an optical impression and a 3Shape X1 used to perform the 3D examination.
- Planning in Implant Studio.
- Straumann TLX NT TiZr SLActive 3.75 x 12.00 mm implant to replace tooth 12.
- 3D printing of the guide designed in Implant Studio and printed in the office on a NextDent 5100 printer with NextDent SG resin.
- Straumann self-locking T-socket made of polyetheretherketone (PEEK) for TLX implants.
- A screw-retained temporary crown, A2 shade, was printed in the office on NextDent 5100 with NextDent Crown & Bridge N1 resin, polymerized in the LC-3D 3D polymerization unit, and stained on an A2 base with an Optiglaze Color Set (GC Europe).
- Variobase SA used for NT crown bonding with Multilink Hybrid Abutment HO.

Assessment of the intervention

- Case treated in **three appointments at the office** (impression and 3D examination, surgery, control at 3 months).
- Final prosthesis made by the referring dentist.

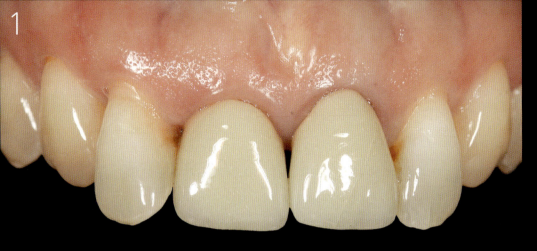

Initial clinical situation with egression and vestibuloversion of 12, associated with type 2 mobility.

3D view of periodontal loss, illustrating the clinical consequences.

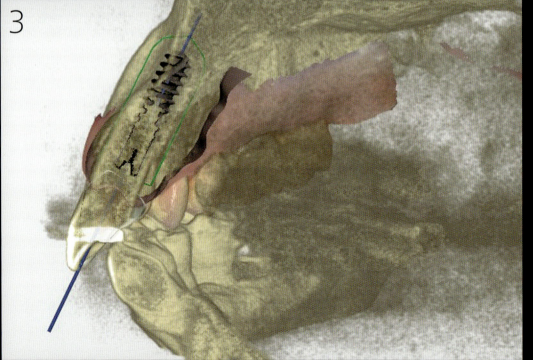

Sagittal section of the plan in Implant Studio. This shows the value of 3D planning, which makes it possible to manage and understand the implant, bone, gingival, and prosthetic volumes. This helps to assess the need for any reconstructions before surgery and to choose the prosthetic abutment best suited to preserving a cosmetic volume that is consistent with an optimal esthetic result.

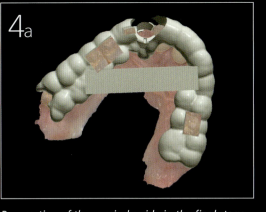
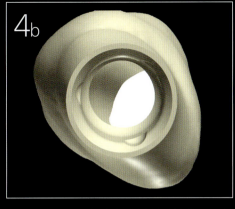
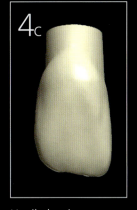
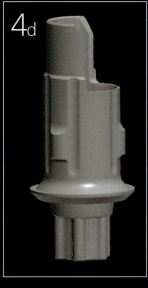

4a Preparation of the surgical guide in the final stage of the planning flow (Implant Studio). A CAD/CAM output file is available with the STL file of the guide; an STL file contains the implant positioning and a PDF file contains the drilling protocol and surgical report. If the tooth has been prepared in Implant Studio, an STL file of the tooth is delivered as a substitute for the "scanwithimplantinfo" file.

4b After exporting the initial CAD/CAM files and intraoral scans from Implant Studio to Dental System, the 12 is made in the office to be printed and bonded to a titanium baseplate. Note the anatomic morphology of the prosthetic CEJ area and the friction grooves and rotational markings for the Variobase NC to be used later.

4c Vestibular view. Note the emergence profile linking the coronal morphology to the platform of the titanium baseplate to be used later.

4d Variobase NC SA for Crown with an asymmetrical screw shaft to allow angulation of the screw axis for use with the SA abutment screwdriver.

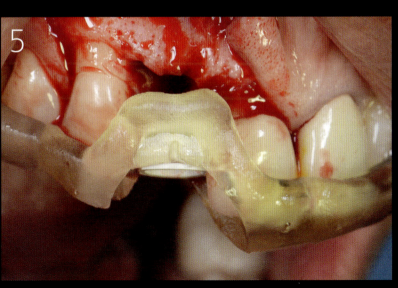

5 Guide in place after extraction and flap elevation. Note the self-locking PEEK sleeve for TLX. The friction of this sleeve was too high and the guide was under a great deal of stress during insertion and removal of the drill handles. The design has since been modified.

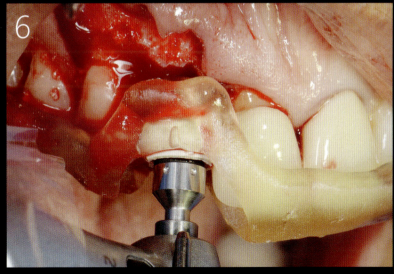

6 Guided placement of the implant with the black line corresponding to the depth H6 and the rotational marker point that needed to be aligned with the groove on the guide. The black line had to be parallel to the edge of the sleeve, confirming the precise axis of guidance.

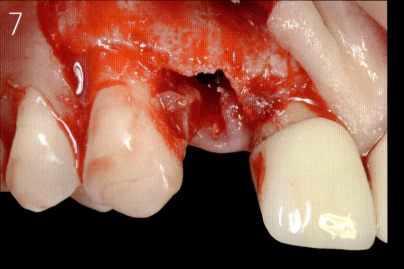

Removal of the guide and subosseous positioning of the TLX.

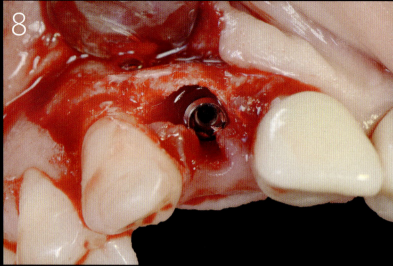

Axial view. Note the mesial bone volume in relation to the implant neck. The TLX range lacks a flaring tool as in the BL and BLX ranges. Its supraosseous design explains this, but in immediate implantation, recommendations and clinical needs may lead to this neck being placed in a subosseous position and having to flare the bone opposite the implant platform.

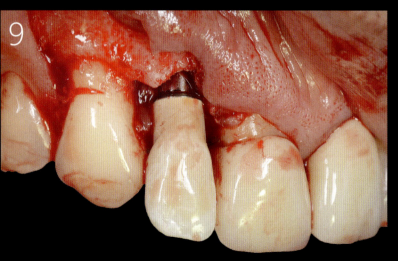

Immediate temporary tooth in place. Note the optimal positioning of the tooth. This confirmed the precision of the guided surgery.

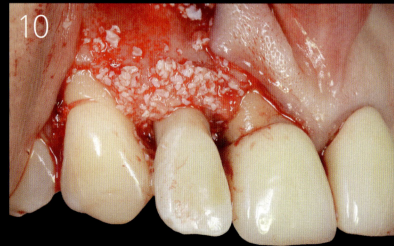

GBR guided by the prosthesis. The filling was made of DBBM (Bio-Oss with fine particles, Geistlich) incubated in the F2 fraction of PRGF (Endoret). This provides easy-to-handle sticky bone and a concentrate of growth factors in the regeneration site.

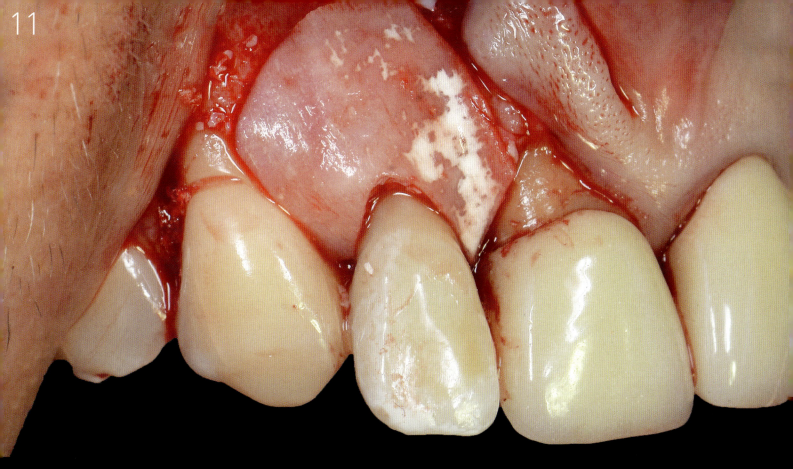

The filling was covered with a resorbable collagen membrane (Bio-Gide Perio).

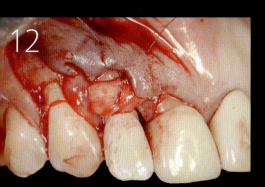
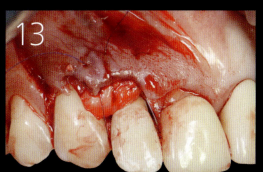
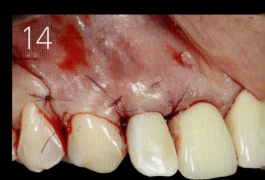

ASAE suture with anchoring of the connective graft. The graft was harvested from the tuberosity, de-epithelialized, and opened

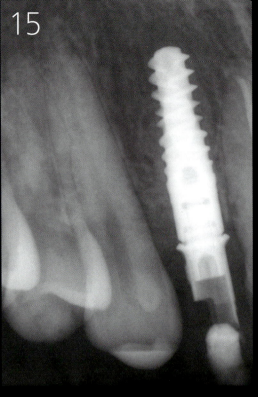

15 Postoperative radiograph. The mesial bone peak prevented optimal seating of the connection on the implant. Biologically, this had no consequence during the provisional phase; however, it can lead to unscrewing of the temporary tooth during the 3 months after bone restructuring. Careful attention must be paid to bone interference when placing the *immediate* denture.

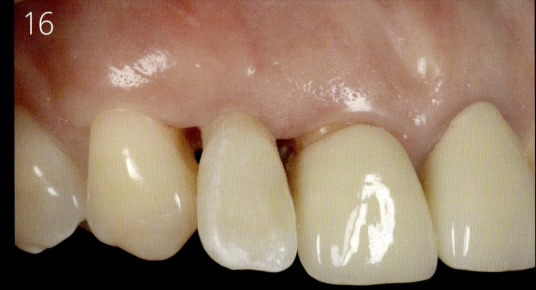

16 Clinical situation at 3 months. Note the level of the collar and the very satisfactory proximal and distal attachment.

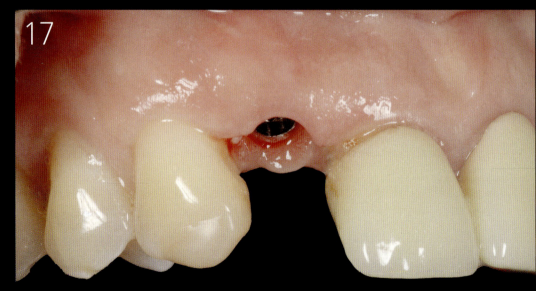

17 Buccal view without the tooth. Note the health of the sulcus and the absence of inflammation due to the smooth surface of the temporary resin (printed or milled) compared to relining in the mouth with a self-curing resin.

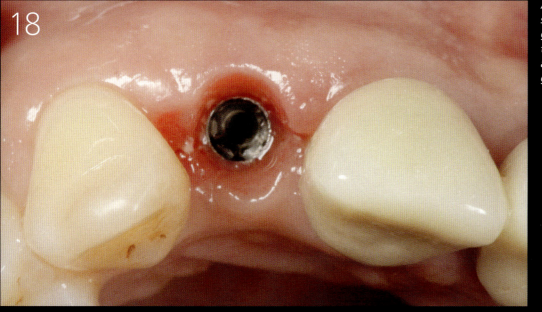

18 Axial view. Note the morphology of the sulcus and the vestibular volume. Bio-Oss granules may still be present. This is due to the fact that cleaning of the site is not always sufficient to eliminate the parasitic granules dispersed after filling.

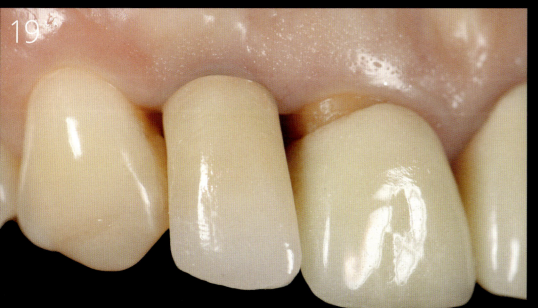

19 Prosthesis made by the treating dental practitioner after 1 year. The esthetic result was questionable, but the periodontal context was satisfactory with a stable peri-implant volume despite the initial losses.

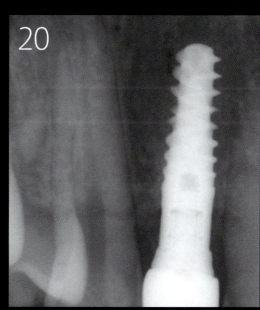

20 The radiographic result at 1 year confirmed good integration of the implant and the good volumetric response of GBR, securing the result.

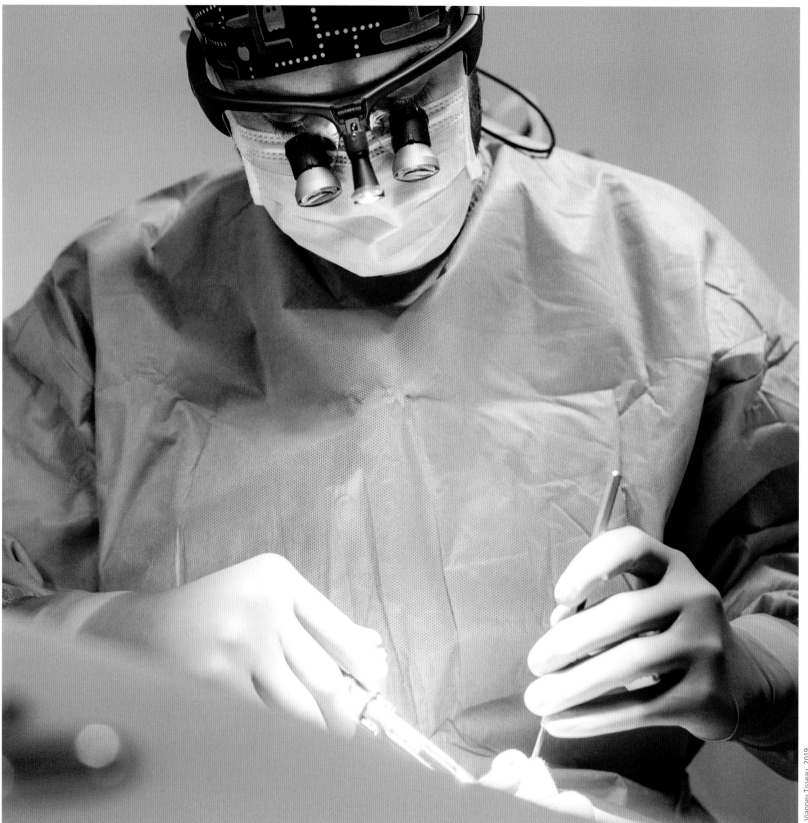
© Vianney Tisseau, 2019.

Single-unit clinical case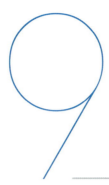

47-year-old patient.

Clinical data

- Middle third root fracture requiring rapid extraction of 11.
- Case processed in November 2022.
- Loss of the vestibular wall on one-third of the root.
- Good mucogingival architecture.

Presurgical treatments

- Trios 4 used to take the optical impression and 3Shape X1 used to perform the 3D examination.
- Planning in Implant Studio.
- Placement of a Straumann TLX SP RT TiZr SLActive 4.5 x 12.0 mm implant.
- 3D printing of the guide designed in Implant Studio, printed in the office on NextDent 5100 with NextDent SG resin and polymerized in the LC-3D 3D polymerization unit.
- Straumann T-socket.
- A screw-retained temporary crown in 11, A2 shade, was printed in the office on a NextDent 5100 printer with NextDent Crown & Bridge N1 resin, polymerized in the LC-3D 3D polymerization unit, and stained on an A2 base characterized with an Optiglaze Color Set (GC Europe).
- Variobase SA used for RT crowns bonded with Multilink Hybrid Abutment HO.

Assessment of the intervention

- Case treated in **four appointments at the office** (impression and 3D examination, surgery, control at 3 months with final impression, crown, and ceramic chips).
- Final prosthesis made in the office (Mathias Berger Laboratory, Lyon, France).

Additional treatments

- In addition to replacement of 11, the diastema was closed at the patient's request with a ceramic chip mesial to 21. This made it possible to rebalance the volumes between 11 and 21, which was not possible with the temporary tooth. When immediate restoration was performed, the diastema was closed using the temporary prosthesis to protect the underlying soft tissue during the healing phase.

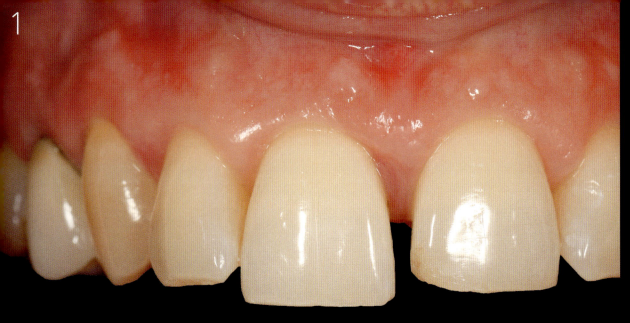

Initial clinical frontal view with egression of 21 related to the horizontal root fracture in the coronal third.

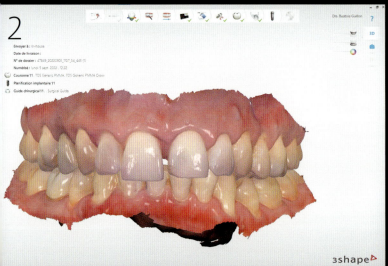

Optical impression taken using the Trios 4 for the planning associated with the 3D radiographic examination during this appointment

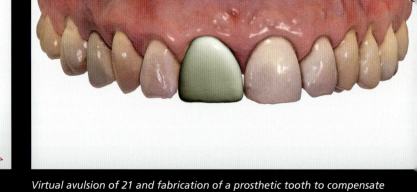

Virtual avulsion of 21 and fabrication of a prosthetic tooth to compensate for the erosion and close the diastema

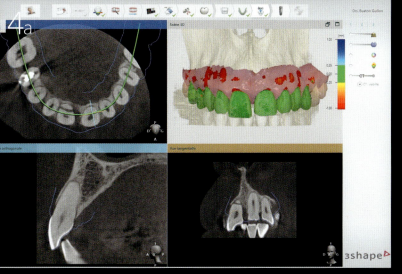
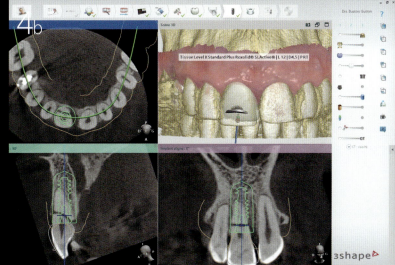

Implant Studio planning software with the fusion of the intraoral STL file generated by the Trios 4 intraoral scanner and the DICOM file from the CBCT. The colorimetric index is used to evaluate the accuracy of the fusion.

3D positioning of a 4.5 x 12 mm TLX SP RT implant. Note the brown lines outlining the gingival contour, and the gray line outlining the prosthetic envelope of the future temporary crown. Immediate implantation was possible as the apicopalatal bone triangle was sufficient to achieve primary stability.

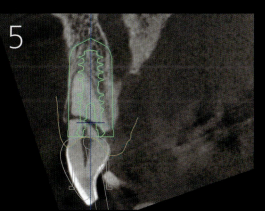
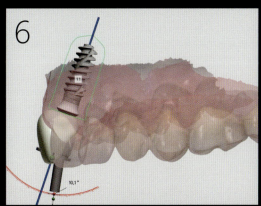
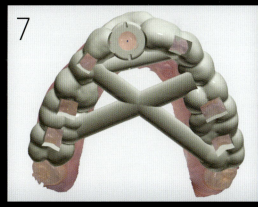

Enlarged view of the sagittal section. Note the adherence to all the International Team for Implantology (ITI) recommended implant positioning parameters in terms of 3D positioning, and the relationship between the smooth neck and the soft tissue and the more apical and palatal positioning of 1 mm that is characteristic of immediate implantation according to Chen et al.

Transparent view of the filters of the necessary modification of the screw shaft axis that would allow screwing in of the prosthesis without changing the optimal bone positioning. A Variobase SA RT for crowns was used.

The finished guide design in Implant Studio prior to export as a STL file for printing. Note the reinforcement bars, inspection windows, recess for the Straumann T-socket, and rotational registration line.

The Quokka protocol

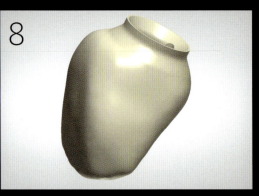

The tooth design in Dental System in the practice.

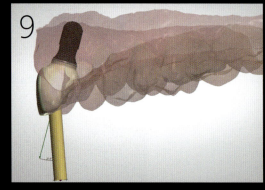

Orientation of the screw shaft axis for correct positioning of the Variobase SA during tooth design.

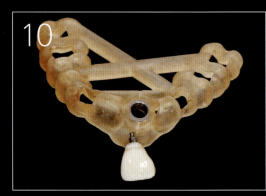

*The guide and **immediate** temporary tooth connected to the Variobase and stained.*

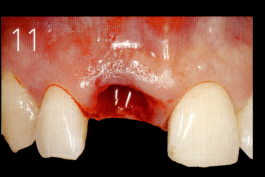

Extracted tooth 11. The site was curetted and rinsed with Betadine.

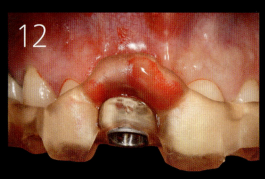

The guide in position.

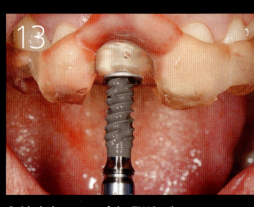

Guided placement of the TLX implant.

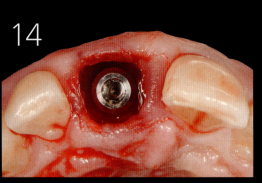

Axial view of the alveolar 3D implant positioning.

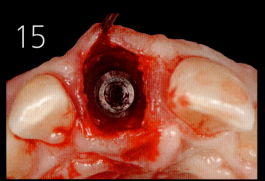

Note the residual vestibular bone wall beyond the coronal third. The vestibular flap was elevated by tunneling. There was sufficient laxity to perform GBR in the coronal third.

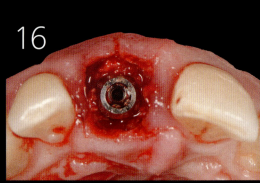

GBR performed with DBBM (Bio-Oss with fine particles) incubated in the F2 fraction of PRGF associated with a resorbable collagen membrane (Bio-Gide Perio).

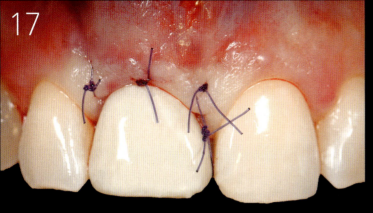
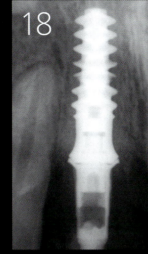

Suturing of the flap with a suspension using the contact point between teeth 11 and 21.

Postoperative radiographic view. Note the volume GBR present in the extraction hiatus in addition to the reconstruction of the vestibular dehiscence. The tooth was not clamped in an optimal manner due to the weaker primary rotational implant stability; however, this delta had no clinical impact.

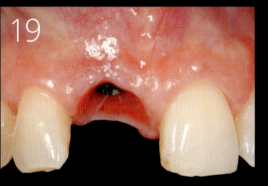
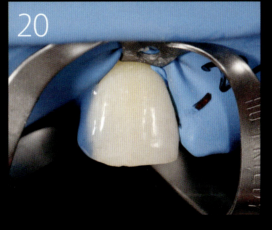

Clinical situation after 3 months, after removal of the temporary crown.

Etching with 37% orthophosphoric acid of tooth 21 before bonding of a ceramic chip on the mesial aspect.

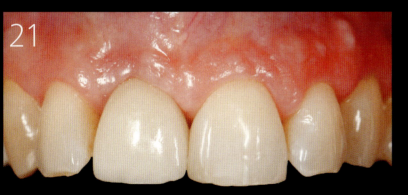
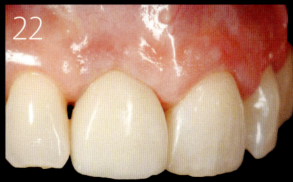

Final view of the ceramic restorations. The diastema was closed at the patient's demand (Mathias Berger Laboratory).

Profile view of the final restorations.

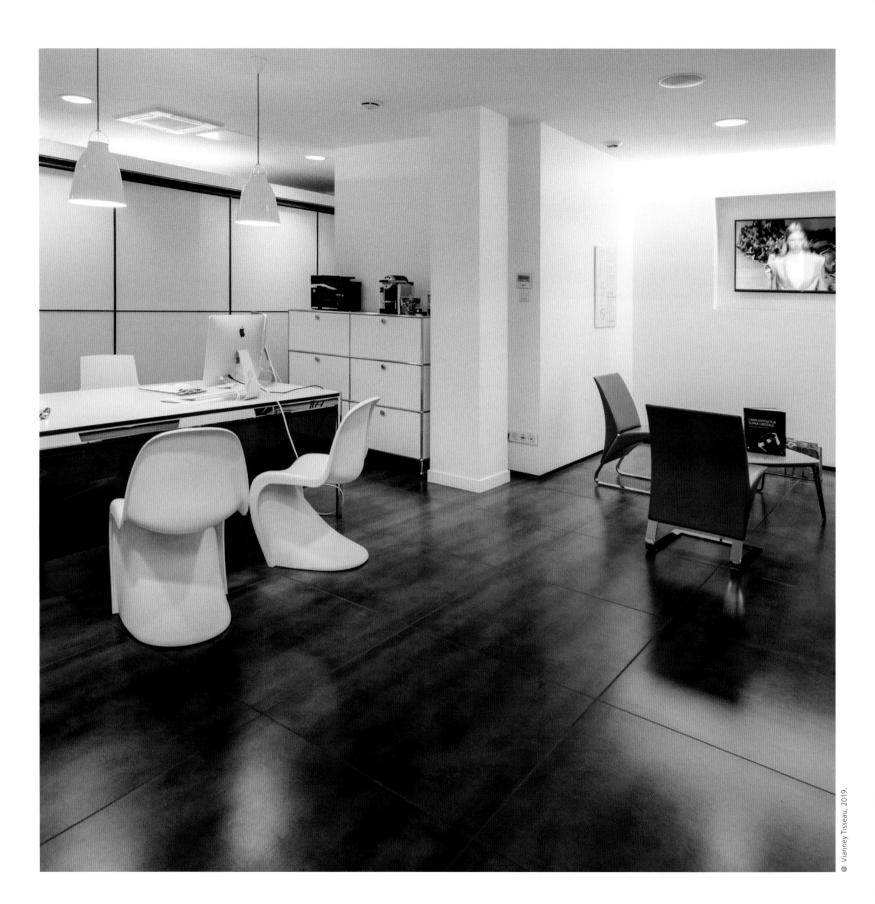

© Vianney Tisseau, 2019.

Single-unit clinical case 10

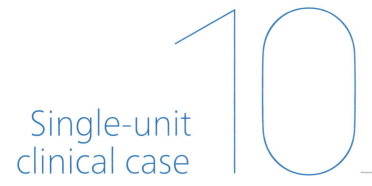

46-year-old man.

Clinical data

- Vertical root fracture in 12.
- Case treated in the office in February 2020.
- Loss of more than one-third of the vestibular bone wall.
- Good mucogingival architecture.

Presurgical treatments

- Trios 3 used to take impressions and Planmeca ProMax used for 3D examination.
- Planning in Implant Studio.
- Straumann BL NC TiZr SLActive 12-mm implant.
- Guide printed by Dentitek Laboratory.
- First-generation Straumann socket.
- Temporary screw-retained crown, A2 shade, milled on a PMMA Ivotion Dent Multi disc on a Roland milling machine (Dentitek Laboratory).
- Variobase NC used for crowns bonded with Multilink Hybrid Abutment.

Assessment of the intervention

- Case treated in **three appointments at the office** (impression and 3D examination, surgery, control at 3 months).
- Final prosthesis made by the referring dentist.

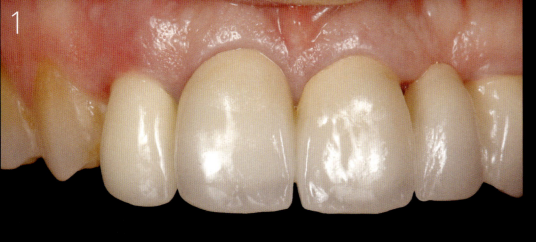

Initial clinical view with erosion of the inflamed tooth 12.

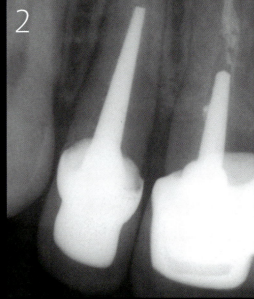

Radiographic view.

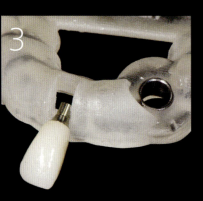

*Radiographic guide and **instant** temporary tooth connected to the Variobase NC for Crown.*

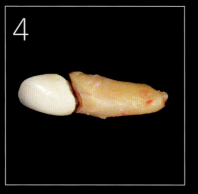

Extracted tooth 12 with root fractures.

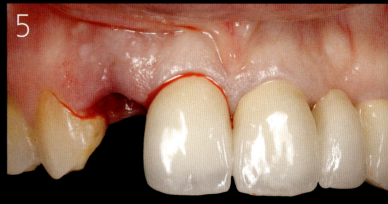

Site curetted with a Lucas curette and rinsed with Betadine.

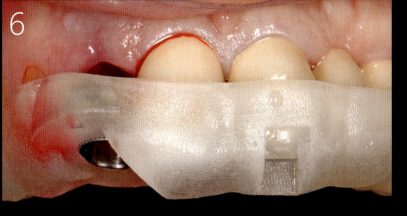

The guide in position.

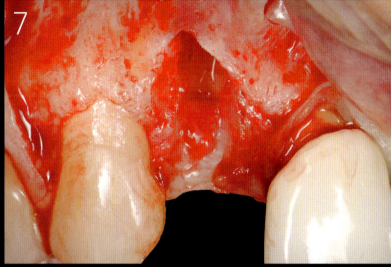

Full-thickness flap with a discharge distal to 13 that exposed the alveolar site and the vestibular and proximal dehiscence.

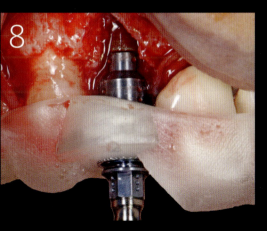

Guided implant placement with rotational and vertical registration.

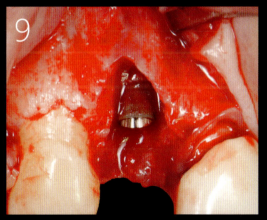

The implant in position. Note the vestibular dehiscence and the proximal defect exposing more than one-third of the root volume.

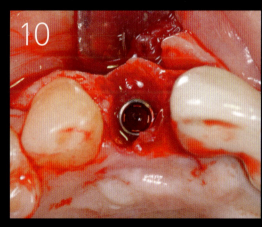

Axial view of the 3D positioning of the implant and the surrounding bone defect.

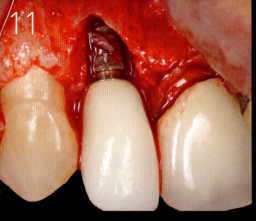

The *immediate* provisional prosthesis in place to serve as a guide for the GBR and sutures.

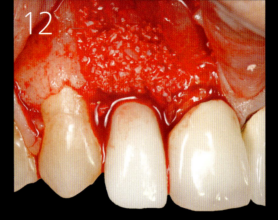

GBR with DBBM (Bio-Oss with fine particles) to reconstruct peripheral and vestibular defects.

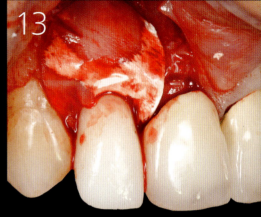

Covering with a resorbable collagen membrane (Bio-Gide).

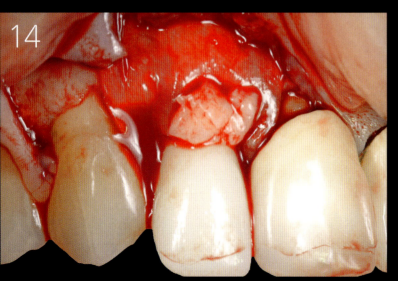

A de-epithelialized tuberous connective tissue graft was removed but left in its full thickness to secure the flap on the midface of the vestibular surface.

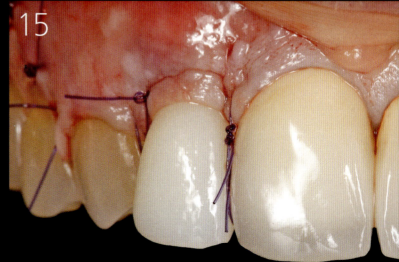

Coronal traction of the flap after a half-thickness incision at the back of the vestibule and placement of an ASAF suture with a suspension on the mesial contact point around 12 and in single stitches on the discharge.

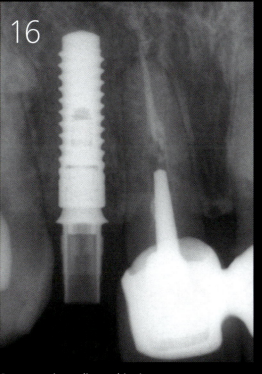

Postoperative radiographic view.

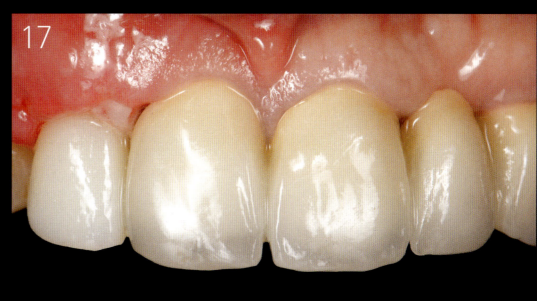

Clinical situation at 7 days. Note the revascularization of the tuberosity graft, which was slower than that of the deep palatal graft because it was more fibrous.

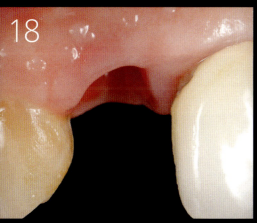

3-month clinical view at follow-up with removal of the temporary tooth. Note the gingival appearance and tissue tone.

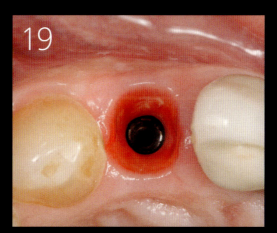

Occlusal view of the implant bed. Note the induced soft tissue morphology and the absence of inflammation. The situation was optimal for a final impression.

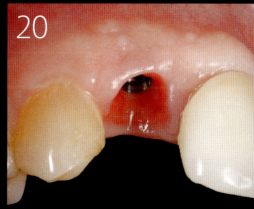

Detailed view of the emergence profile.

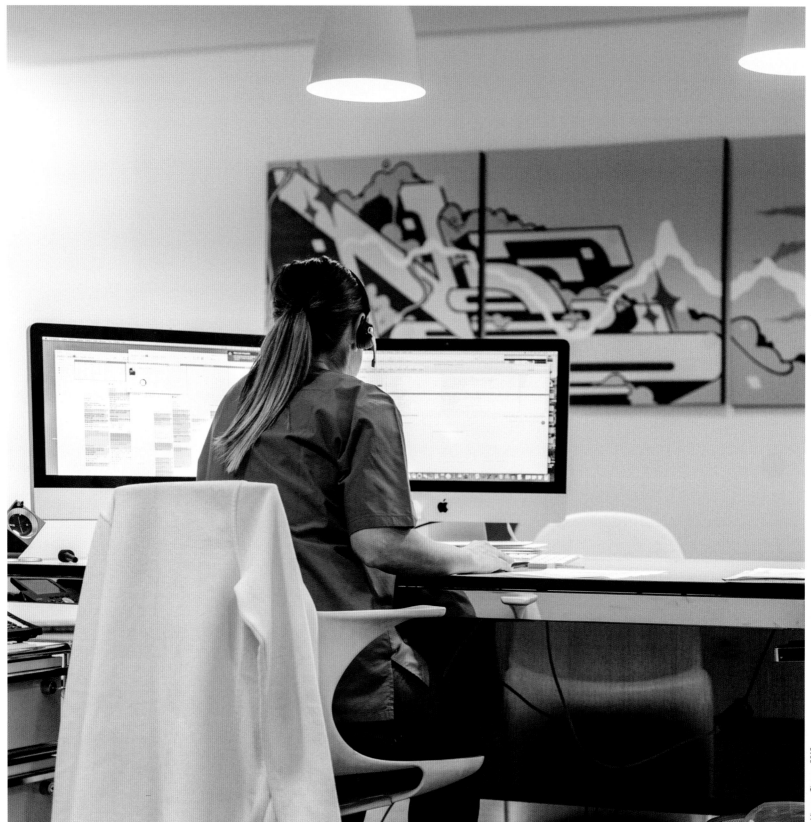

Single-unit clinical case 11

41-year-old woman.

Clinical data

- Loss of 21 by horizontal fracture following a fall.
- Case treated in November 2017.
- Vestibular dehiscence not exceeding two-thirds of the residual root managed by GBR (Bio-Oss and Bio-Gide).
- Good mucogingival architecture, but gingival reinforcement was performed with a connective tissue substitute (Fibro-Gide membrane, Geistlich).

Presurgical treatments

- Trios 3 used for optical impressions and Planmeca ProMax used for 3D examination.
- Planning in Implant Studio.
- Placement of a Straumann BL guided implant RC TiZr SLActive 4.1 x 12.0 mm to replace tooth 21.
- 3D printing of the guide designed in Implant Studio (Dentitek Laboratory).
- First-generation Straumann socket.
- Provisional screw-retained crown, shade A3, milled on a PMMA Ivotion Dent Multi disc on a Roland milling machine (Dentitek Laboratory).
- Variobase RC used for crowns bonded with Multilink Hybrid Abutment.
- Emax crown screwed on Variobase RC fabricated at 4 months (JC Allègre Laboratory).

Assessment of the intervention

- Case treated in **four appointments at the office** (impression and 3D examination, surgery, 4-month check-up associated with the final impression, final prosthesis).

Additional treatments

- In addition to the fracture to be managed as an emergency, the difficulty was in preserving the site of 11. Indeed, 11 and 21 had been treated 2 years earlier with coronal positioning of two Miller type 1 recessions with crown repositioning at 3 months in 11. Tunneling with preservation of the papilla between 11 and 21 was chosen to minimize the periodontal trauma in 11.

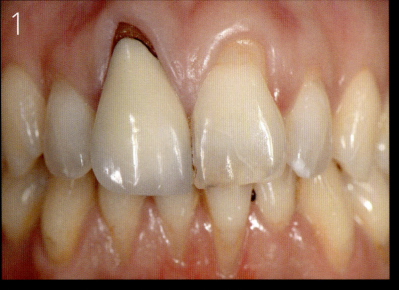

Clinical situation 2 years earlier, in November 2016.

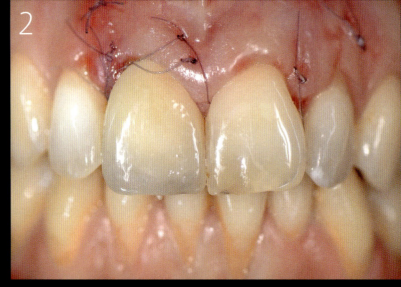

Correction of the two recessions with a coronal positioning flap associated with a buried connective band.

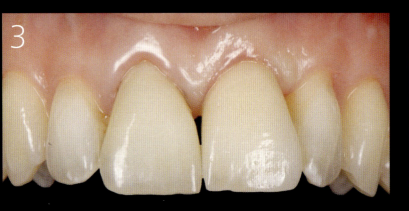

Situation on the day of placement of the two final ceramic crowns, 4 months after surgery (e-max crowns, JC Allègre Laboratory).

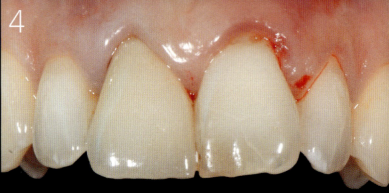

Clinical situation in 2018 following a fall with horizontal fracture of 21.

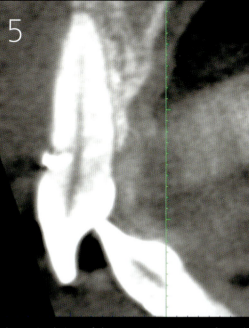

The sagittal view of the 3D examination confirmed a sufficient bone triangle to consider immediate implantation.

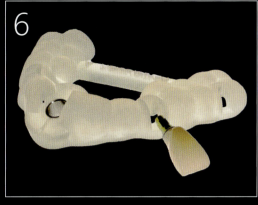

The surgical guide and *immediate* provisional tooth fabricated after planning in Implant Studio.

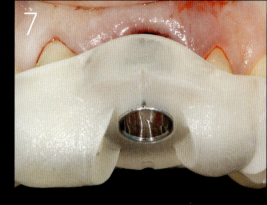

Fitting of the guide.

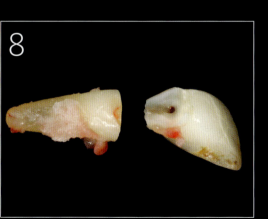

Tooth 21 with its horizontal fracture.

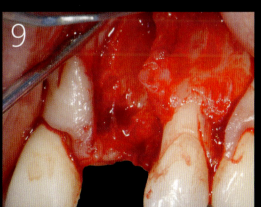

Elevation of a full-thickness flap opposite teeth 21 and 22 by sulcular incision in 21 and 22, papillary preservation between 21 and 11, and distal unloading of 22.

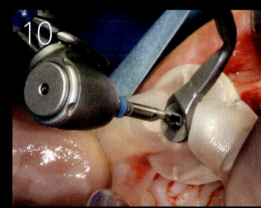

Guided drilling performed according to the guidance protocol published by Implant Studio.

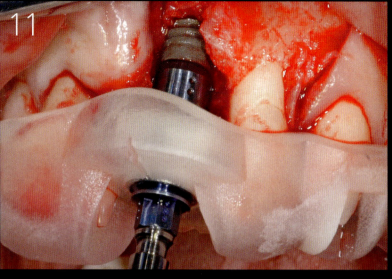

Guided placement of the BL implant with vertical (H6) and rotational registration. Note the positioning of the implant platform 3 to 4 mm apical to the gingival margin of 11. The vertical position was in accordance with the recommendations for a juxta-osseous implant.

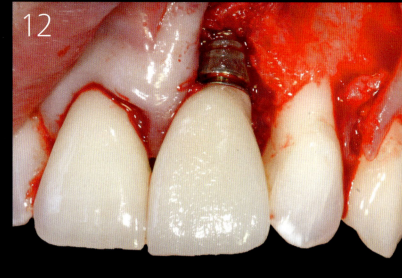

The **immediate** temporary tooth in position.

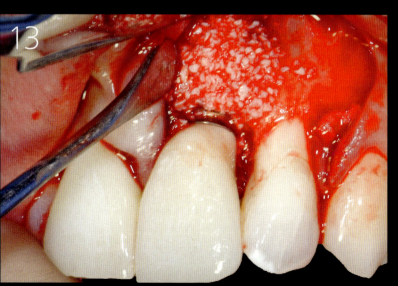

Filling of the vestibular dehiscence with GBR material (Bio-Oss with fine particles).

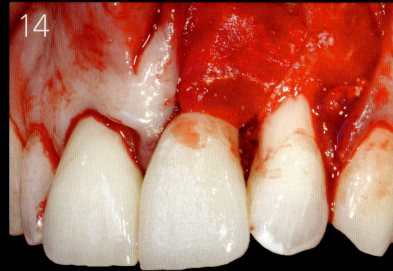

The DBBM filling was covered with a resorbable collagen membrane (Bio-Gide Perio).

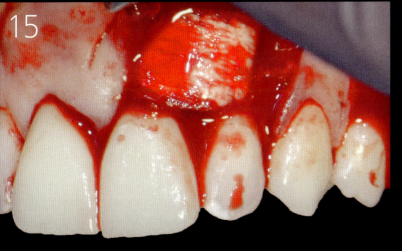

Placement of a collagenous connective graft substitute (Fibro-Gide, Geistlich) to thicken and secure the vestibular flap.

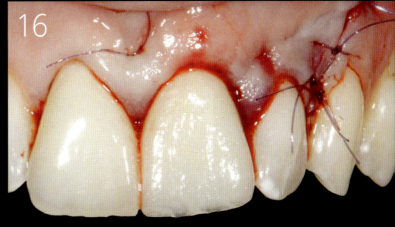

ASAF suture completed with single stitches on the distal discharge. Note the need for an occlusal touch-up on the palatal margin of 21 to avoid contact in propulsion.

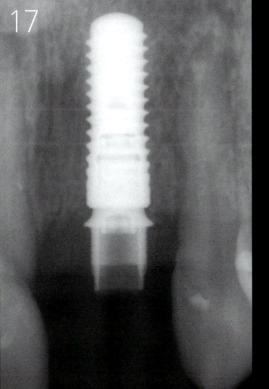

Clinical situation in frontal view at 3 months. Note the optimal periodontal integration and the good preservation of the gingival level in the immediate implant, but also on 11.

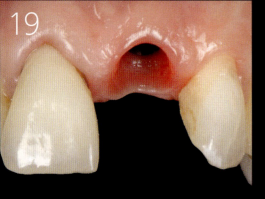

Frontal view without the temporary tooth. Note the quality of the sulcus and the absence of inflammation.

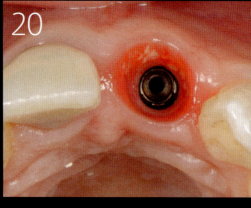

Occlusal view of the emergence profile, which again confirmed the anatomic and tissue quality of the prosthesis-guided healing.

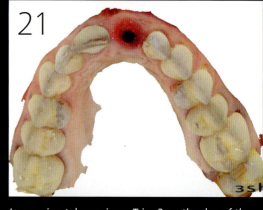

Impression taken using a Trios 3 on the day of the implant check-up with the gingival maturation being completed. This is one of the advantages of the Quokka protocol.

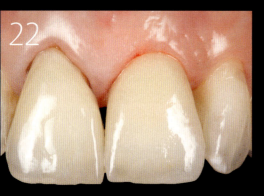

Vestibular view of the final prosthesis on the day of insertion (screw-retained e-max crown, JC Allègre Laboratory).

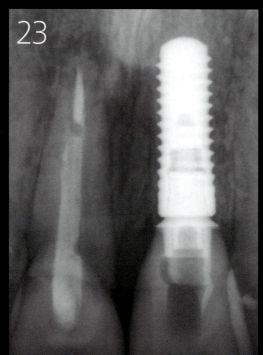

Lateral view of the emergence profile to highlight the quality of the hard and soft tissue management during immediate implantation.

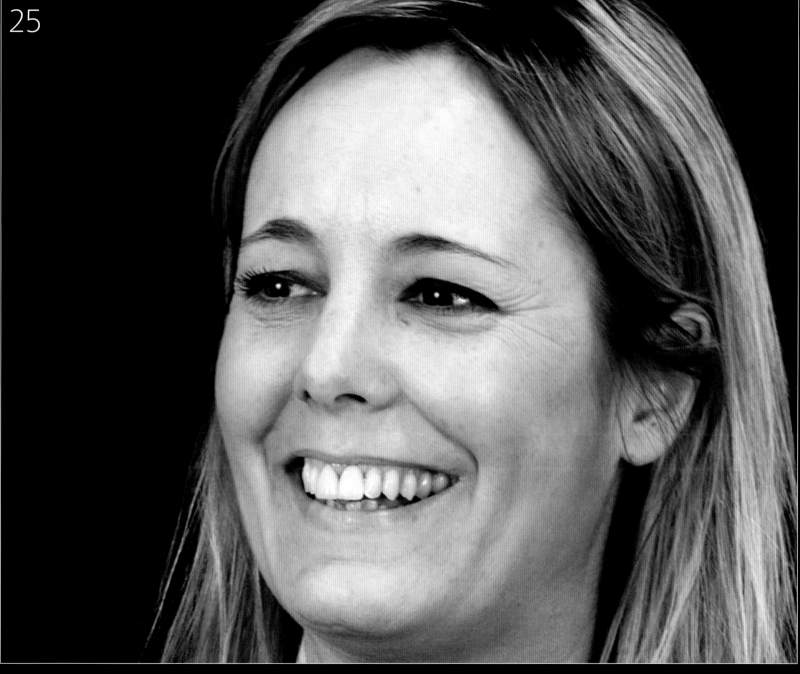

A harmonious result that integrated into the patient's smile.

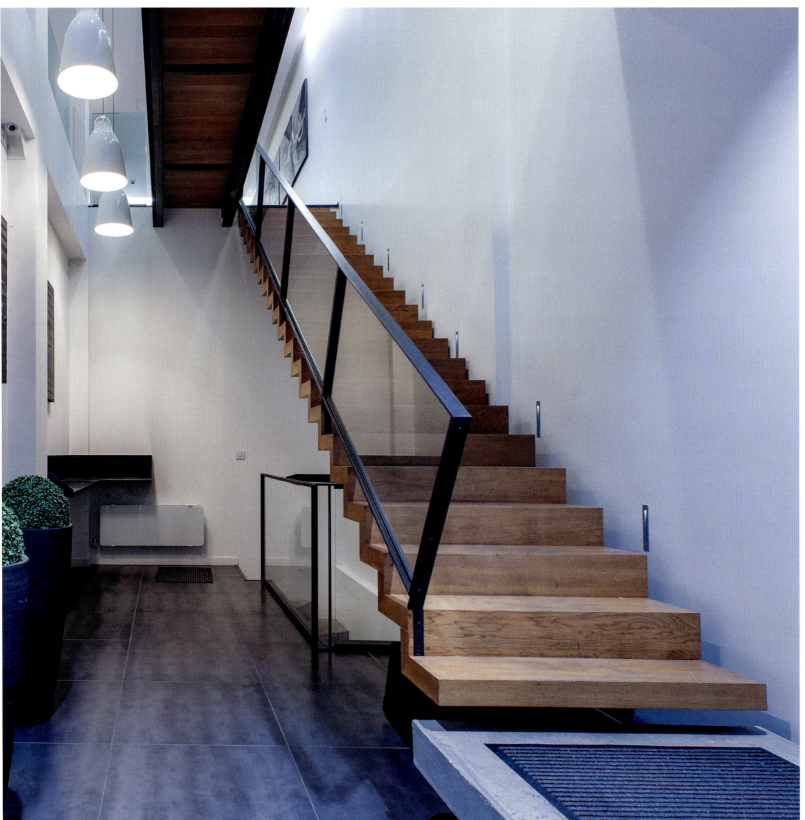

© Vianney Tisseau, 2019.

Single-unit clinical case 12

62-year-old woman.

Clinical data

- Fracture of 13 with loss of ceramic crown on post.
- Case treated in the office in December 2019.
- Vestibular bone wall with a loss of more than two-thirds of the root volume.
- Good mucogingival architecture.

Presurgical treatments

- Trios 3 used to take impressions and Planmeca ProMax used to perform 3D examination.
- Planning in Implant Studio.
- Placement of a 12-mm Straumann TL RN guided implant TiZr SLActive.
- 3D printing of the guide designed in Implant Studio (Dentitek Laboratory).
- First-generation Straumann socket.
- Provisional screw-retained crown, A3 shade, milled on a PMMA Ivotion Dent Multi disc on a Roland milling machine (Dentitek Laboratory).
- Variobase RN for crowns bonded with Multilink Hybrid Abutment.

Assessment of the intervention

- Case treated in **three appointments at the office** (impression and 3D examination, surgery, control at 3 months).
- Final prosthesis made by the referring dentist.

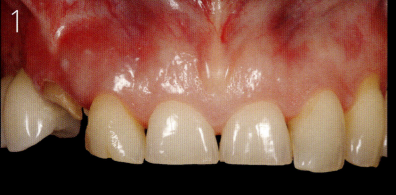

Initial clinical frontal view with the loss of the post and crown on 13.

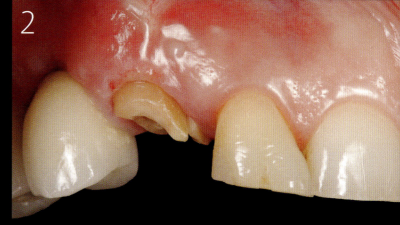

Detailed view of 13. The mucogingival architecture was favorable. Note the presence of a posterior implant rehabilitation. The fracture was visible, but the thick periodontium generally masked the clinical inflammation.

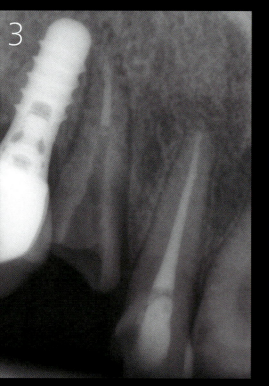

Radiographic view with the presence of a TL RN implant placed a few years earlier. The dental situation was heterogeneous.

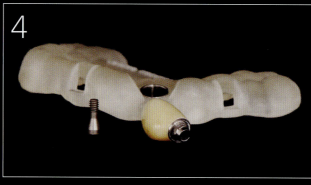

The guide and **immediate** temporary tooth connected to the Variobase RN for Crown before surgery.

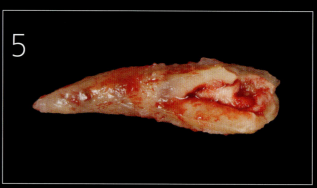

Extracted tooth 13 with the bevelled root fracture.

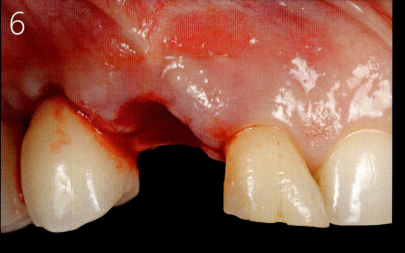

Clinical view after extraction, curettage of the site with a Lucas curette, and rinsing with Betadine.

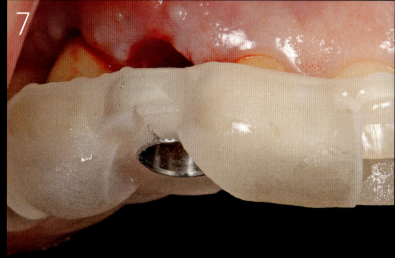

The surgical guide in place with optimal adaptive control (via inspection windows) and rotational registration grooves.

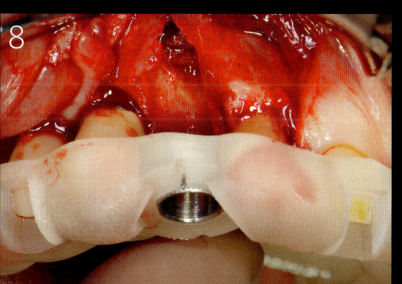

Elevation of a full-thickness flap with a mesial dehiscence of 12. The dehiscence was more than two-thirds of the coronal volume. This situation is the riskiest for immediate implantation. Note the very good bone stability around the TL SP RN implant in 14, placed 6 years earlier in the office.

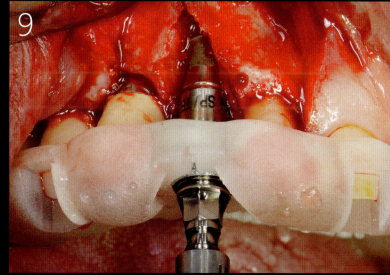

Guided implant placement. Note the similarity in vertical position between the two TL RN implants.

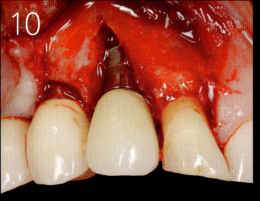

The **immediate** temporary tooth in place. The enlarged view shows a very slight gap due to interference of the emergence profile of the provisional with the mesial bone wall. Ideally, ridge flares should be used for immediate implant placement with TL or TLX implants as with BL implants.

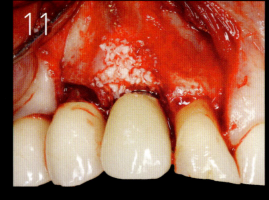

Filling of the vestibular dehiscence and the proximal and palatal hiatus with DBBM (Bio-Oss with fine particles).

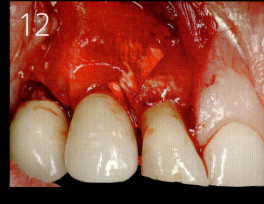

Covering with a resorbable collagen membrane (Bio-Gide Perio).

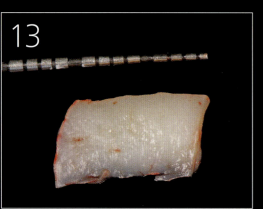

Harvesting of a palatal epithelioconjunctival graft measuring 10 × 5 mm.

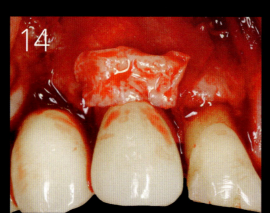

Placement of the de-epithelialized graft in the vestibular region to secure the flap opposite the large, filled dehiscence.

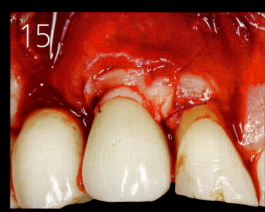

Stabilization of the graft with single sutures in the palatine.

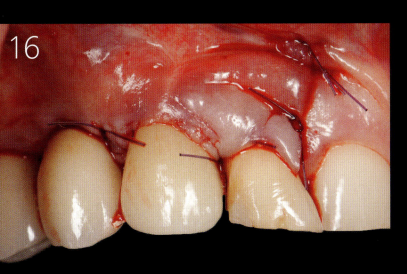

Half-thickness incision at the back of the vestibule from 14 to 12 for a coronal laxity. The flap was sutured with single sutures.

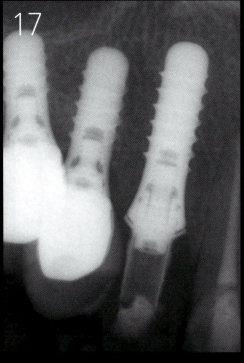

Radiographic view. Note the good density of GBR. The gap between the implant neck and the Variobase was visible but had no biologic impact. It did, however, increase the risk of tooth loosening with mesial bone reshaping.

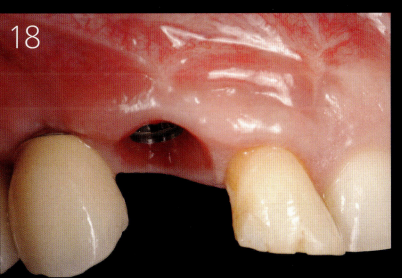

Clinical appearance at 3 months with good periodontal integration and maintenance of the collar level despite immediate implantation in an unfavorable bone context.

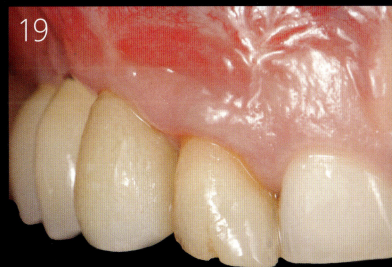

Clinical appearance of the implant bed of a TL implant. Note the absence of inflammation at 3 months after extraction of a fractured tooth and the extensive reconstruction of the peripheral bone site.

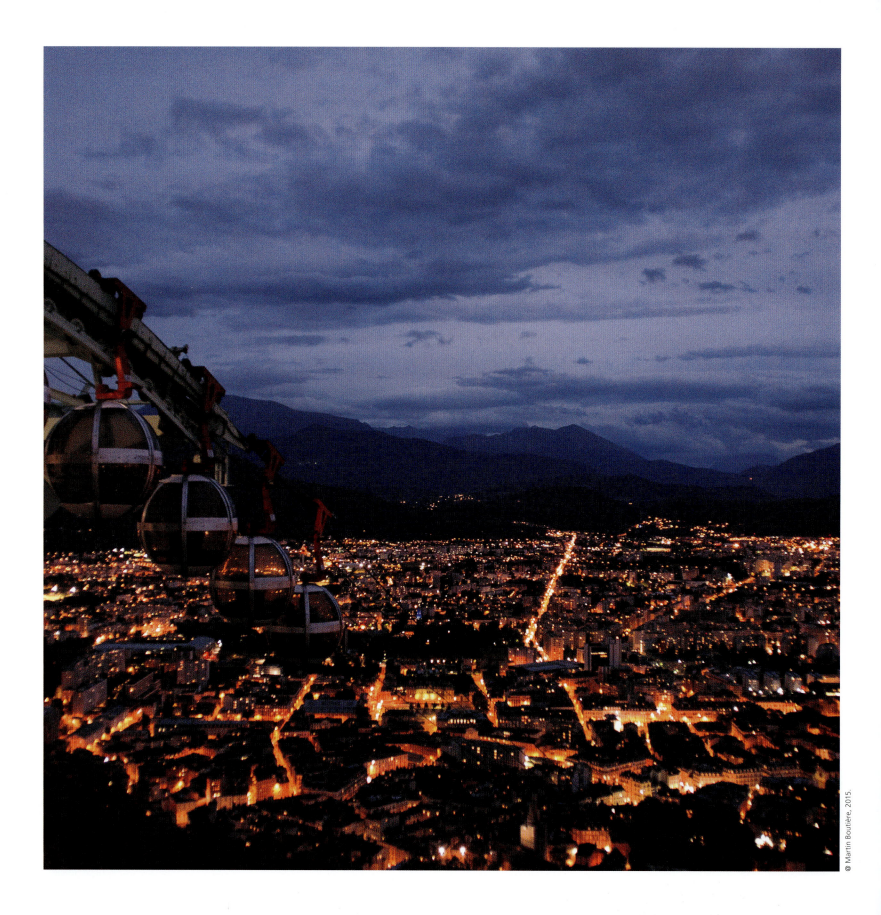

© Martin Boutière, 2015.

Single-unit clinical case 13

48-year-old woman.

Clinical data

- Loss of 12 by bevel fracture under crown.
- Case treated in June 2019.
- Vestibular bone wall had a dehiscence greater than two-thirds of the alveolus which would be managed by GBR (Bio-Oss and Bio-Gide).
- Good mucogingival architecture.

Presurgical treatments

- Trios 3 used for the optical impression and Planmeca ProMax used for the 3D examination.
- Planning in Implant Studio.
- Straumann BL NC TiZr SLActive 12-mm implant to replace tooth 12.
- 3D printing of the guide designed in Implant Studio (Dentitek Laboratory).
- First-generation Straumann socket.
- Provisional screw-retained crown, A3 shade, milled on a PMMA Ivotion Dent Multi disc on a Roland milling machine (Dentitek Laboratory).
- Variobase NC used for crowns bonded with Multilink Hybrid Abutment.

Assessment of the intervention

- Final prosthesis was made by the referring dentist.

The Quokka protocol

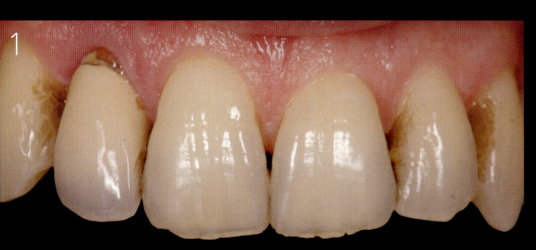

Initial clinical situation.

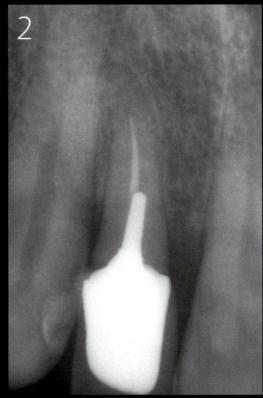

Preoperative radiograph.

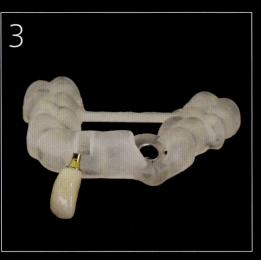

The surgical guide and **immediate** temporary tooth from the plan. The guide was printed and the tooth was milled in the Dentitek Laboratory.

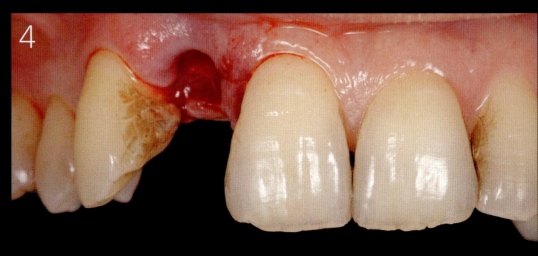

The extracted tooth at the beginning of surgery.

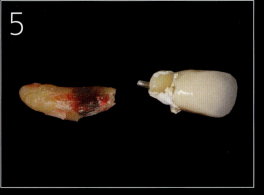

The fractured tooth 12.

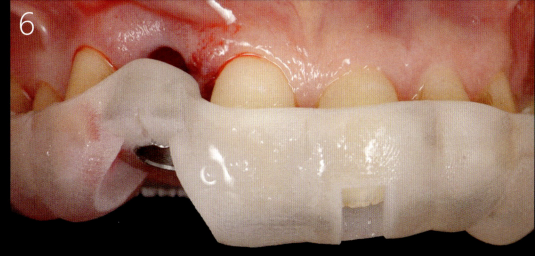

Fitting of the guide with the inspection windows.

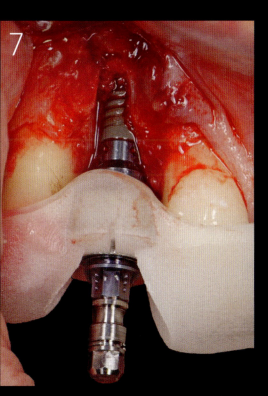

Guided implant placement, still with vertical (H6) and rotational registration (one-sixth turn offset with BL implants in the 3Shape ecosystem).

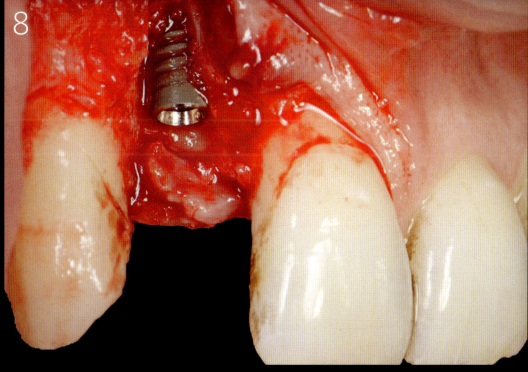

The implant in place with a vestibular dehiscence of more than two-thirds of the root. Note the 1-mm implant platform apical to the palatal wall. Intact proximal bone peaks were present.

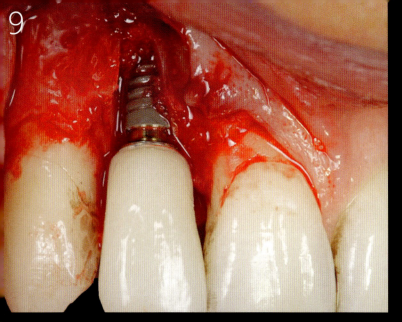

The **immediate** temporary tooth in an optimal position.

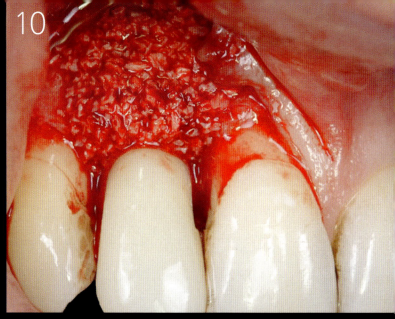

Filling of the vestibular dehiscence with GBR material (Bio-Oss with fine particles). Overcorrection was guided by the prosthesis.

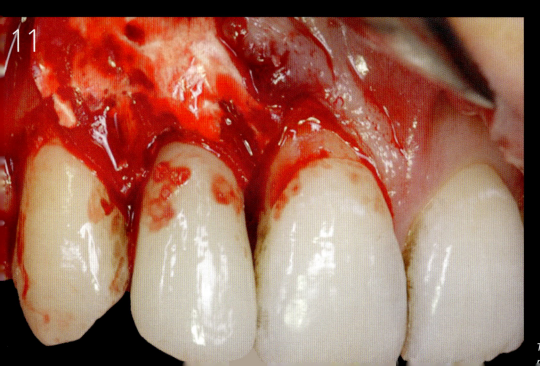

The filling was covered with a resorbable collagen membrane (Bio-Gide) stabilized by an apical pin.

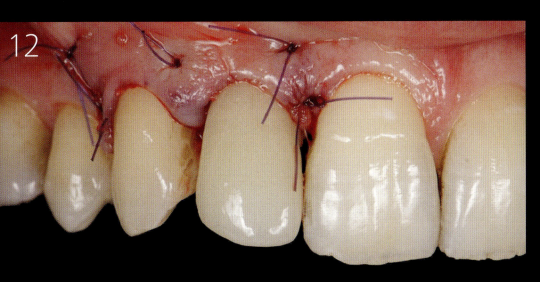

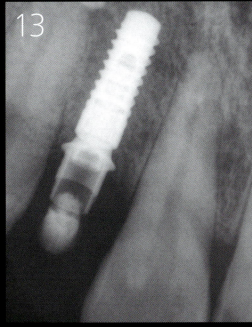

Suturing of the flap after a half-thickness incision at the back of the vestibule with an ASAF suture.

Postoperative radiographic view.

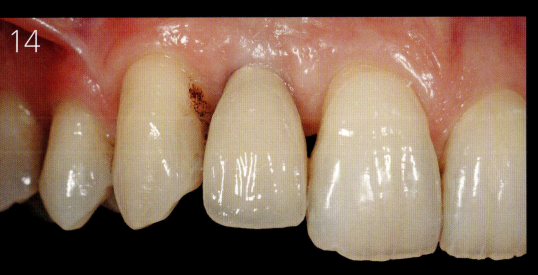

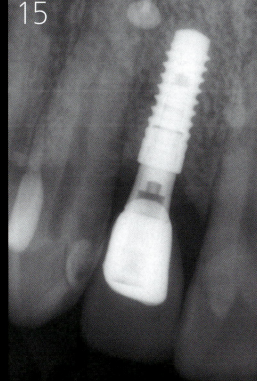

Final prosthesis placed at 1 year by the corresponding dental practitioner. A gray halo was present at the collar. The vestibular flap should have been thickened with a connective graft.

Radiographic view confirming good bone integration of the implant. The grayed-out appearance of the collar was due to the customized titanium intermediate abutment for a cemented crown where a laminated zirconia crown screwed onto a 1-mm-high titanium base would have been more appropriate.

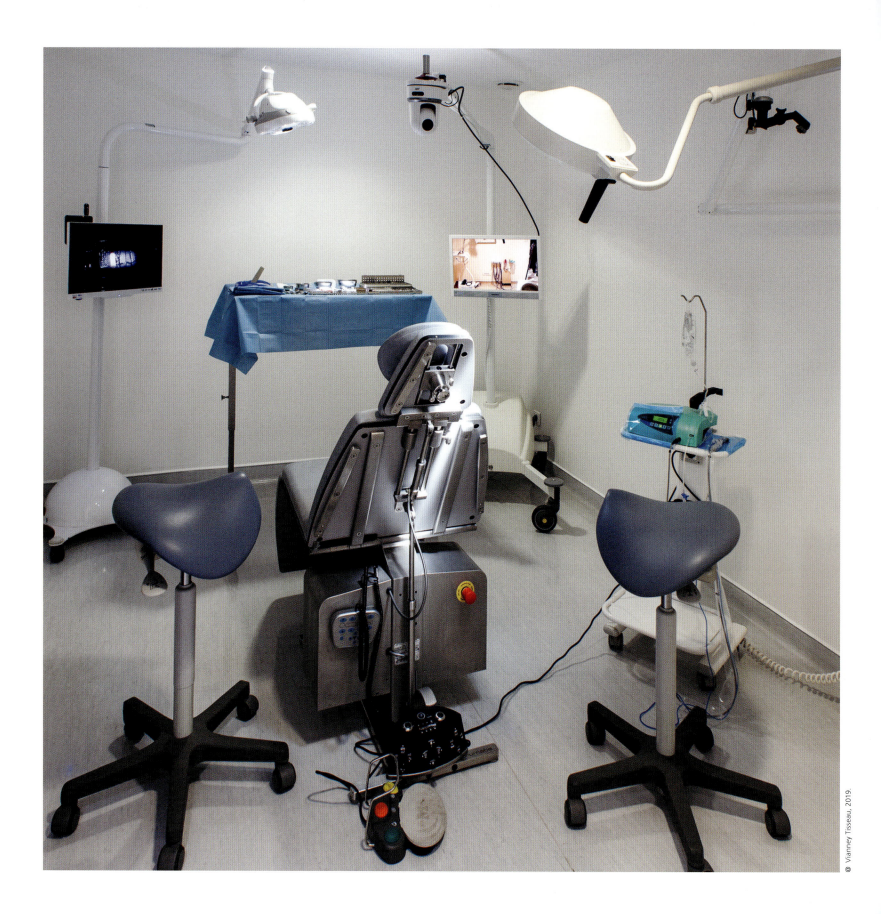

© Vianney Tisseau, 2019.

Single-unit clinical case 14

68-year-old woman.

Clinical data

- Periodontal loss of 23 with a 10-mm pocket mesial to 23.
- Case processed in October 2022.
- Loss of the vestibular and mesial bone wall of more than two-thirds of the alveolus to be managed by open flap GBR.
- Mucogingival architecture was to be corrected by coronal repositioning of the flap without a connective graft. Flap thickness was greater than 2 mm.

Presurgical treatments

- Trios 4 used for optical impressions and 3Shape X1 used for 3D examination.
- Planning in Implant Studio.
- Placement of a Straumann TLX SP RT TiZr SLActive 4.5 x 12.0 mm implant to replace tooth 23.
- 3D printing of the guide designed in Implant Studio and printed in the office on a NextDent 5100 printer with NextDent SG resin.
- Straumann T-socket, non-self-locking.
- Screw-retained temporary crown, A2 shade, printed in the office on a NextDent 5100 printer with NextDent Crown & Bridge N1 resin, polymerized in the LC-3D 3D polymerization unit, and stained on an A2 base with an Optiglaze Color Set.
- Variobase SA used for RT crowns bonded with Multilink Hybrid Abutment HO.

Assessment of the intervention

- Final prosthesis made by the referring dentist.
- The patient had been treated in the office in 2012 with two implants for four teeth from 12 to 22. A 10-mm periodontal pocket with a history of suppuration in 23 required urgent management in view of the proximity of the implant in 22 to preserve the present BLT implant. The option of immediate implantation and loading was validated by the patient in view of the precariousness of her tooth. Periodontitis was located on 23.

The Quokka protocol

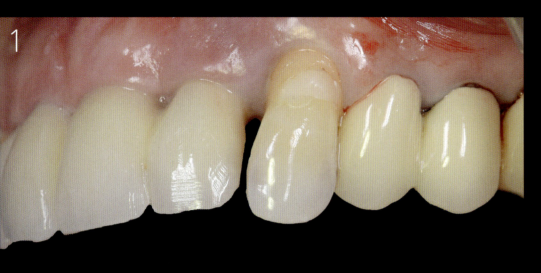

1. Initial clinical view with extrusion of 23 and inflammatory infiltration of the surrounding gingiva, especially mesially, where a 10-mm pocket was present.

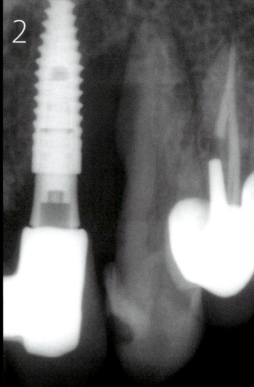

2. Radiographic view confirming deep periodontal damage mesial to 23 with endangerment of the BLT implant. As is often the case, the patient waited for the damage to become more advanced before deciding to consult, despite having had similar experiences previously.

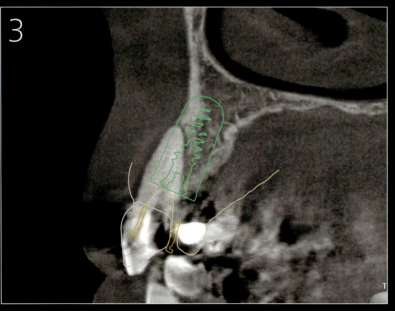

3. Sagittal view of the 3D examination required for planning, confirming the possibility of immediate implantation thanks to the presence of an apical and palatal bone triangle. The examination confirmed major bone loss.

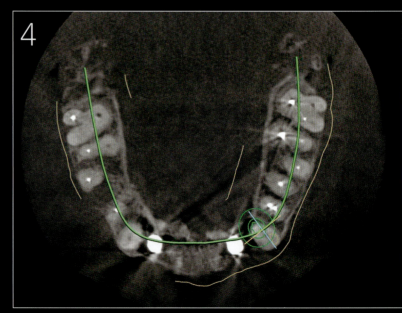

4. Axial view.

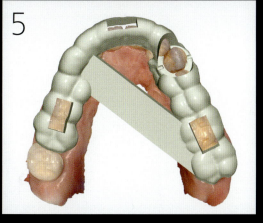

Design of the radiographic guide in the final planning stage in Implant Studio with the inspection windows and the recess for the Straumann T-sleeve as well as the groove for rotational marking.

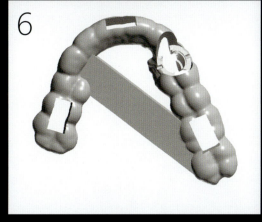

STL file of the guide for printing in the office.

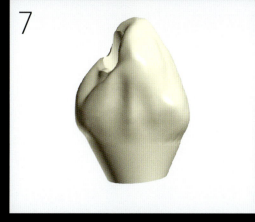

STL file of the provisional tooth designed in Dental System to be exported to the 3D printing software for printing in the practice.

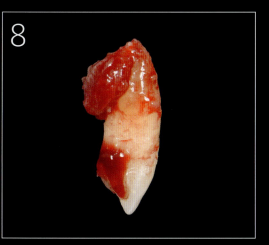

Extracted tooth 23 with a large inflammatory granuloma.

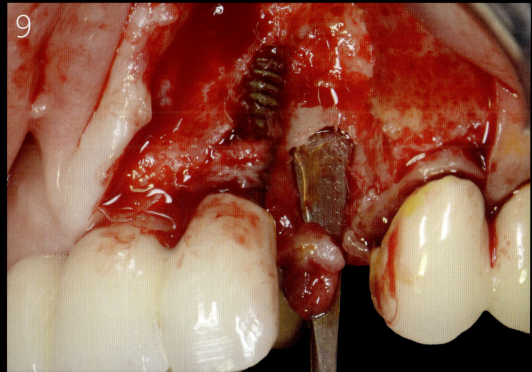

Clinical situation after extraction and elevation of a full-thickness vestibular and palatal flap. Exposure of the defect. Rinse thoroughly with Betadine.

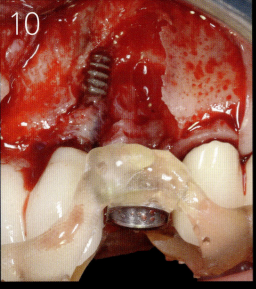

10 The surgical guide in place with inspection windows. The drilling and guided placement protocol could be performed.

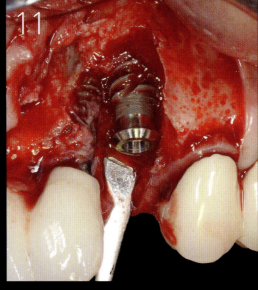

11 The TLX SP RT 4.5 x 12.0 mm implant in place with its vertical positioning dictated by the palatal wall.

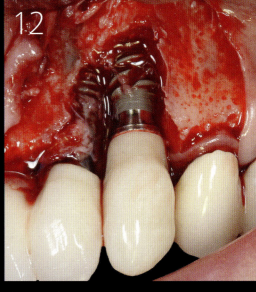

12 The **immediate** temporary tooth in an optimal position.

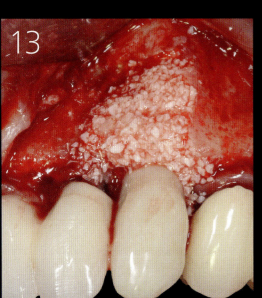

13 Filling of the proximal and vestibular defects with DBBM (Bio-Oss with fine particles) incubated in the F2 fraction of PRGF.

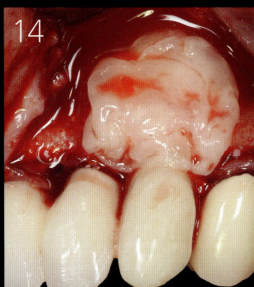

14 Vestibular and palatal coverage by a fibrin membrane derived from the F1 fraction of PRGF, the site of delayed release of growth factors via the alpha granules.

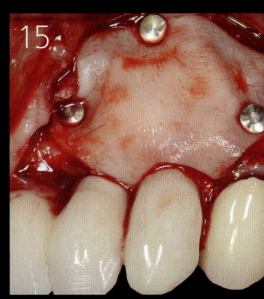

15 Covering with a resorbable collagen membrane stabilized using three pins (Bio-Gide Perio). Note the architecture of GBR guided by the **immediate** prosthesis.

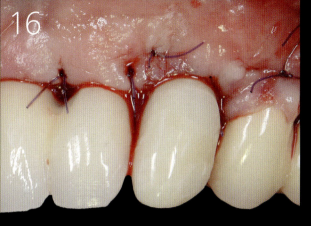

16 The flap was repositioned coronally following half-thickness incisions at the back of the vestibule, stabilized, and then plated with an ASAF suture and simple stitches on the distal discharge.

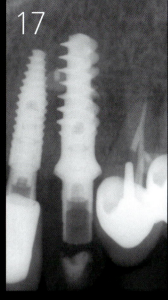

17 Postoperative radiographic view. Note the filling present between the TLX and the BLT implant.

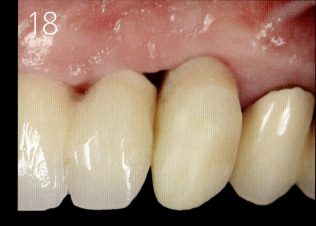

18 3-month status confirming vertical gain at the neck level of 23. The texture and gingival maturation were satisfactory. Proximal probing at 3 mm and without bleeding was very promising.

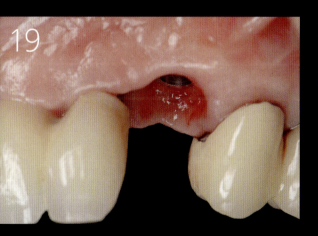

19 Very healthy appearance of the sulcus.

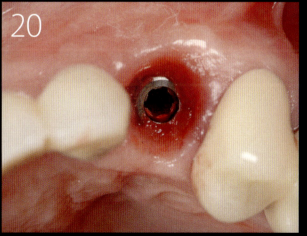

20 Axial view of the sulcus.

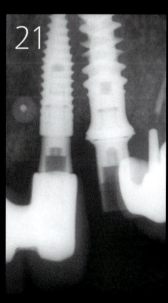

21 Radiographic view at 3 months.

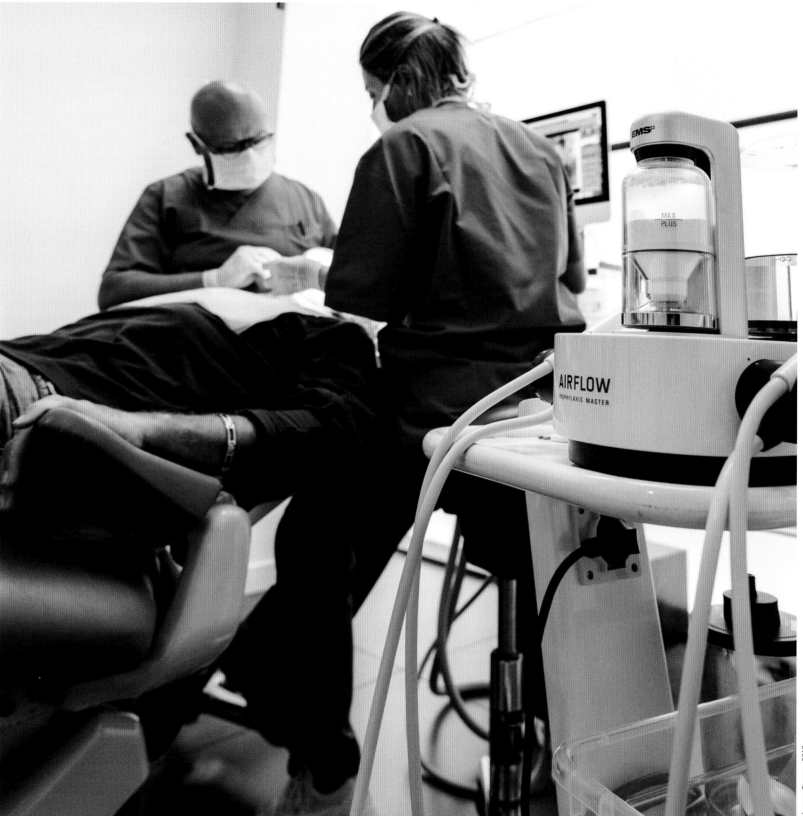

Single-unit clinical case 15

50-year-old man.

Clinical data

- Periodontal loss of tooth 11, which present with external root resorption. History of trauma on this tooth.
- Case treated in the office in October 2022.
- Major bone loss.
- Altered mucogingival architecture.

Presurgical treatments

- Impressions with Trios 4 and 3D examination using 3Shape X1.
- Planning in Implant Studio.
- Placement of a Straumann TLX SP RT TiZr SLActive 4.5 x 12.0 mm implant.
- 3D printing of the guide designed in Implant Studio, printed in the office on a NextDent 5100 printer with NextDent SG resin and polymerized in an LC-3D 3D polymerization unit.
- Straumann TLX T-socket.
- Screw-retained temporary crown in 11, A3 shade, printed in the office on a NextDent 5100 printer with NextDent Crown & Bridge N1 resin, cured in an LC-3D 3D curing unit, and stained on an A3 base with an Optiglaze Color Set.
- Variobase SA used for RT crowns bonded with Multilink Hybrid Abutment HO.

Assessment of the intervention

- Case treated in **three appointments at the office** (impression and 3D examination, surgery, control at 3 months).
- Prosthesis made by the referring dentist.

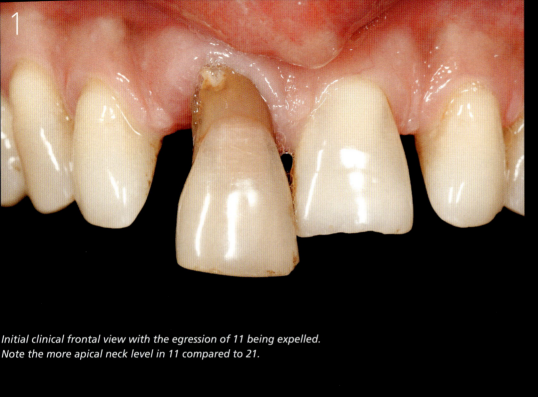

Initial clinical frontal view with the egression of 11 being expelled. Note the more apical neck level in 11 compared to 21.

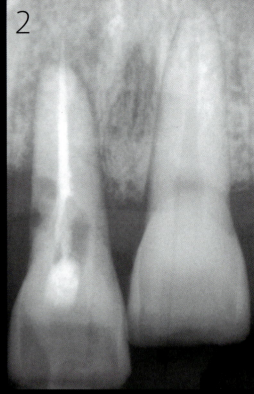

Radiographic view with internal rhizomes.

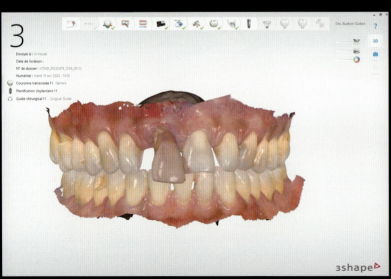

Intraoral digital impression in Implant Studio combined with a CBCT examination in the same 3Shape flow.

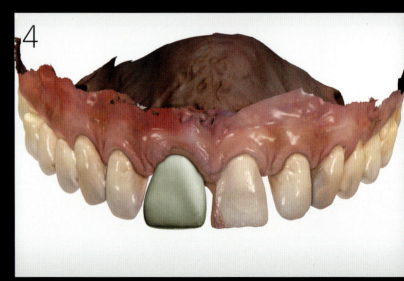

Virtual avulsion of 21 and creation of the virtual crown and prosthetic guide for implant planning.

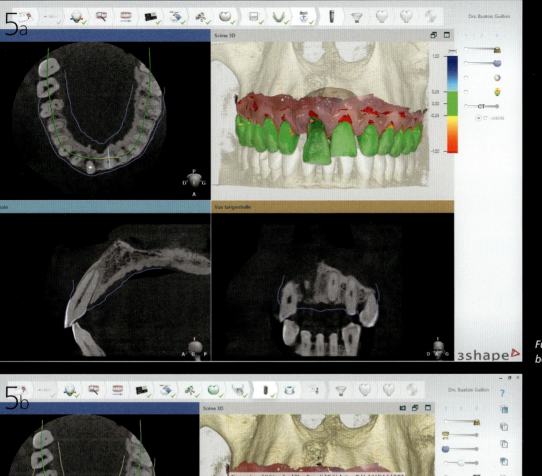

Fusion of STL and DICOM files before implant planning.

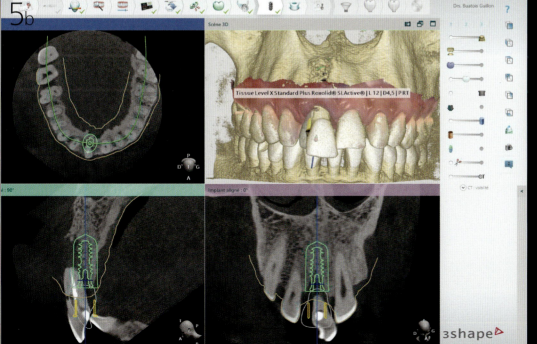

3D positioning of the RT implant in a weak bone context. We were within the limits for immediate implantation. The alternative would have been preimplant bone grafting if extraction took place with a conventional healing time of 3 months.

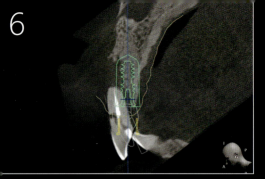

Magnified view showing the relationship between the residual bone volume, future prosthetic volume, and existing gingival environment.

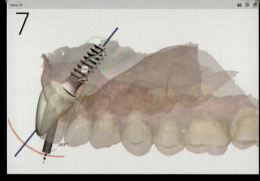

In Implant Studio, variations in the axis of the abutments can be simulated to allow visualization of the screwing-in required for **immediate** restoration.

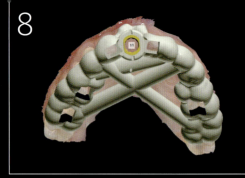

Design of the surgical guide in Implant Studio after validation of the plan.

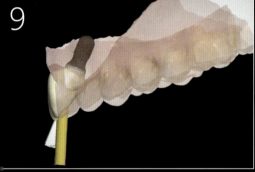

After validation of the protocol in Implant Studio, the STL files could be exported to Dental System for fabrication of the prosthesis. The crown is shown with the positioning of the Variobase SA RT for Crown allowing angulation of the screw axis.

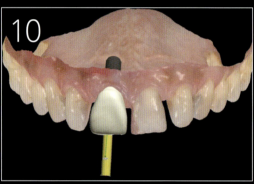

Frontal view of the different filters in the file.

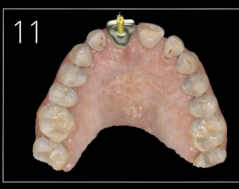

Occlusal view confirming the position of the screw hole without altering the incisal edge and the solidity of the buccal surface, while respecting the bone constraints.

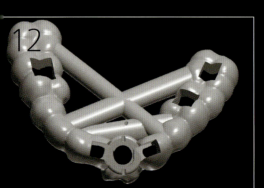

STL file of the surgical guide exported from Implant Studio for in-office printing.

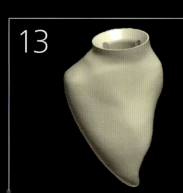

STL file of the tooth from Dental System

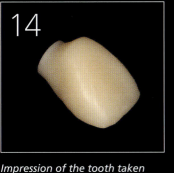

Impression of the tooth taken on a NextDent 5100 printer with NextDent Crown & Bridge N1 resin.

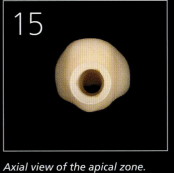

Axial view of the apical zone.

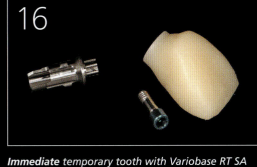

***Immediate** temporary tooth with Variobase RT SA for Crown and screw before connection.*

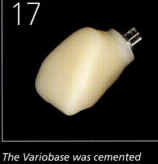

The Variobase was cemented to the temporary tooth.

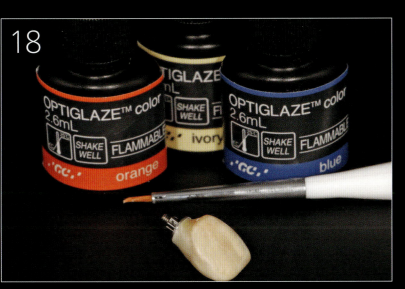

Optiglaze staining kit (GC Europe).

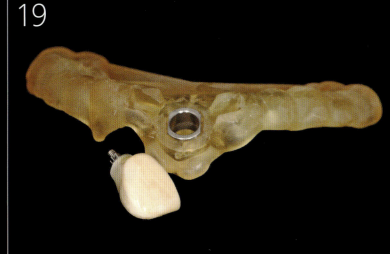

*The guide and the **immediate** temporary tooth.*

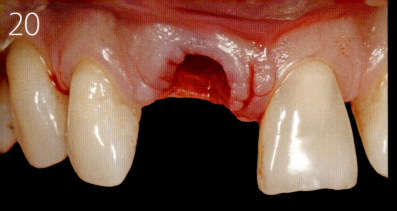

Clinical view after extraction, curettage of the socket with a Lucas curette, and rinsing with Betadine.

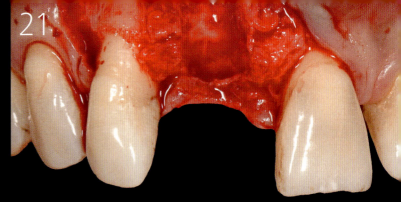

Elevation of a full-thickness flap from 21 to 12 with distal unloading of 12. Note the 3D bone defect involving more than two-thirds of the root volume.

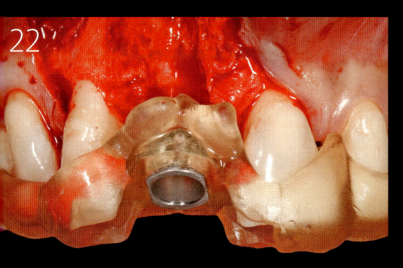

The guide in place with all controls validated.

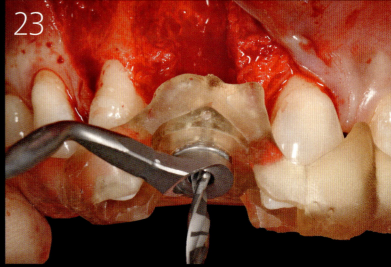

Guided drilling for TLX implants.

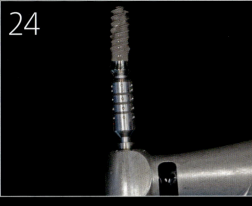

TLX SP RT implant (4.5 x 12.0 mm) on the TLX SP gripper.

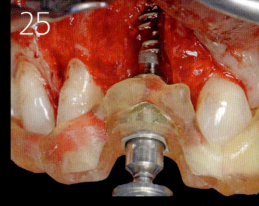

Final insertion of the implant with the hand gripper for tightening beyond 50 Ncm (motor torque), confirming excellent primary stability of the implant in the dense residual bone and the aggressive design of the TLX coils.

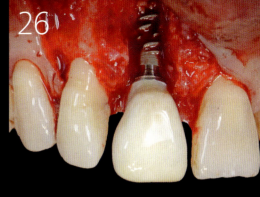

Placement of the **immediate** temporary tooth on the implant with an optimal fit.

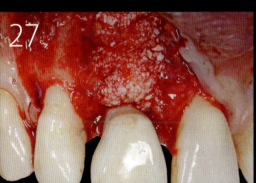

Filling of the dehiscence with DBBM (Bio-Oss with fine particles) incubated in the F2 fraction of PRGF. Sticky bone is easier to handle. The concentration of growth factors brings biological activity to the osteoconductive matrix of DBBM.

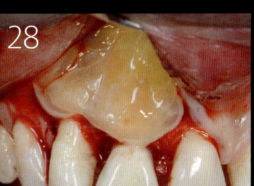

Overlay of a fibrin membrane from the F1 fraction of PRGF. Fibrin releases growth factors remotely via the alpha granules.

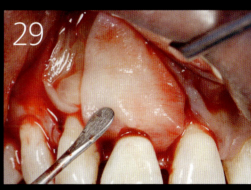

Overlay with a moistened resorbable collagen membrane in the F2 fraction of the PRGF.

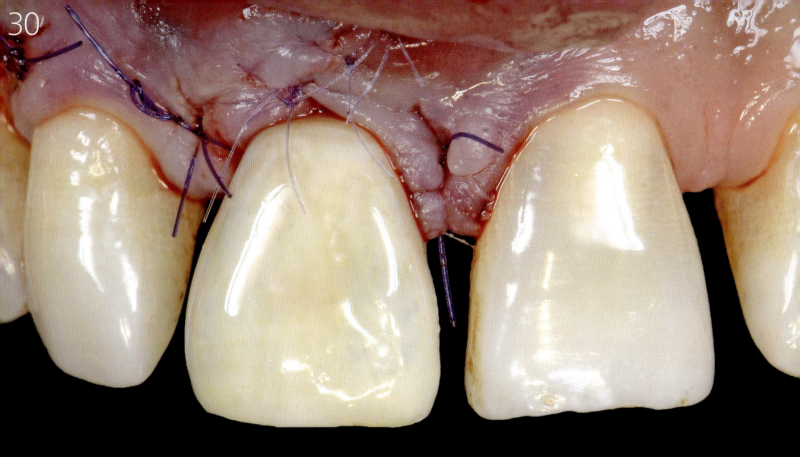

30 After the half-thickness incision and coronal traction, the flap was sutured with an ASAF suture combined with simple papillary sutures and in the distal discharge.

31 Radiographic view. Flaring of the bone would have removed an interference between the generally palatal or proximal walls and the emergence profile of the provisional tooth. It is difficult to judge these small hiatuses during surgery.

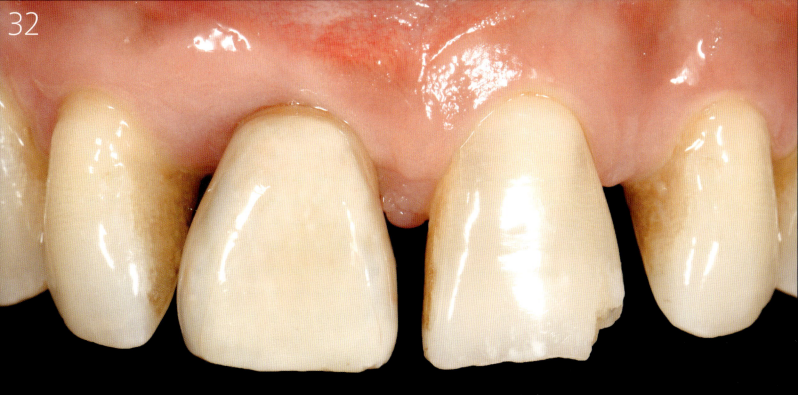

Clinical view at 3 months. Note the good periodontal integration, and especially the vertical gain in the neck of 11.

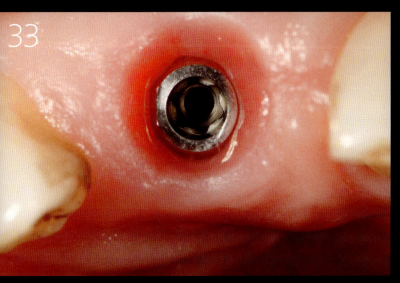

Axial view of the implant bed with a non-inflammatory sulcus.

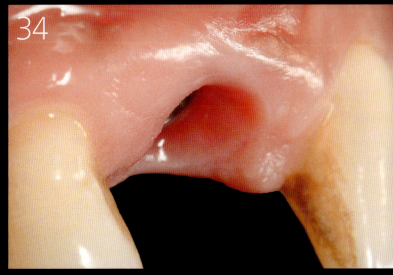

The implant bed with optimal support from the tonicity of the surrounding periodontal tissues due to adequate perimplant reconstruction.

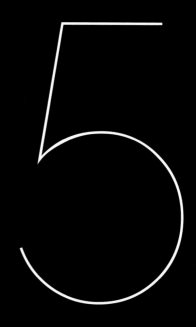

Clinical applications for partially edentulous patients

Two to three anterior teeth
Plural-unit cases 16 and 17 185

Two to three posterior teeth
Plural-unit cases 18 and 19 199

Four anterior teeth
Plural-unit cases 20 and 21 211

Six teeth or more
Plural-unit cases 22 to 24 231

One implant for two teeth
Plural-unit case 25 259

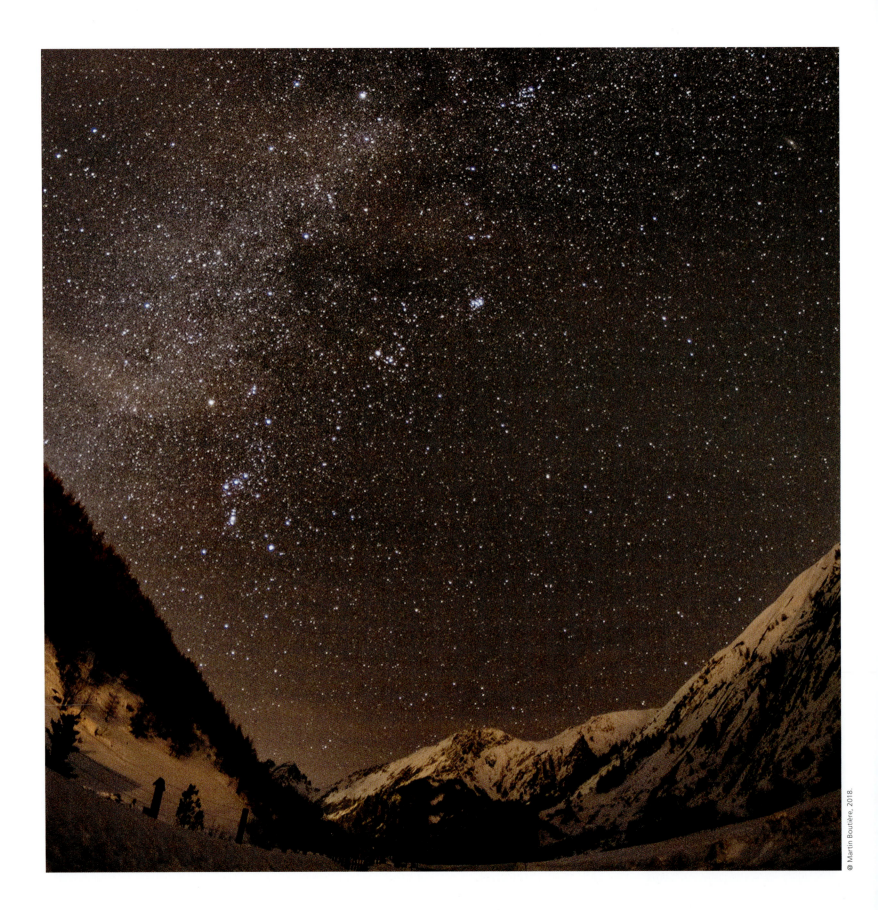

Plural-unit clinical case 16

60-year-old woman.

Clinical data

- Loss of the teeth from 21 to 12, which had become mobile due to caries lesions, apical infection, and periodontal damage. Teeth 12, 11, and 21 had to be extracted for implant-prosthetic rehabilitation of two implants replacing three teeth. The patient opted for immediate implantation in 12 and 21 and **immediate** restoration of 12 to 21.
- Case treated in April 2022.
- Vestibular bone wall present in 12, altered in two thirds in 11 and 21.
- Good mucogingival architecture, but very inflammatory.

Presurgical treatments

- Optical impression taken using Trios 4 (3Shape, Copenhagen, Denmark) and 3D examination using a 3Shape X1.
- Planning using Implant Studio.
- Placement of a Straumann TLX SP NT 3.75 x 12.00 mm implant in 12 and RT 3.75 x 12.00 mm in 21 (Basel, Switzerland).
- 3D printing of the guide designed in Implant Studio and printed in the office on a NextDent 5100 printer (Utrecht, The Netherlands) with NextDent SG resin and polymerized in an LC-3D 3D polymerization unit.
- Straumann TLX T-socket, non–self-locking.
- Temporary fixed/removable partial denture of three teeth, screwed in 12 and 21, shade A3, printed in the office on a NextDent 5100 printer with NextDent Crown & Bridge N1 resin, polymerized in a LC-3D 3D polymerization unit and stained on an A3 base with an Optiglaze Color Set (GC Europe, Leuven, Belgium).
- Variobase SA used for RT crowns in 21 and NT in 12, bonded with Multilink Hybrid Abutment HO (Ivoclar Vivadent, Schaan, Lichtenstein). There is currently no Variobase SA for fixed/removable partial denture work in the Straumann range.

Assessment of the intervention

- Case treated in **three appointments at the office** (impression and 3D examination, surgery, control at 3 months).
- Prosthesis made by the referring dentist.

Additional treatments

- Presence of suppuration which, in addition to the classic antibiotic treatment (2g amoxicillin/day for 8 days, treatment started 48 hours before the operation), was cleaned in situ by extracting the teeth, cleaning the granuloma, and rinsing abundantly with Betadine. The screw hole in 21 was closed with flowable composite.

The Quokka protocol

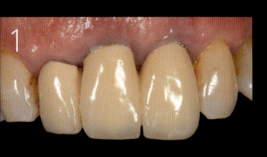

Initial clinical view. Note the inflammatory state and suppuration requiring extraction of these three teeth.

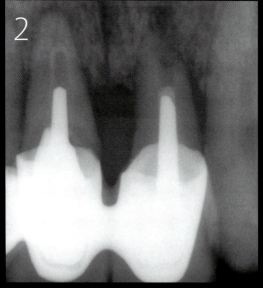

Retroalveolar radiograph of 11 and 21.

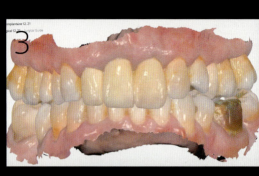

Optical impression taken with a Trios 4 with the 3D examination in the same 3Shape flow with the X1.

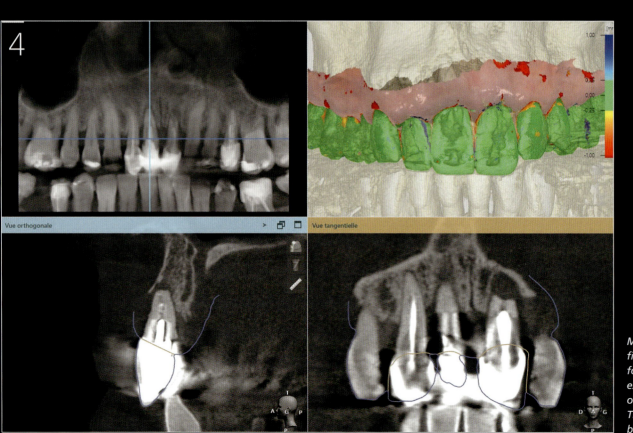

Merging of the STL and DICOM files with the colorimetric index for precision control. On the bone examination, note the degree of damage to these three teeth. The gingival contour is delimited by the brown line.

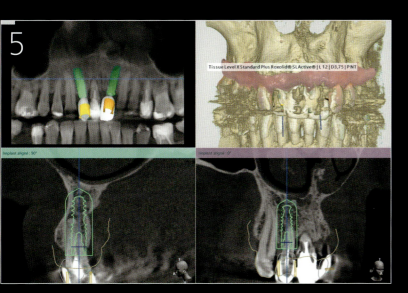

Implant planning in 12. Note the bone, gingival, and prosthetic relationships (gray line on the future prosthesis) to standardize the theoretical 3D position from the literature. The NT neck conformed to the emergence profile of a lateral incisor.

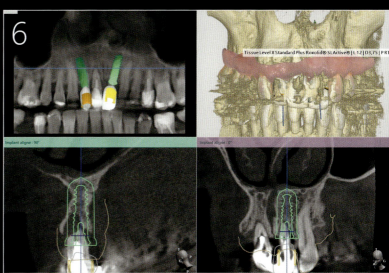

Implant planning in 21. Note the bone, gingival, and prosthetic relationships (gray line on the future prosthesis) to standardize the theoretical 3D position from the literature. The RT neck conformed to the emergence profile of a central incisor.

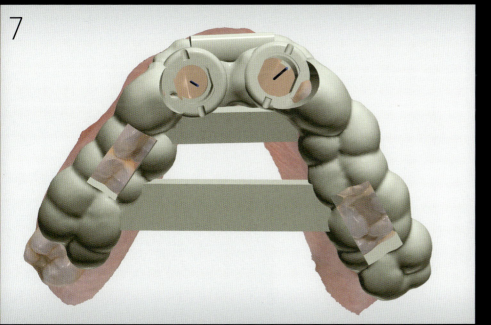

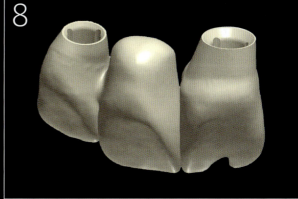

STL file of the provisional partial denture designed in Dental System in the office. Note the screw hole on the incisal edge in 21.

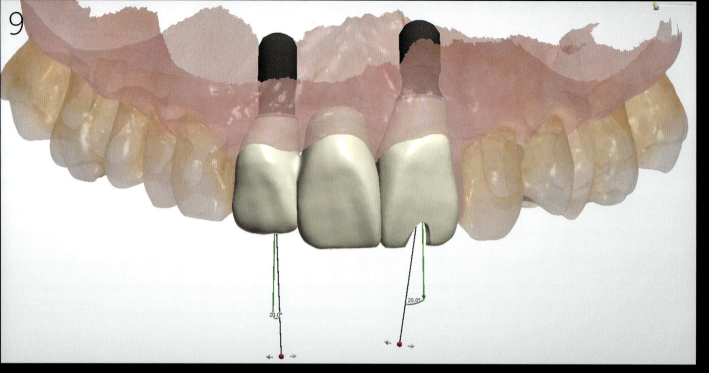

A set of filters in Dental System for angulating the screw axis and correctly positioning the Variobase SA for NT and RT crowns. Variobase crown restorations had to be used since there is no Variobase SA partial denture restoration in the Straumann product range. This made it difficult to insert the partial denture.

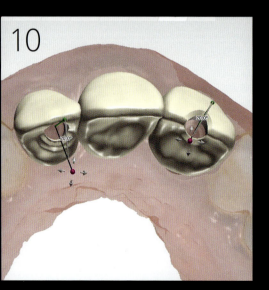

Occlusal view.

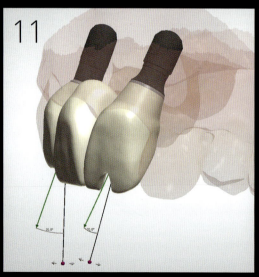

Side view.

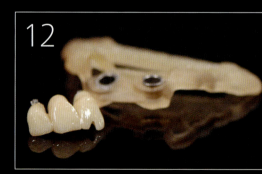

Surgical guide and partial denture with connected Variobase crowns before surgery.

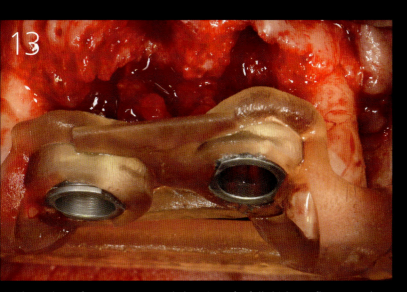

Guide in place after extractions and elevation of a full-thickness flap. Note the controls on the fit of the guide, and the bone defects present after curettage and Betadine flushing.

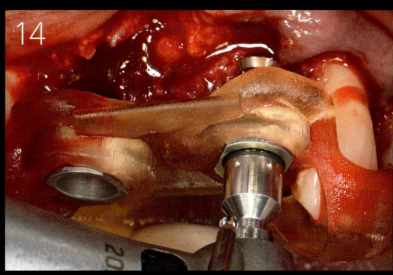

Guided implant placement.

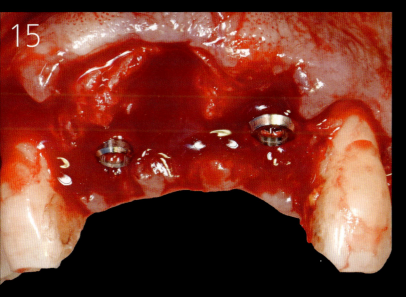

TLX implants in place.

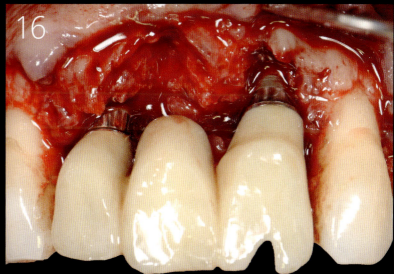

Immediate provisional fixed/removable partial denture in place despite the engaging connections. Note the design of the prosthetic CEJ conforming to the adjacent teeth, which serve as a guide for the GBR and the flap sutures. Also note the design of the pontic in 11 made to form a deep pontic bed at 3 months, generating pseudopapillae.

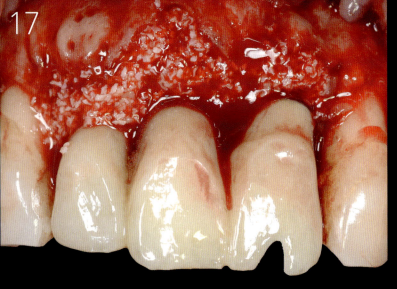

17 3D bone reconstruction with DBBM (Bio-Oss with fine particles) incubated in the F2 fraction of PRGF (Endoret, BTI France).

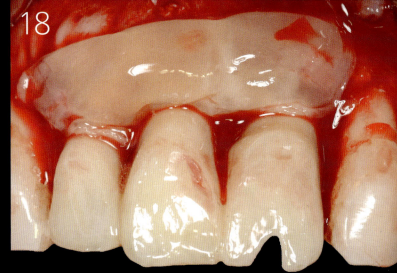

18 Overlay with PRGF fraction F2 and a fibrin membrane from PRGF fraction F1.

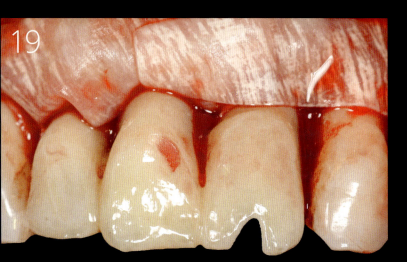

19 Covering of the fillings with a resorbable collagen membrane (Bio-Gide Perio) soaked in the F2 fraction.

20 After a half-thickness incision was made at the back of the vestibule from 13 to 23, coronal traction of the flap and suturing in two ASAF sutures around 12 and 21 and single papillary sutures.

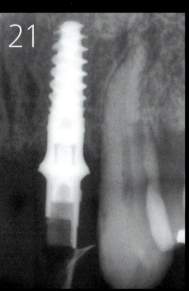

Radiographic view of tooth 21.

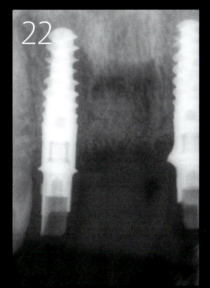

Radiographic view of tooth 12 after final tightening of the partial denture to close the small gap present at the time of insertion. The flexibility of the resin and the viscoelastic properties of the bone allowed this terminal adaptation. Note the good density

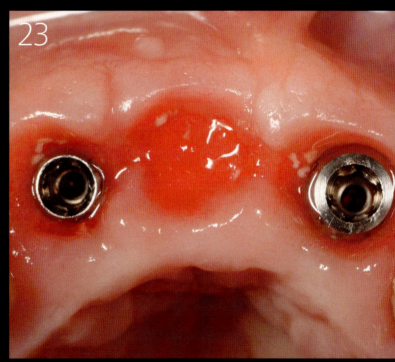

Occlusal view of the implant beds and pontic bed at 3 months during the implant check-up. Note the adapted vestibular volumes.

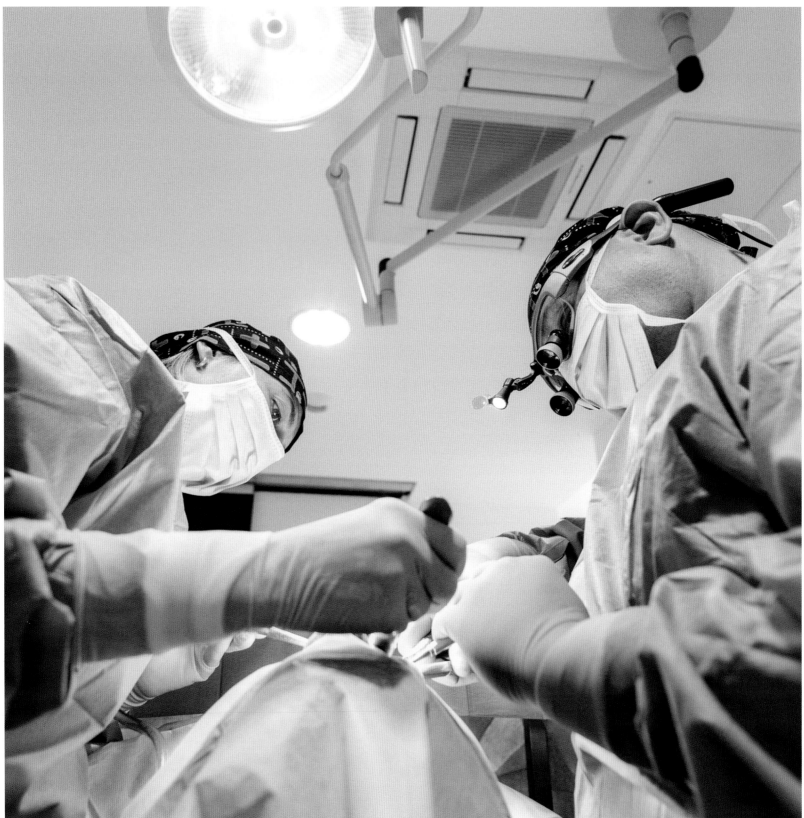

© Vianney Tisseau, 2019.

Plural-unit clinical case 17

58-year-old woman.

Clinical data

- Advanced mobility of teeth 12, 11, and 21 in a context of reduced but healthy periodontium.
- Case treated in March 2018.
- Vertical bone loss of two-thirds of the roots of 12, 11, and 21.
- Altered mucogingival architecture (loss of attachment of more than 6 mm).

Presurgical treatments

- Optical impression taken using Trios 3 and 3D examination performed using Planmeca ProMax (Helsinki, Finland).
- Planning using Implant Studio.
- Placement of a Straumann BL NC Roxolid SLActive 3.3 x 12.0 mm implant in 12 and RC 4.1 x 12.0 mm implant in 21.
- 3D printing of the guide designed in Implant Studio (Dentitek Laboratory).
- First-generation Straumann socket.
- Temporary fixed/removable partial denture was milled in polymethyl methacrylate (PMMA) (Ivotion Dent Multi, Ivoclar Vivadent) (Dentitek Laboratory).
- Variobase NC and RC used for fixed/removable partial dentures bonded with Multilink Hybrid Abutment.

Assessment of the intervention

- Case treated in **four appointments at the office** (impression and 3D examination, surgery, control at 3 months and final impression, placement of the prosthesis).
- Final prosthesis made in the office (JC Allègre Laboratory).
- This case illustrates the benefit of advanced implantology with reconstruction and immediate implantation compared to deferred implantology with poor positioning or at least poor management of the periodontal volumes. The stability and integration of an implant without taking into account the periodontal volumes gives a very limited esthetic result.

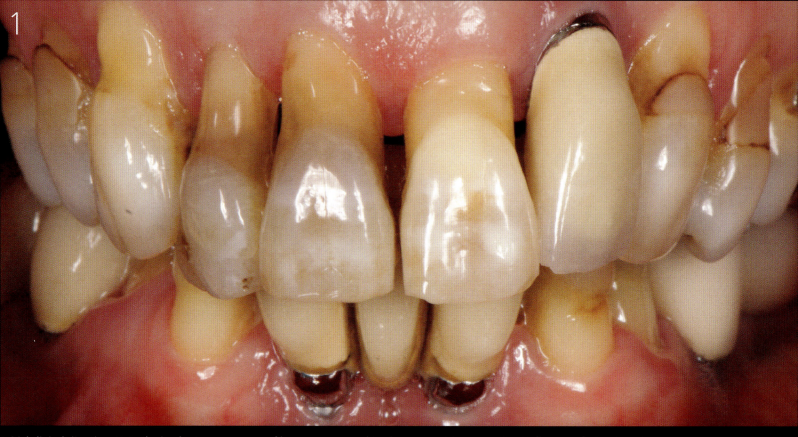

Initial clinical situation. Note the implant emergence profiles present around implants placed 4 years earlier. Unfortunately, implantology cannot be limited to a titanium screw in a bone crest.

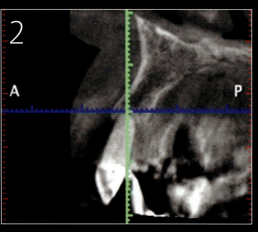

Sagittal section of the CBCT scan in 12.

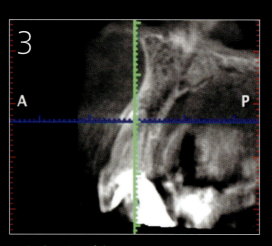

Sagittal section of the CBCT scan in 11.

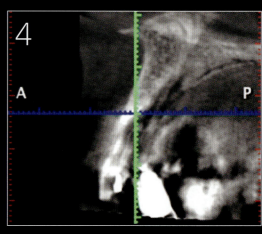

Sagittal section of the CBCT scan in 21.

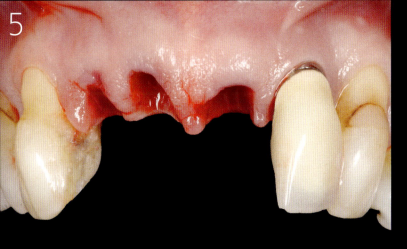

5 The patient accepted the option of immediate GBR implantation and restoration, planning, surgical guide development, and the **immediate** temporary partial denture for three teeth that was screw-retained in 12 and 21.

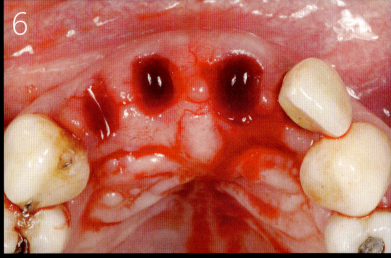

6 Axial view of the extraction site. Note the periodontal volume still present on the day of extractions in relation to the area of 22 delayed implantation.

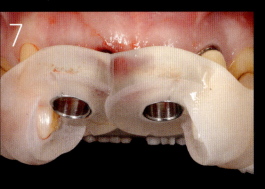

7 The surgical guide in place (inspection windows). Rotational registration was optional since we were using Variobase for partial denture work.

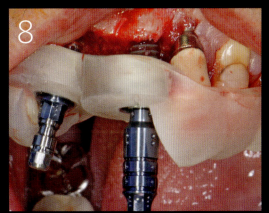

8 Guided placement of BL guided implants. The first generation of BL and TL guided surgery implants were delivered with the gripper guided and screwed onto the implant. This made it possible to leave the gripper in place to lock the guide and thus secure possible movements of the guide. The evolution of concepts and experience has made it possible to phase out use of this type of gripper.

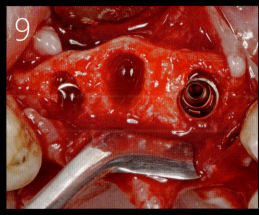

9 Axial view of the implants in place. The positioning, 1 mm more apical and 1 mm more palatal, was in accordance with the recommendations for immediate implantation as defined in the literature.

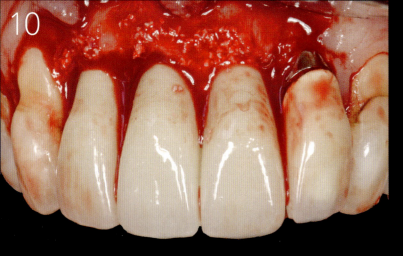

Vestibular view of the **immediate** temporary partial denture in place with the compensatory GBR at the extraction site hiatus.

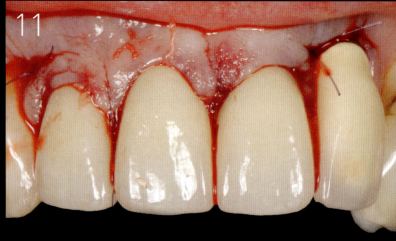

Flap positioned coronally after the half-thickness incision and immobilized and plated with hanging sutures and single papillary sutures.

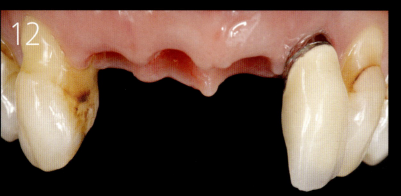

Clinical situation at 3 months when the implant osseointegration was checked and before the digital impression was taken. Note the pontic bed and the resulting pseudopapillae, and the maintenance of the periodontal volume.

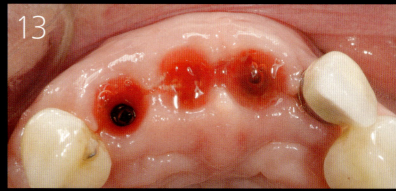

Axial view confirming the value of periodontal volume maintenance with immediate implantation and GBR.

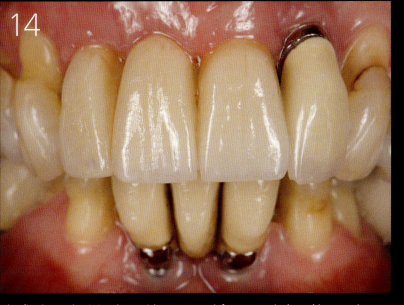

The final prosthesis in place with a more satisfactory periodontal integration of the implant-prosthetic rehabilitation.

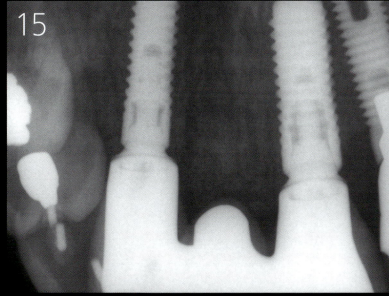

Radiographic view. Good density of the GBR material at the level of the ridge preservation in the pontic area to secure the volume under the partial denture pontic over time.

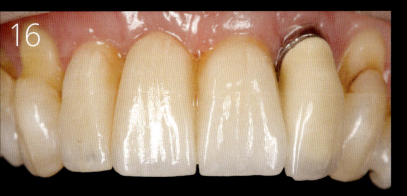

Good periodontal integration of the implant-prosthetic rehabilitation.

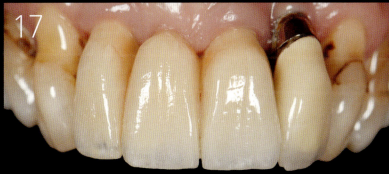

Clinical situation at 5 years. Despite reduced periodontal evolution, the esthetic integration and stability of the pontic area remained satisfactory. Note the evolution of the emergence profile in 22.

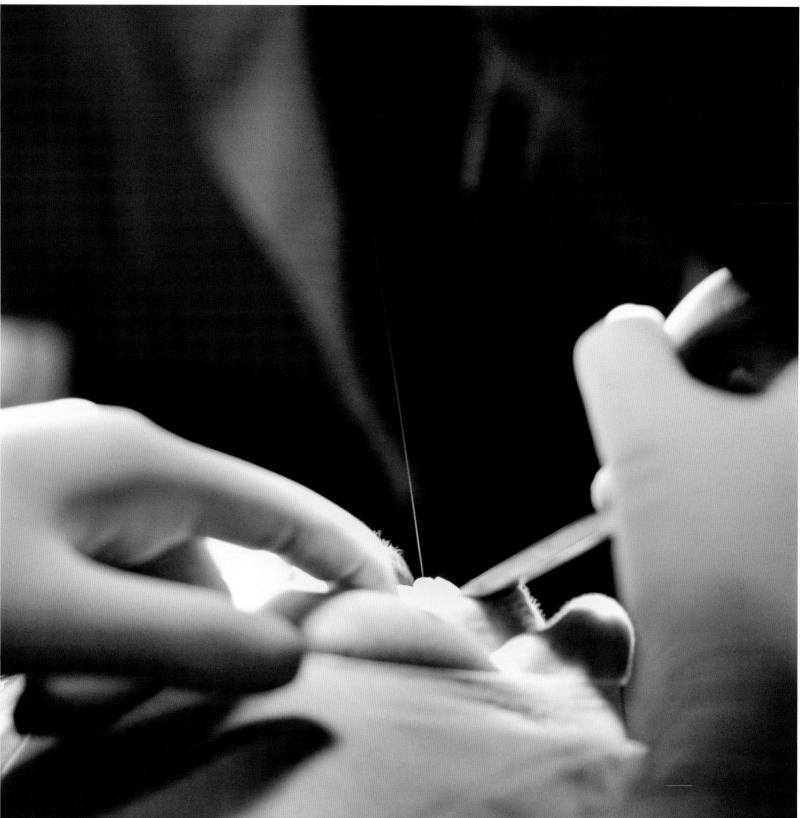

© Vianney Tisseau, 2019.

Plural-unit clinical case 18

66-year-old woman.

Clinical data

- Advanced mobility of teeth 12, 11, and 21 in a context of reduced but healthy periodontium.
- Case treated in January 2019.
- Edentulous area with the need for a sinus graft in the area of 25 and 26. Partial denture replacing 14, 15, 24, 25, and 26.
- Good mucogingival architecture.

Presurgical treatments

- Optical impression taken using Trios 3 and 3D examination performed using Planmeca ProMax 3D.
- Planning using Implant Studio.
- Straumann TiZr SLActive 12-mm RC guided BLT in 14, 10-mm RC guided BLT in 25 and 26, 8-mm RC guided BLT in 15, and 10-mm NC guided BLT in 24.
- 3D printing of the guide designed in Implant Studio (Dentitek Laboratory).
- First-generation Straumann.
- Temporary partial denture milled in PMMA (Dentitek Laboratory).
- Variobase NC and RC used for partial dentures bonded with Multilink Hybrid Abutment.

Assessment of the intervention

- Case treated in **four appointments at the office** (impression and 3D examination, surgery, control at 3 months and final impression, placement of the prosthesis).
- Final prosthesis made in the office (JC Allègre Laboratory).
- In this case, the Quokka protocol allowed the patient to come to the office with a removable appliance and leave with fixed teeth and a left sinus lift. The Quokka protocol uses digital technology to perform the procedures in a single step with prosthesis management during surgery.
- This was an advanced procedure on a motivated patient who could no longer stand her appliance. We opted to perform rehabilitation using one implant per tooth to secure the loading of an implant engaged in a sinus graft zone. In our learning curve, we tried to work on BL implants with direct connection, by placing the implants as parallel as possible to facilitate insertion of the partial denture.

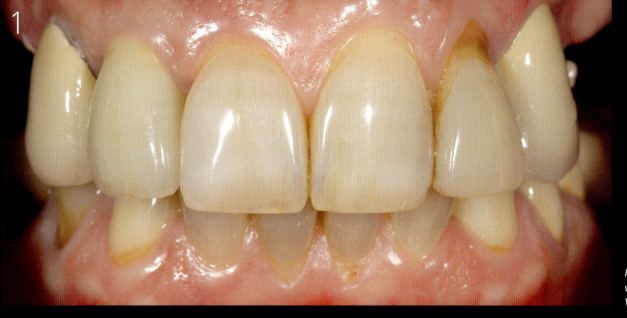

Initial clinical view of the patient without her partial denture. Very good periodontal context.

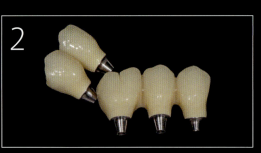

*Milled **provisional** partial dentures connected to the Variobase for partial denture work in the BL series.*

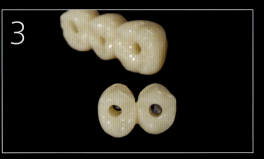

Occlusal view of optimally centered screw holes with prosthesis-guided implant planning.

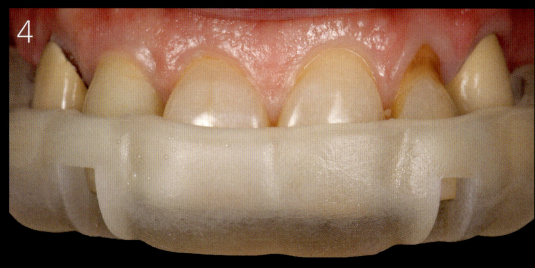

Fitting the surgical guide in place with the inspection windows prior to any incisions being made.

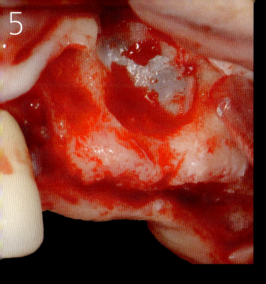

Full-thickness flap from 24 to 27 and preparation of a 17-mm-long by 10-mm-high sinus access window centered at 25 and 26.

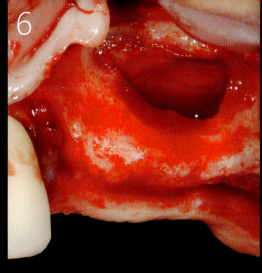

The sinus membrane was lifted without any particular difficulty. The membrane was tested for optimal sealing prior to filling.

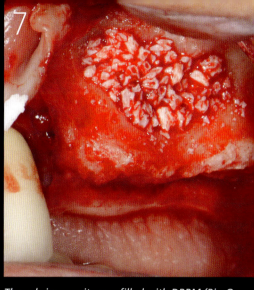

The subsinus cavity was filled with DBBM (Bio-Oss with large particles). Filling was done exceptionally prior to preparation of the implant beds due to the surgery and guided implant placement.

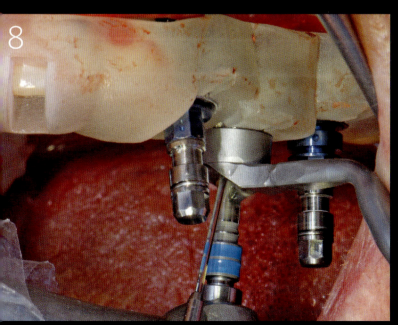

Drilling and guided placement of BL guided implants in sites 24, 25, and 26.

Drilling and guided placement of BL guided implants in sites 14 and 15.

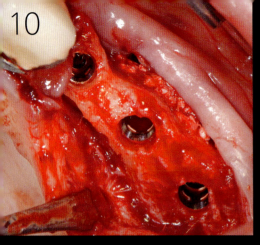

BL implants in an infracrestal position in sites 24, 25, and 26.

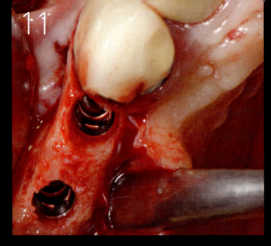

BL implants in an infracrestal position in sites 14 and 15.

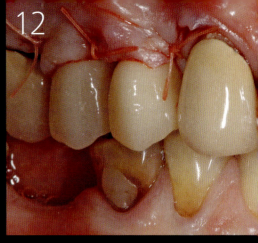

Immediate temporary partial denture in place in sites 14 and 15.

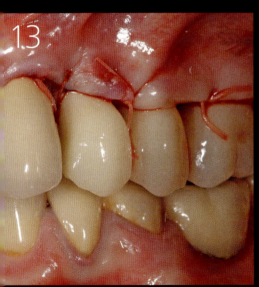

Immediate temporary partial denture in place in sites 24, 25, and 26.

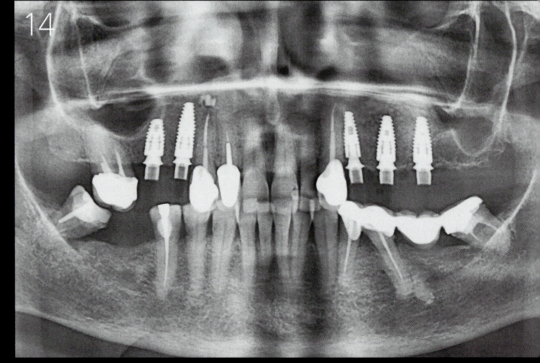

Postoperative panoramic radiograph. Note the partial insertion of the Variobase in 24. The implant in 24 was slightly divergent and therefore limited the insertion passivity. This had no clinical impact but confirmed that the direct implant to BL or BLX connection is not reproducible for an *immediate* provisional approach. SRA intermediate abutments are required for such an approach on BL, BLX, or BLT implants.

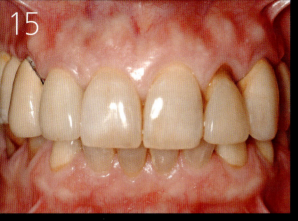

Clinical appearance at 6 months (sinus graft).

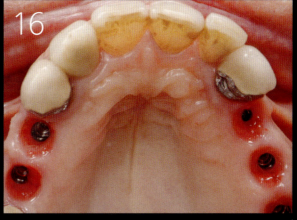

Axial view of the implant beds after removal of the provisional partial dentures for implant control. Osseointegration was very good and the architecture and health of the implant beds were quite satisfactory.

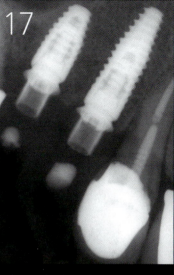

Radiograph of the final prostheses at 4 years in sites 14 and 15. The referring dentist replaced tooth 13 with an implant.

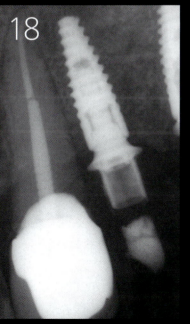

Radiograph of the final prostheses at

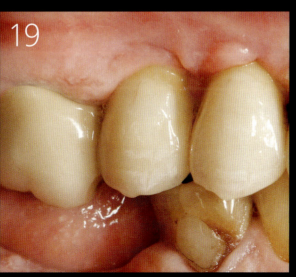

Clinical appearance of sector 1 at 4 years.

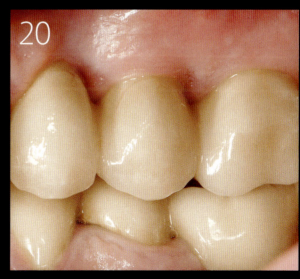

Clinical appearance of sector 2 at 4 years.

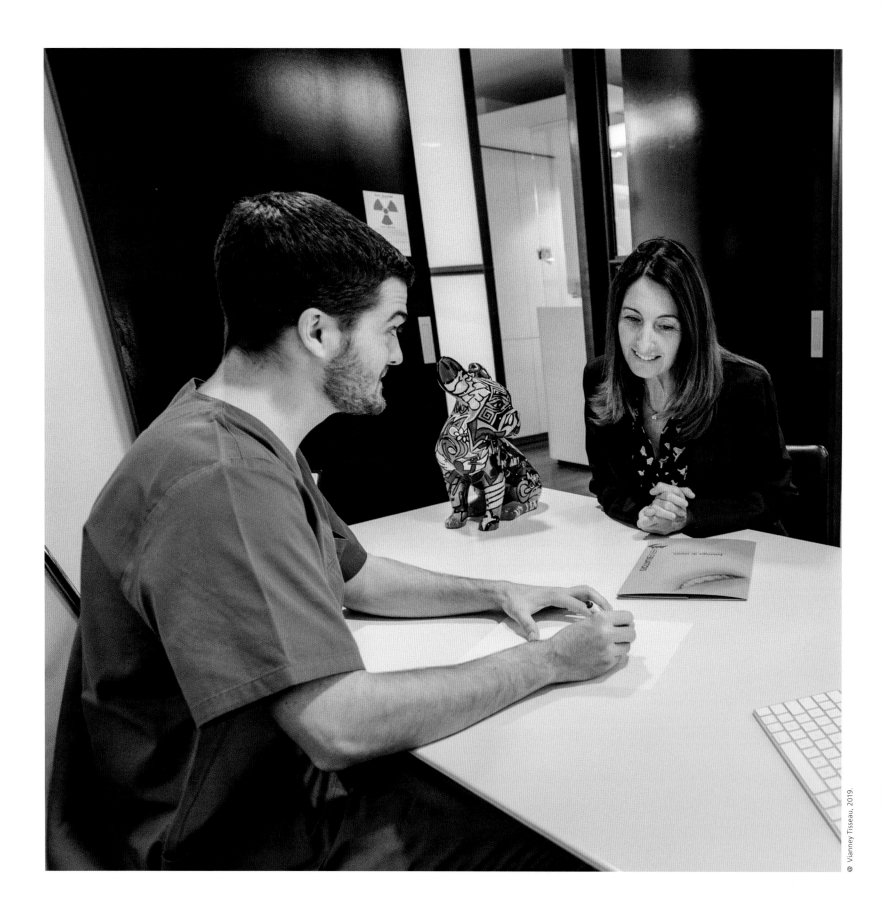

© Vianney Tisseau, 2019.

Plural-unit clinical case 19

73-year-old woman.

Clinical data

- Teeth 16, 15, and 14 were to be extracted.
- Case treated in January 2022.
- Suitable bone context in a guided surgery setting.
- Good mucogingival architecture.

Presurgical treatments

- Trios 4 used to take the optical impression and 3Shape X1 used to perform the 3D examination.
- Planning using Implant Studio.
- Placement of Straumann TLX SP NT 3.75 x 8.00 mm implants in 14, NT 3.75 x 8.00 mm implants in 15, and RT 4.5 x 8.0 mm implants in 16. The choice of NT diameters and necks in 14 and 15 was related to mesiodistal management of the implant emergence profiles guided by the prosthesis.
- 3D printing of the guide designed in Implant Studio, printed in the office on a NextDent 5100 printer with NextDent SG resin, and polymerized in a LC-3D 3D polymerization unit.
- Straumann TLX polyetheretherketone (PEEK) self-locking sockets.
- Temporary partial denture for three teeth, screwed in 14, 15, and 16, in shade A1, printed in the office on a NextDent 5100 printer with NextDent Crown & Bridge N1 resin, polymerized in an LC-3D 3D polymerization unit and stained on an A1 base with an Optiglaze Color Set.
- Variobase for NT used in 14 and 15 and RT in 16, bonded with Multilink Hybrid Abutment HO.

Assessment of the intervention

- Case treated in **four appointments at the office** (impression and 3D examination, surgery, control at 3 months and impression, placement of the prosthesis).
- Prosthesis made in the office (Mathias Berger Laboratory).
- The patient came to us for a consultation. She wanted a second opinion on an approach that called for extractions, a sinus graft at 2 months and placement of three implants at 6 months before the final prosthesis 2 months after. We suggested a single procedure with fixed temporaries during surgery and placement of the final prosthesis in two appointments at 3 months.

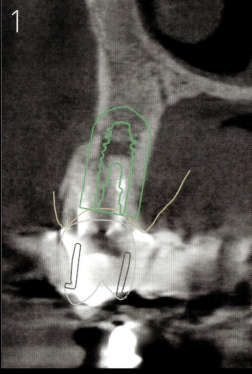

Implant planning in site 14. Note the more apical and palatal positioning of the NT. Also note the correlation between the implant axis and prosthetic axis, and the relationship between the gingiva and the implant neck.

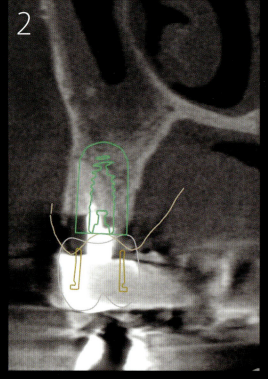

Planning of the NT implant in site 15.

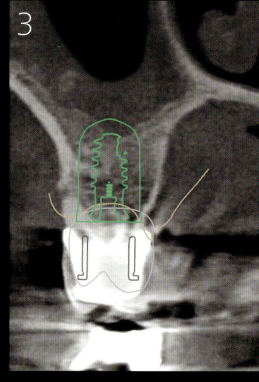

Planning of the RT implant in site 16.

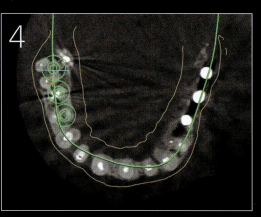

Axial view showing the more palatal position.

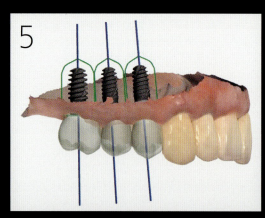

*Demonstration of the implant-prosthetic and gingival relationship with the design of the **immediate** temporary partial denture.*

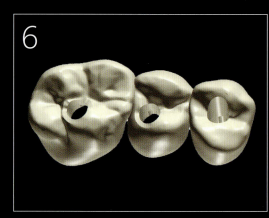

STL file of the provisional partial denture to be imported into 3D Sprint software (3D Systems, Rock Hill, SC, USA) for printing.

7

Implant position	Implant Art. No.	Implant	Sleeve Art. No.	Sleeve	Sleeve height	Sleeve position	Basic implant bed preparation		
							Milling cutter	Guided drill	Cylinder of drill handle
14	035.3008S	TLX SP ø3.75 NT, SLActive® 8mm, RXD	034.299V4	Ø 5.0 mm T-Sleeve, self-locking	5 mm	H6	Ø 3,50 mm	≡ Medium 20 mm Soft ○2.8 Medium ○3.2 ●(3.7) Hard ●3.5 (3.7)	• +1 mm
15	035.3008S	TLX SP ø3.75 NT, SLActive® 8mm, RXD	034.299V4	Ø 5.0 mm T-Sleeve, self-locking	5 mm	H4	Ø 3,50 mm	≡ Medium 20 mm Soft ○2.8 Medium ○3.2 ●(3.7) Hard ●3.5 (3.7)	••• +3 mm
16	035.3508S	TLX SP ø4.5 RT, SLActive® 8mm, RXD	034.299V4	Ø 5.0 mm T-Sleeve, self-locking	5 mm	H4	Ø 4,20 mm	≡ Medium 20 mm Soft ○2.8 Medium ●3.7 Hard ●4.2	••• +3 mm

Warning: The VeloDrill™ drill tip is up to 0.5 mm longer than the insertion depth of the implant.

Note: Guided handles are compatible up to Ø 4.2 mm. For drills larger than Ø 4.2 mm remove the template for freehand drilling.

BLX and TLX implant in medium and hard bone requires coronal widening. Follow the sleeve position/implant length matrix for coronal widening.

Note: The drill size in brackets is used for depths of 4 mm (for implant lengths of 6-8 mm) and 6 mm (for implant lengths of 10+ mm) for widening the coronal segment of the implant bed.

Note: Avoid planning 6 mm and 8 mm BLX and TLX implants in the H2 sleeve position, since 4 mm of guided drilling is not possible in the H2 position. Instead, remove the template and continue drilling using conventional procedures.

	Implant length	Coronal widening implant 6-8 mm	Coronal widening implant 10+ mm
Sleeve position	H2 2mm		Short drill − +3 handle •••
	H4 4mm	Short drill − +3 handle •••	Short drill − +1 handle •••
	H6 6mm	Short drill − +1 handle •	Medium drill ≡ +3 handle •••

Drilling protocol output by Implant Studio after validation of the plan. Once validated, the planning flow was locked to prevent errors.

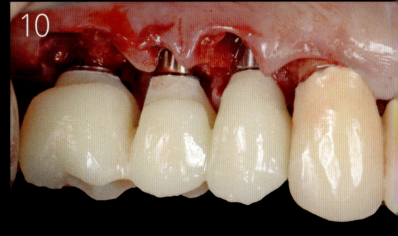

8

3D printing of the bridge and guide using a NextDent 5100. Self-locking PEEK sleeves bonded to NexTDent SG resin in the guide slots, Variobase connected to the bridge before surgery.

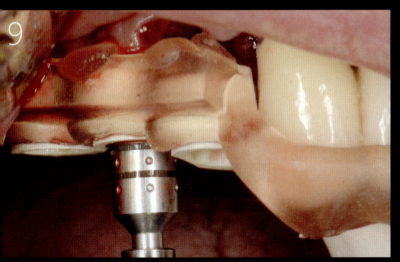

9

After guided drilling, guided placement of the implant was performed in site 15.

10

Immediate partial denture in place on all three implants.

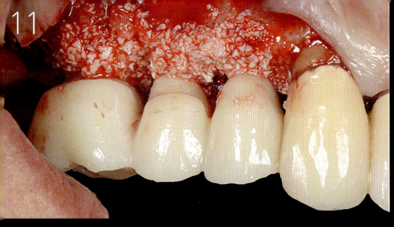 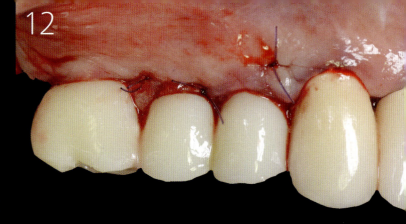

Filling of extraction gaps with DBBM (Bio-Oss with fine particles) incubated in the F2 fraction of PRGF (Endoret, BTI France). This filling was covered by a fibrin membrane from the F1 fraction of PRGF plasma.

Flap suturing using ASAF sutures.

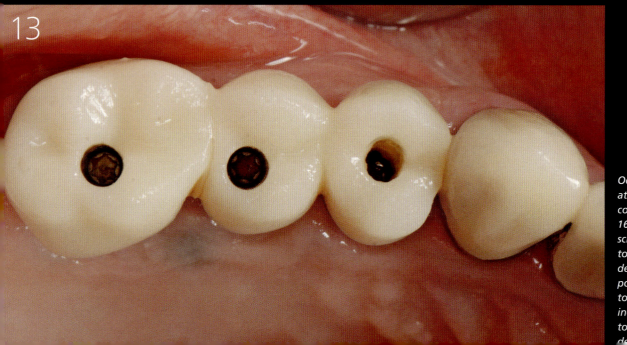

Occlusal view of the partial denture at 3 months. Note the crack in the connector between teeth 15 and 16, probably due to tension during screwing. The "one implant–one tooth" relationship makes the partial denture less flexible in relation to pontic areas. It is therefore better to use an implant and a pontic to increase the flexibility of the resin to ensure the passivity of the partial denture.

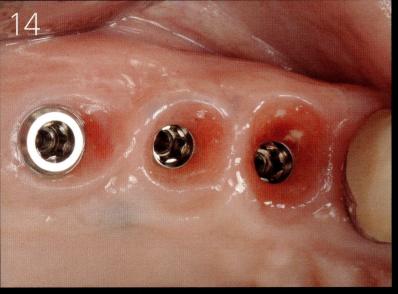

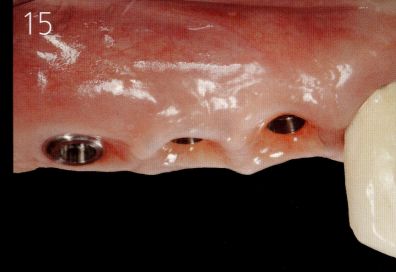

Occlusal view with good osseointegration of the implants and healthy anatomic implant beds. Note the maintenance of a good vestibular periodontal volume despite the extractions.

Vestibular view with the presence of pseudopapillae.

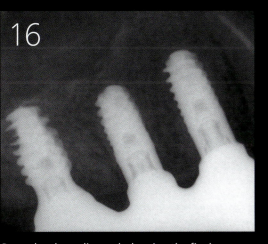

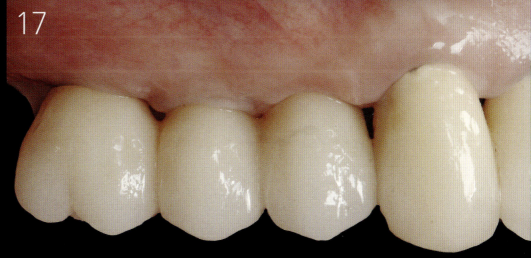

Retroalveolar radiograph showing the final partial denture in place, demonstrating good implant placement, sub-sinus management, and GBR integration. This one-step approach avoided the need for a perimplant sinus graft in the event of a delayed implant approach.

Final partial denture placed in a fourth appointment after the radiographic elements and the initial planning impression were taken. This was 3.5 months after the start of treatment (Mathias Berger Laboratory).

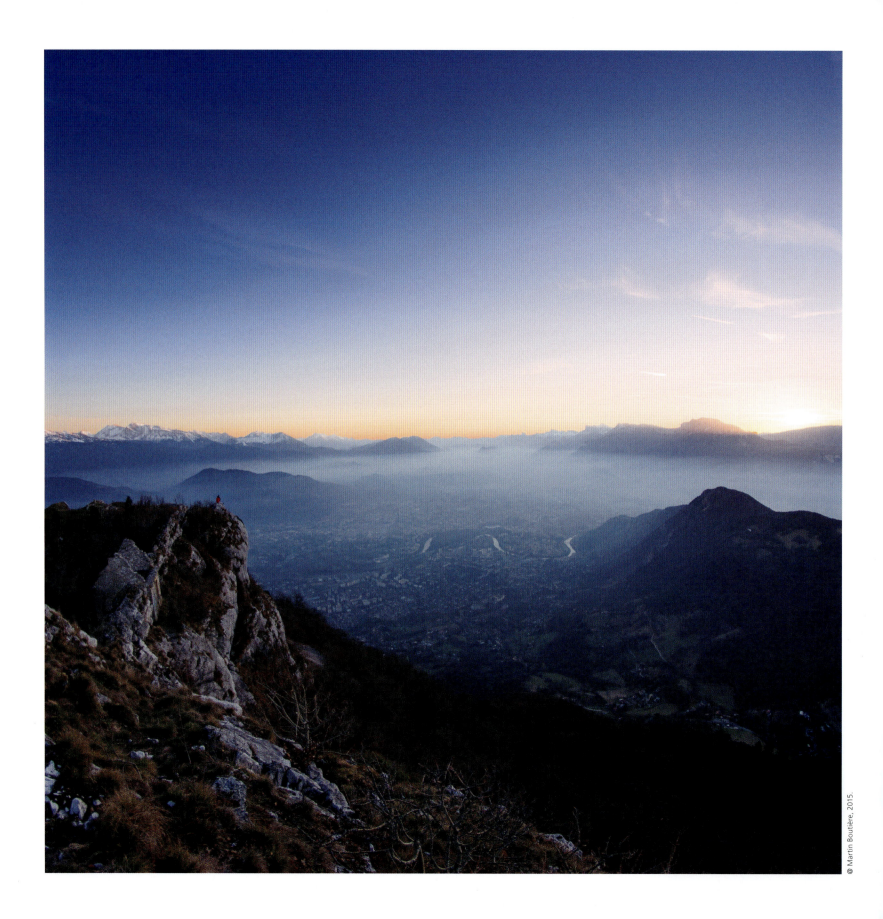
© Martin Boutière, 2015.

Plural-unit clinical case 20

52-year-old woman.

Clinical data

- Teeth 12, 11, 21, and 22 were to be extracted, sequelae of stabilized aggressive periodontitis.
- Case treated in May 2022.
- Suitable bony context in a context of generalized horizontal bone loss.
- Mucogingival architecture with significant horizontal bone loss.

Presurgical treatments

- Trios 4 used to take the optical impression and 3Shape X1 used to perform the 3D examination.
- Planning using Implant Studio.
- Placement of Straumann TLX SP NC implants (3.75 x 12.00 mm) in 12 and 22.
- 3D printing of the guide designed in Implant Studio, printed in the office on a NextDent 5100 printer with NextDent SG resin and polymerized in a LC-3D 3D polymerization unit.
- Straumann T-sockets.
- Temporary partial denture for four teeth screwed in 12 and 22, A3 shade with pink false gingiva, milled in PMMA (Ivotion Dent Multi) (Dentitek Laboratory).
- NT Variobase TLX for Bridgework used in 12 and 22, bonded with Multilink Hybrid Abutment HO.

Assessment of the intervention

- Case treated in **five appointments at the office** (impression and 3D examination, surgery, control at 3 months and impression, validation index, placement of the prosthesis).
- Prosthesis made in the office (Dental Art Technology Laboratory, Richard Demange, Nice, France).

Additional treatments

- The patient came to us to find a solution to the unsightly migration of their maxillary incisors. She presented with advanced periodontitis with an aggressive component. First, the periodontal disease was treated with a 1-year protocol of nonsurgical surfacing (GBT, EMS) combined with antiseptic treatments (mouthrinse and brushing), antibiotic therapy followed by a re-evaluation at 2 months, and a bimonthly periodontal maintenance follow-up. After 1 year, in view of the stability of the site (pocket depth [PD] less than or equal to 4 mm and bleeding on probing [BOP] less than 10%), we moved forward with implant treatment on this reduced, fragile, but healthy periodontum.

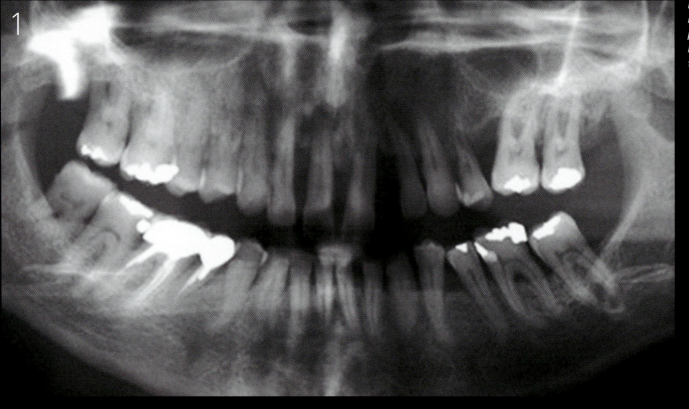

Initial panoramic radiograph that the patient brought with her on the day of the consultation.

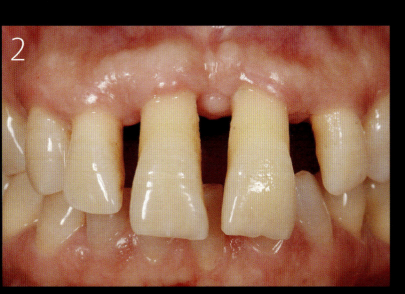

Frontal view of the clinical situation after periodontal treatment at 1 year. The patient was followed up with bimonthly maintenance (GBT, EMS).

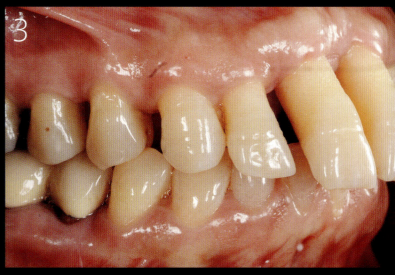

Lateral clinical view showing the vestibular migration of the incisors.

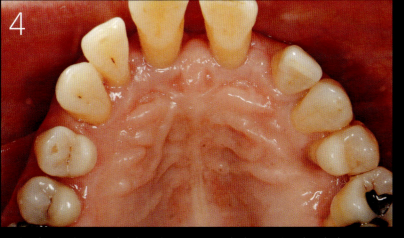

Occlusal view showing the dental migrations which, associated with the attachment loss, complicated the esthetic potential of the final rehabilitation.

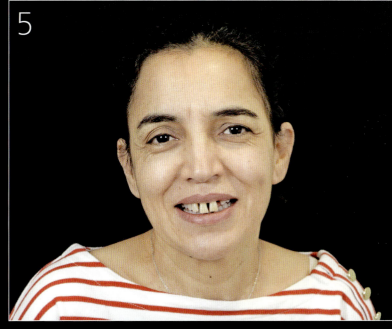

Assessment of dental disorder in relation to the entire smile and face.

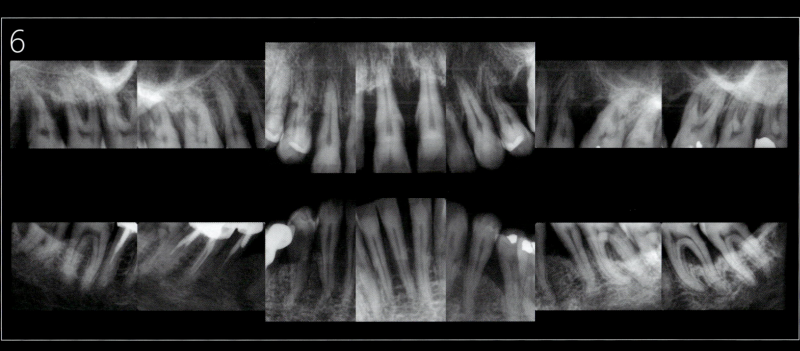

Retroalveolar radiographic assessment of the long cone anterior to periodontal treatment.

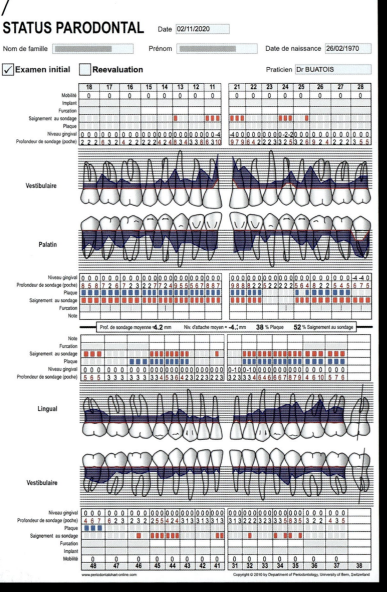

Initial periodontal status.

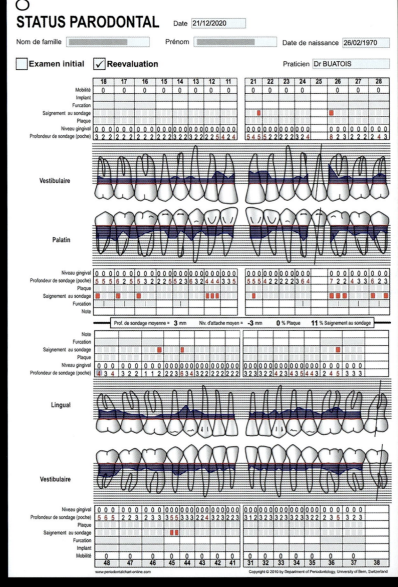

Periodontal status of 2-month re-evaluation post-surfacing. Three pockets between 5 and 6 mm deep remained. A decision was made to perform active

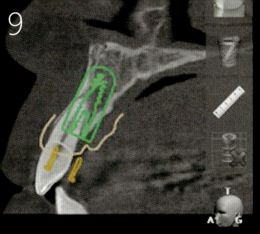

Implant Studio plan for the implant in site 12 in sagittal view.

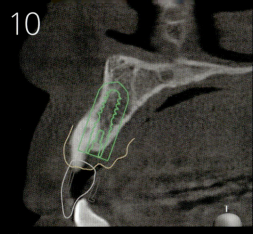

Plan for the implant in site 22 in sagittal view.

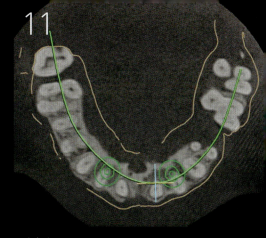

Axial view.

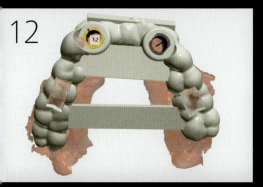

Design of the surgical guide with the reinforcements, sleeve pockets, and inspection windows.

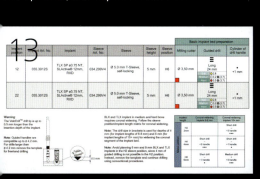

Drilling protocol delivered by Implant Studio.

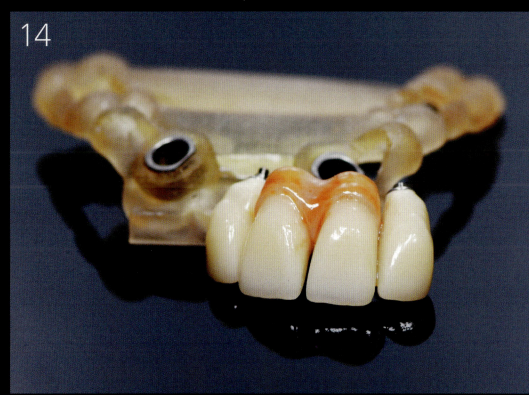

Printed surgical guide and partial denture with milled false gingiva.

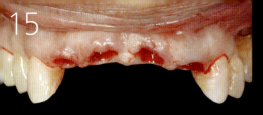
Extraction of the four maxillary incisors.

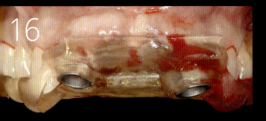
Fitting of the surgical guide in place after extraction of the four incisors.

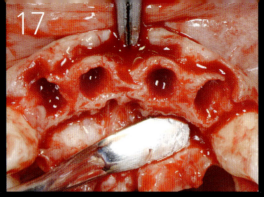
Occlusal view of the bone crest after flap removal.

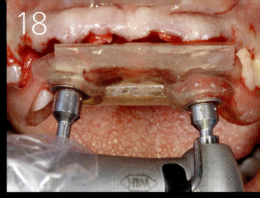
Guided placement of the two implants with vertical registration. Rotational registration was not useful here since we were using Variobase partial denture work.

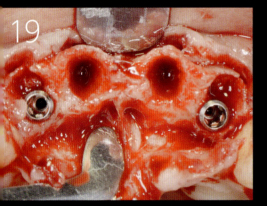
Axial view of the inserted implants. Note their more palatal and apical positioning in the sockets according to the recommendations given in the literature.

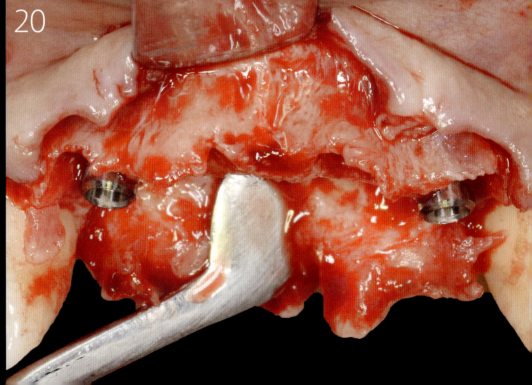
Frontal view with 1.0 to 1.5 mm more apical positioning

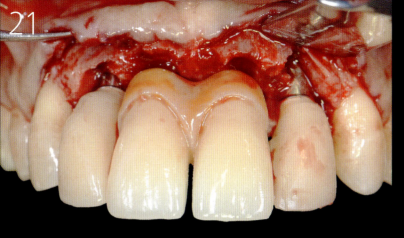

Immediate temporary partial denture in place with false gingiva around teeth 11 and 21. In addition to managing vertical volumes, this allowed the presence of diastemas to distribute the volumetric ratios of the incisors harmoniously.

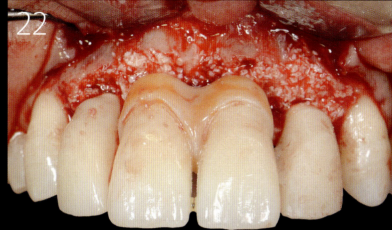

Filling of extraction gaps in 12 and 22 and ridge preservation in 11 and 21 with DBBM (Bio-Oss with fine particles) incubated in the F2 fraction of plasma (PRGF, Endoret, BTI France).

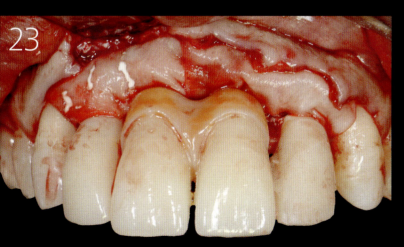

Covering with a resorbable collagen membrane (Bio-Gide).

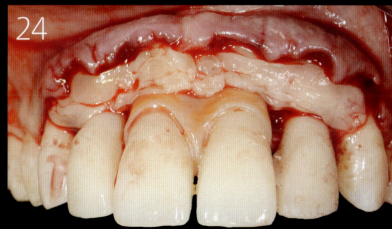

Covering of the whole using a fibrin membrane from the F1 fraction of the plasma (PRGF).

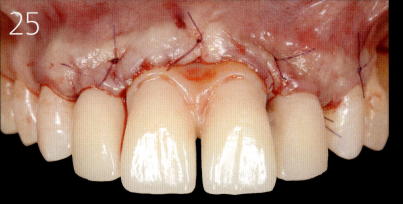

25 ASAF suture in place with wrapping of the base of the pontic to provide a pontic bed that allowed for easier working of the gingival and false gingival transition.

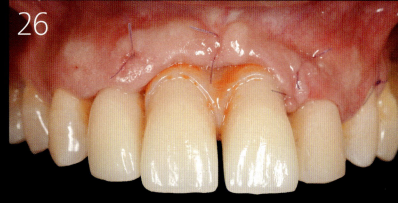

26 Clinical situation at 8 days.

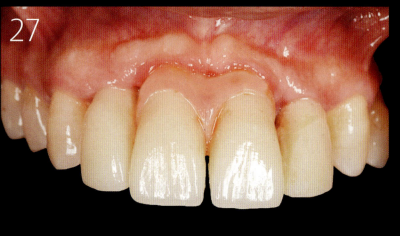

27 Clinical situation at 3 months.

28 Analysis of the smile. Note the slight frontal tilt to be corrected in the final partial denture.

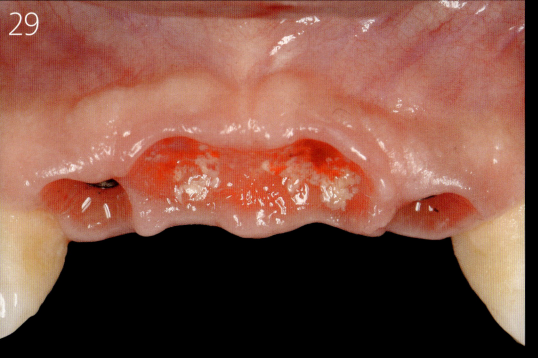

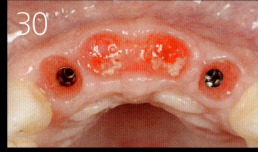

Occlusal view. Note the quality of the implant beds in 12 and 22 and the pontic bed in 21 and 11.

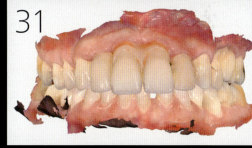

Impression taken with a Trios 4 pre-preparation scanner.

Frontal view of the clinical situation 3 months after removal of the provisional partial denture when implant osseointegration was checked.

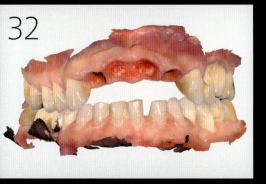

Computed tomography (CT) scan of the gingival profile.

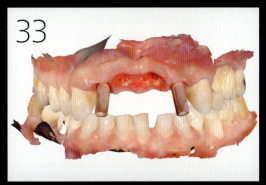

Scanner with the scan bodies in 12 and 22.

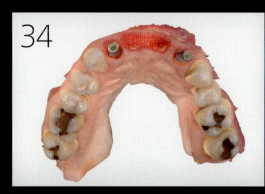

Occlusal view of the scanner with the TLX scan bodies.

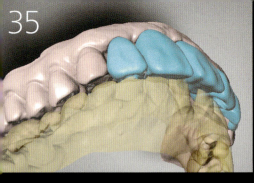
Importation into the Dental Wings ecosystem at the Dental Art Technology Laboratory (Richard Demange).

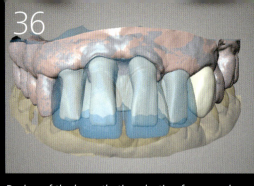
Design of the homothetic reduction framework according to the modified wax-up after analysis of the photos in 3Shape Smile Design software.

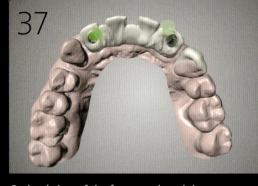
Occlusal view of the framework and the screw axes.

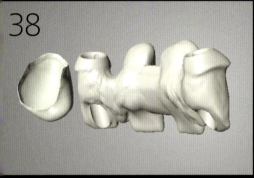
STL file of the partial denture and veneer in 23 to close the excessive diastema between teeth 22 and 23. The file was sent for zirconia machining with Metoxit disks (Createch Medical).

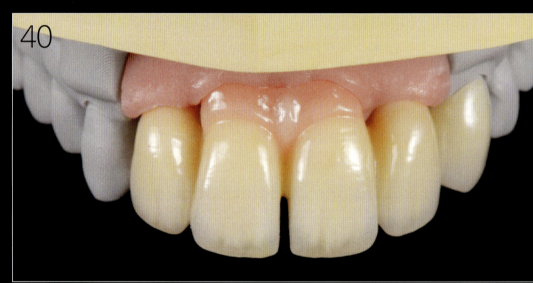
Finished partial denture on the printed laboratory model (Shera).

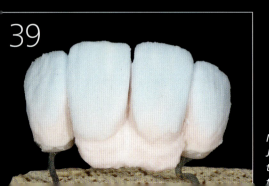
Mounting of the ceramic (CZR; Noritake, Nagoya, Japan) on the zirconia framework. Note that this is the first step involving physical work on the model since the beginning of treatment.

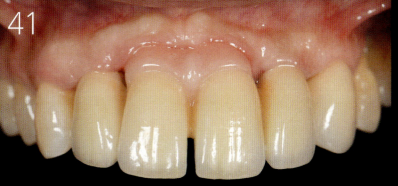

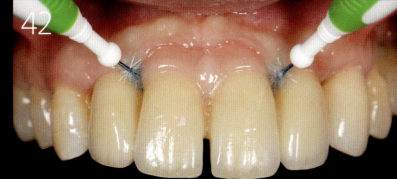

Partial denture in place with the veneer bonded in 23 (Panavia). Note the horizontal butt joint support of the false gingiva facilitating the fusion of the two pink layers.

Interdental spaces calibrated to 1.2 mm in the laboratory and checked in the mouth.

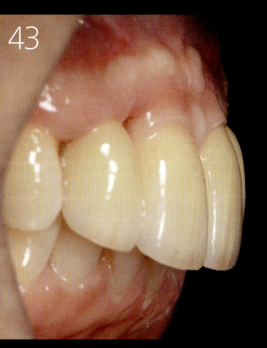

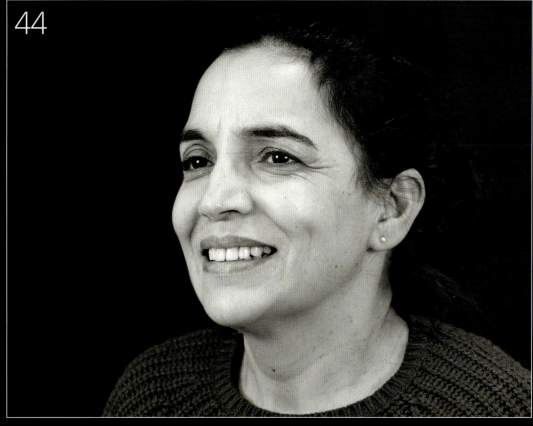

Profile view of the emergences. Note the butt joint support of the false gingiva.

Overall esthetic result.

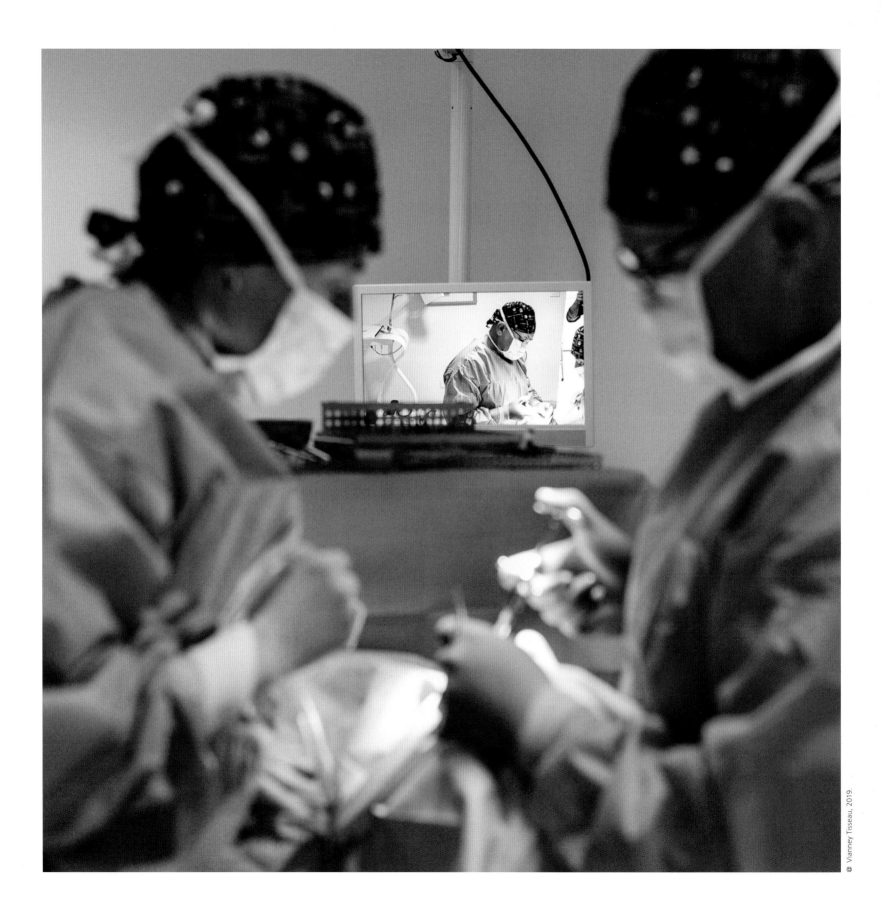

© Vianney Tisseau, 2019.

Plural-unit clinical case 21

63-year-old man.

Clinical data

- Terminal mobility of 12 to 22 on stabilized periodontal terrain.
- Case treated in January 2022.
- Favorable bone context.
- Good mucogingival architecture.

Presurgical treatments

- Trios 4 used to take the optical impression and 3Shape X1 used to perform the 3D examination.
- Planning using Implant Studio.
- Placement of Straumann TLX SP NT 3.75 x 10.00 mm implants in 12 and 22 for a four-tooth partial denture.
- 3D printing of the guide designed in Implant Studio, printed in the office on a NextDent 5100 printer with NextDent SG resin and polymerized in a LC-3D 3D polymerization unit.
- Straumann TLX PEEK self-locking sockets.
- Temporary partial denture for four teeth, screwed in 12 and 22, shade A4, printed in the office on a NextDent 5100 printer with NextDent Crown & Bridge N1 resin, polymerized in a LC-3D 3D polymerization unit and stained on an A4 base with an Optiglaze Color Set.
- NT Variobase for Bridge used in 12 and 22, bonded with Multilink Hybrid Abutment HO. The screw shaft in 22 was incisal as there is currently no Variobase SA for partial denture work.

Assessment of the intervention

- Case treated in **three appointments at the office** (impression and 3D examination, surgery, control at 3 months).
- The patient moved to Brittany, so the final prosthesis was fabricated remotely based on the control in the patient's new home.

Additional treatments

- This patient was followed for 4 years for the sequelae of periodontal disease, which was stabilized by his referring dentist. The maxillary posterior sectors had already been implanted 4 years prior. The already present mobility from 12 to 22 had increased and required intervention in this area.

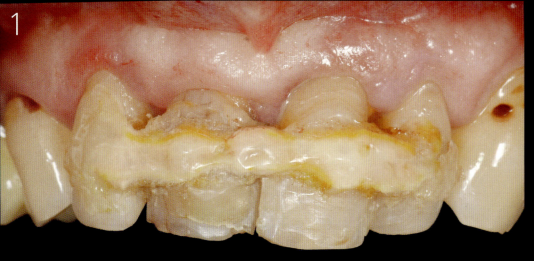

Initial clinical situation in January 2022 with the temporary retainer having been made in December to hold the teeth in place and avoid the need for an immediate removable appliance.

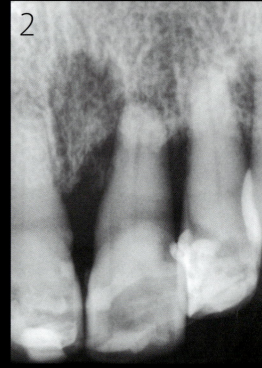

Radiographic view, particularly of teeth 21 and 22.

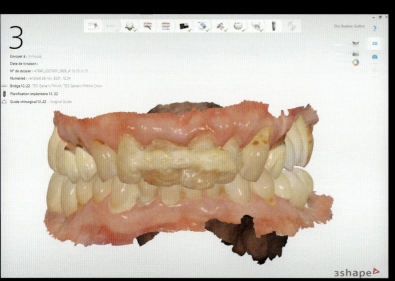

Intraoral optical impression taken with a Trios 4. Note on the upper bar the complete 3Shape flow using the CBCT X1 scanner, the teeth to be extracted are removed, the design of the new teeth, the merging of the STL and DICOM files, and the implant planning after which the radiologic guide was drawn.

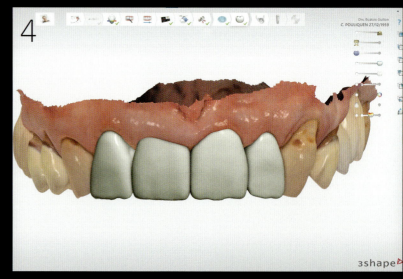

Design of the future partial denture that was to be transferred to Dental System and finalized.

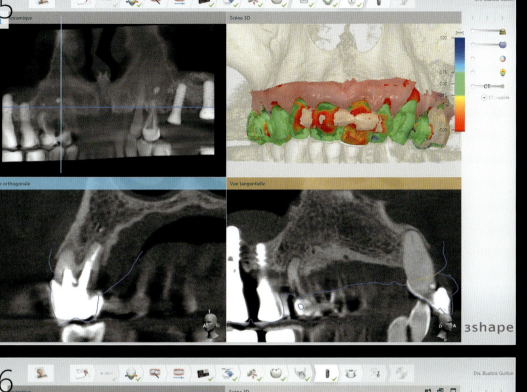

Merging of STL and DICOM files. The colorimetric index allowed the accuracy of the surfacing to be evaluated. Note that the composite restraint on 12 was not radiopaque, which resulted in a zone of inconsistency in the fusion at this level. Also note the blue line showing the dental and gingival contours on the CBCT file.

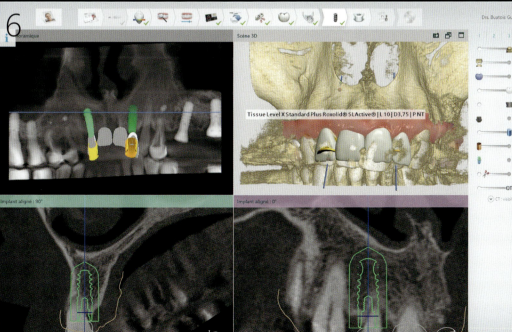

Planning of site 12. Note the correction of the egressions between the prosthetic project and the actual position of the teeth on the CBCT scan.

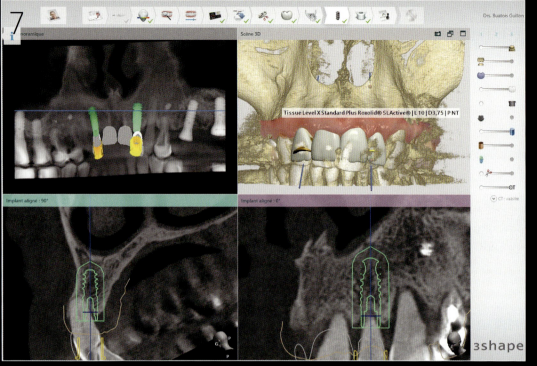

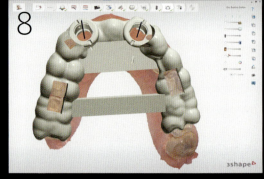

Design of the surgical guide with the usual inspection windows, reinforcement bars, socket pockets, and rotational marking (optional here since we were using Variobase for Bridge).

Planning of site 22.

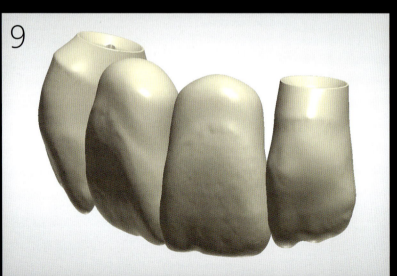

STL file with emergence profiles and bonding boxes for the Variobase, delivered by Dental System after the design phase.

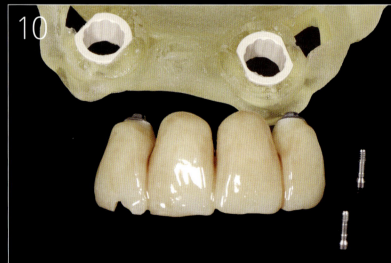

Printed surgical guide and a provisional partial denture for four teeth printed and stained. Note that we were at the limit of the indication for printing on a four-unit prosthesis. It would be better to mill more than three teeth but to do the full case chairside we opted for printing. Also noteworthy is the incisal screw

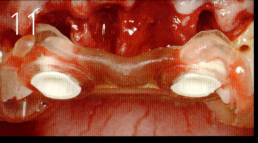

Guide in place after extractions.

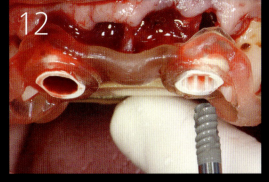

Presentation of the 3.75 x 10.00 mm NT implant after guided drilling.

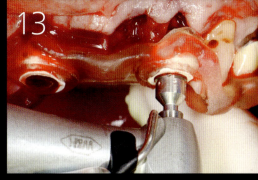

Guided implant placement with a vertical marking at H6.

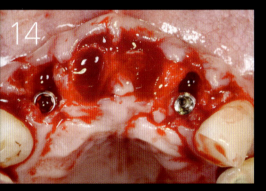

Occlusal view of the implants in place immediately in the extraction sockets, positioned 1 mm more palatally and apically.

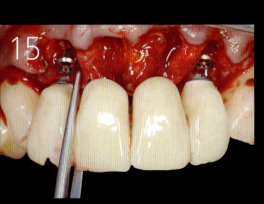

Presentation of the **immediate** temporary partial denture.

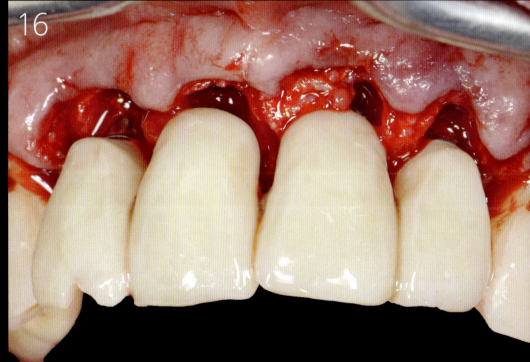

Partial denture in place, seated optimally on the two NT implants. Note the relationship of the pontics to the sockets in 11 and 21.

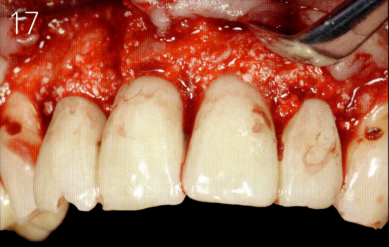
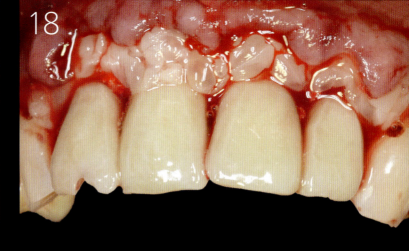

Compensatory GBR in extraction hiatus in 12 and 22 and in ridge preservation in 11 and 21. Filling was performed with DBBM (Bio-Oss with fine particles) sticky bone incubated in the F2 fraction of plasma.

Covering of the filling zone with a fibrin membrane from the F1 fraction of the plasma (PRGF).

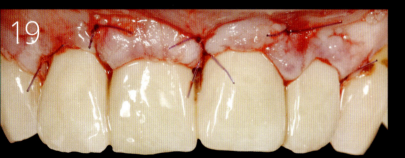
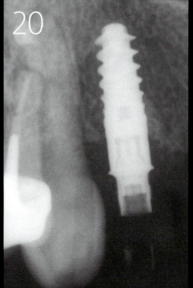
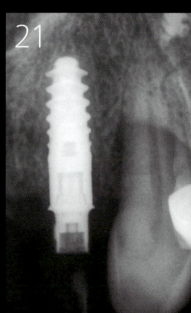

Flap suture with ASAF sutures at 12, 11, 21, and 22. Note the favorable thickness of the gingival tissue. The screw hole in 12 was closed with EverGlow flowable composite (Coltene, Altstätten, Switzerland) after the screw heads were protected with Teflon plugs.

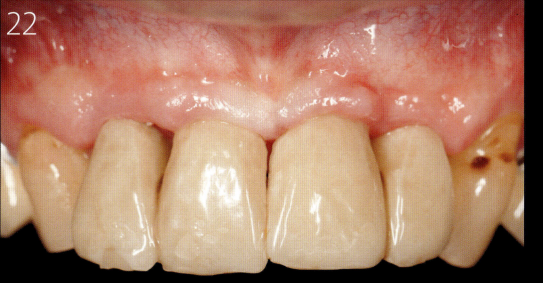

Clinical situation at 3 months with the **immediate** temporary partial denture in place.

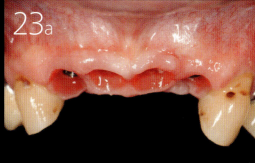

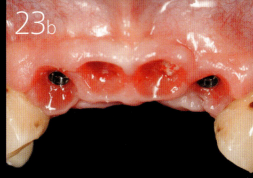

Vestibular view of the implant and pontic beds.

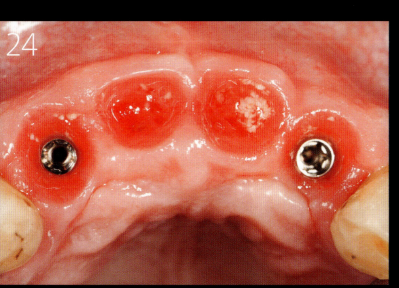

Occlusal view of the anatomic emergence profiles induced by healing around the **immediate** partial denture. The situation was esthetically and biologically

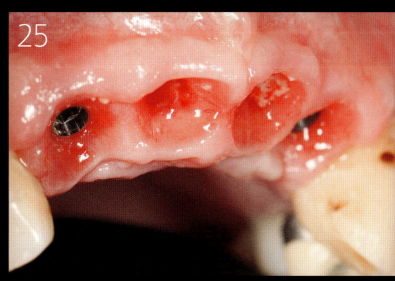

View of the sulci. Note the gingival health at 3 months after immediate implantation and compensatory GBR.

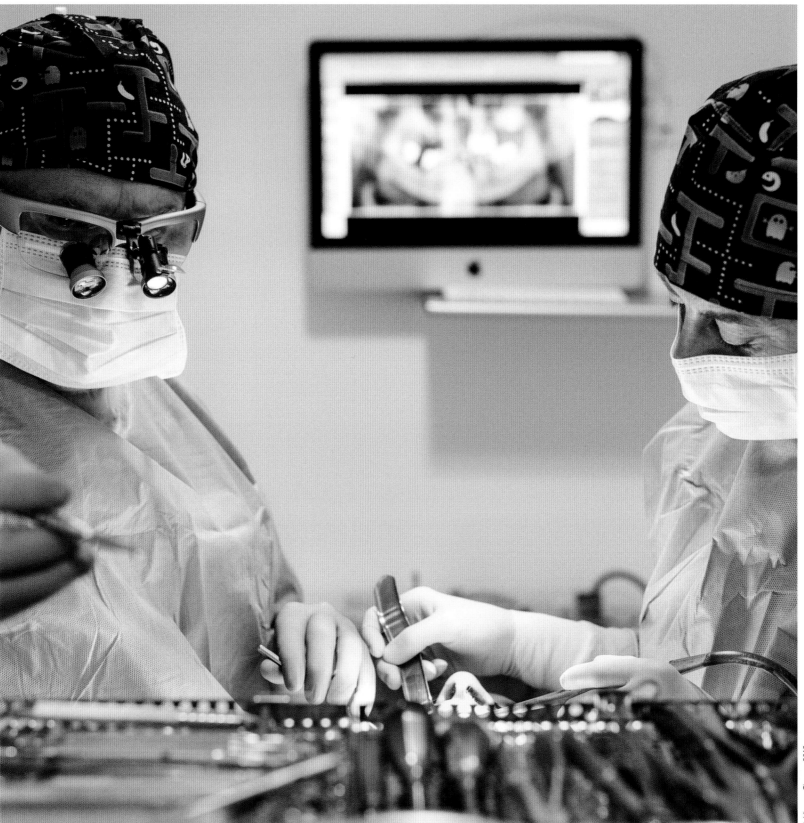

© Vianney Tisseau, 2019.

Plural-unit clinical case 22

66-year-old woman.

Clinical data

- Both implants had been lost in 24 and 26 due to peri-implantitis in the context of active periodontal disease, resulting in the loss of teeth 22 and 23 and condemning 13, 12, and 11.
- Case treated in May 2022.
- Altered bony context with generalized horizontal bone loss.
- Mucogingival architecture with significant horizontal bone loss.

Presurgical treatments

- Trios 4 used to take the optical impression and a 3Shape X1 used to perform the 3D examination.
- Planning using Implant Studio.
- Placement of Straumann TLX SP RT 3.75 x 8.00 mm implant in 26, RT 3.75 x 10.00 mm implant in 24, and two NT 3.75 x 12.00 mm implants in 12 and 22.
- 3D printing of the guide, designed in Implant Studio, printed in the office on a NextDent 5100 printer with NextDent SG resin and polymerized in an LC-3D 3D polymerization unit.
- Straumann T-sockets.
- Temporary partial denture for nine teeth, screwed in 12, 22, 24, and 26 (extension in 13) in shade A3 with pink false gingiva, milled in PMMA (Dentitek Laboratory).
- NT Variobase TLX for Bridgework in used 12 and 22 and RT in 24 and 26, bonded with Multilink Hybrid Abutment HO.

Assessment of the intervention

- Case treated in **five appointments at the office** (impression and 3D, surgery, control at 3 months and impression, validation key, placement of the prosthesis).
- Prosthesis made in the office (Dental Art Technology Laboratory, Richard Demange).

Additional treatments

- The patient presented 7 years after implant treatment for both maxillary posterior sectors. At that time, two sinus grafts were performed with four implants placed in 24, 26, 14, and 16 (WN in 16 and 26 and RN in 14 and 24). The final prosthesis was made in the office 6 months after surgery. The patient preferred to be followed up for periodontal maintenance in another practice. Follow-ups were not done and the recurrence of periodontitis challenged the clinical status quo at that time.

The Quokka protocol

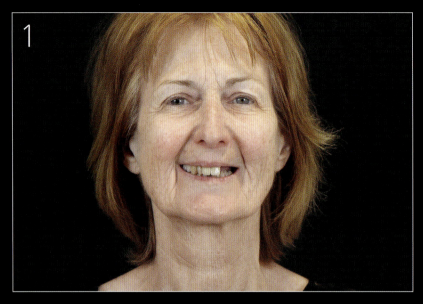

*Photographs of the smile taken during the esthetic analysis appointment to gather the elements required for the prosthetic project in view of implant planning and the design of the **immediate** temporary prosthesis.*

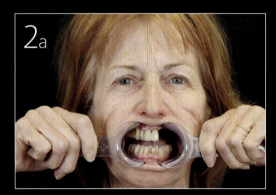

Second photo with retractor. These two photos were superimposed in the Smile Design module within the Trios scanner.

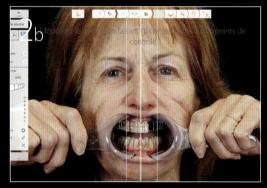

Smile template selected from a large library of templates.

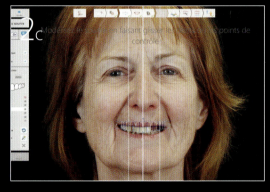

Same template integrated into the smile.

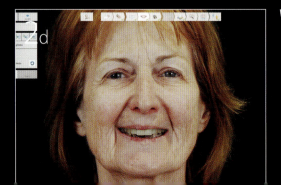

Volume setting of the selected teeth.

Final page of the Smile Design module with the ability to slide from the "before" situation to the "after" situation. This can be used as a communication aid to replace the resin mask in the mouth. The specifications given by the patient were integrated in this assembly

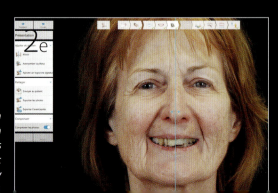

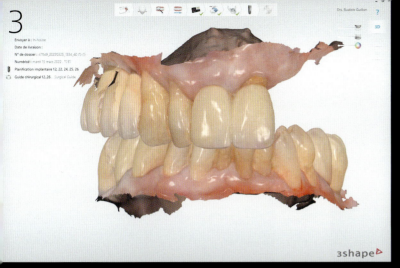

ntraoral optical impression.

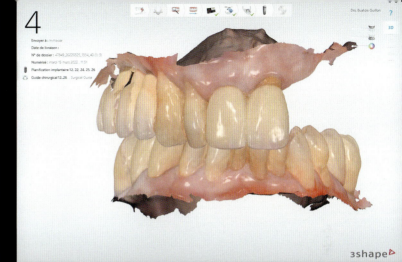

Maxilla with the presence of a laminated impression in quadrant 1 that was not ideal and should have been corrected during entry.

Digital wax-up of the assembly according to the project elaborated in Smile Design software.

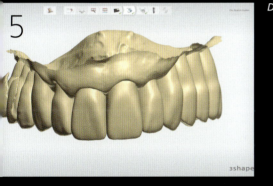

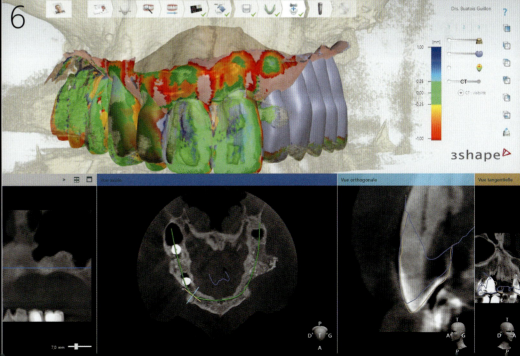

As the different STL files were elaborated in the same coordinate system (the same ecosystem within the same workflow), they could be merged in an optimal manner during the planning phase. We thus had the present intraoral situation at the time, merged with the DICOM file of the CBCT scan of the same clinical situation, always with the colorimetric index of control, upon which was superimposed on the STL file of the digital wax-up of the prosthetic project. The brown line indicates the existing dental volume and the blue line

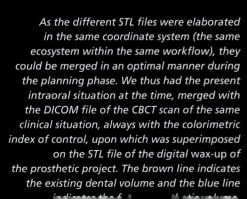

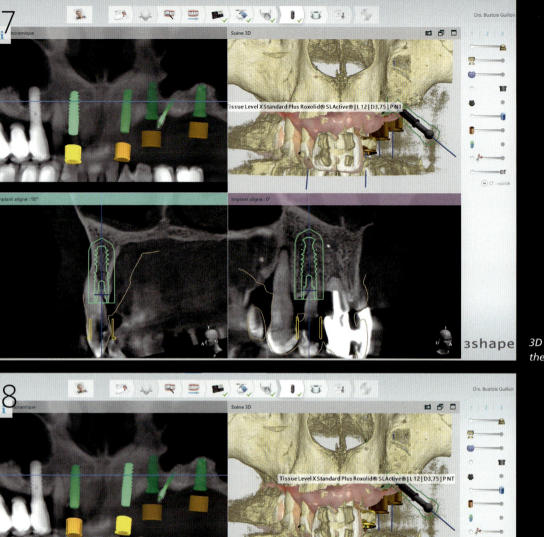

3D bone-guided implant planning in 12. Note the terminal damage in 13, 12, and 11.

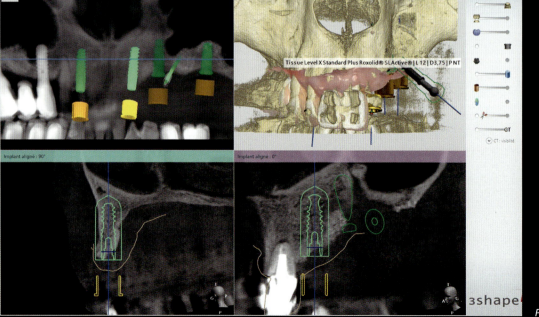

Planning in 22.

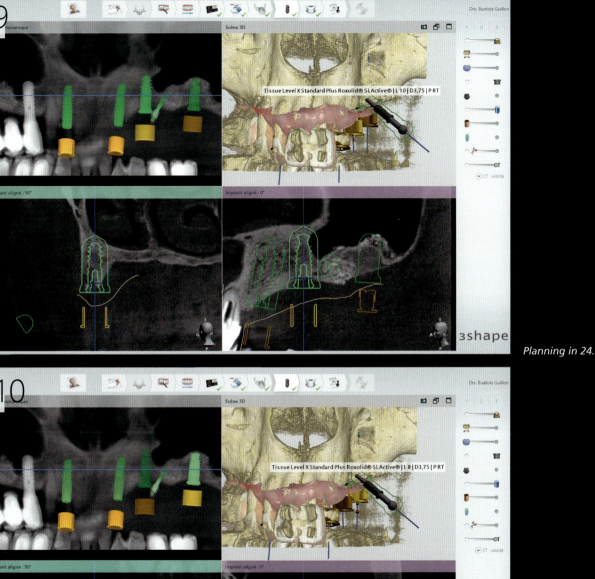

Planning in 24.

Planning in 26. Note the preservation of bone gain by the sinus graft performed 7 years earlier despite the loss of the Straumann WN implant in site 26 due to peri-implantitis.

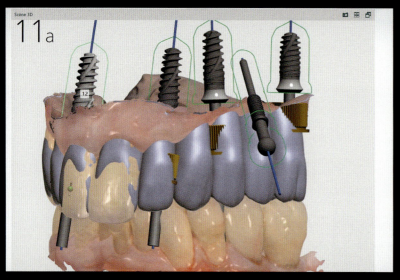
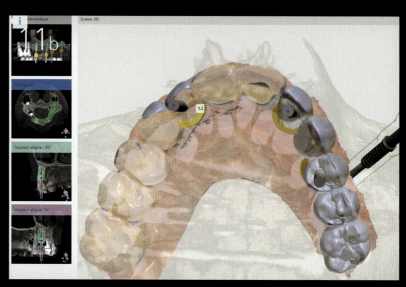

Overview of implant planning within the intraoral files and the prosthetic project without the DICOM file. A key was planned in 25 to stabilize the surgical guide in this area, which was not supported by dental restorations.

Axial view. The different windows and the set of filters help to visualize the plan in relation to the different parameters.

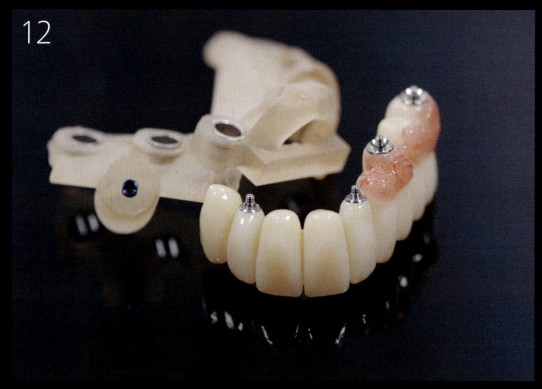

Printed surgical guide, including positioning of a sleeve for insertion of the stabilization pin.

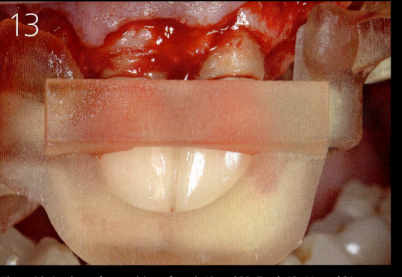

The guide in place after avulsion of teeth 12 and 22. Teeth 13, 11, and 21 were retained to support the guide in addition to the existing partial denture from teeth 14 to 16.

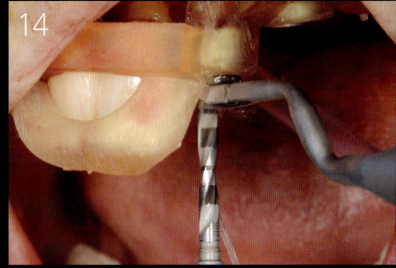

Guided drilling.

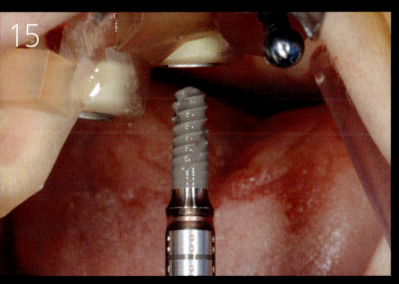

The Straumann TLX SP NT 3.75 x 12.00 mm implant on the guided implant holder prior to insertion.

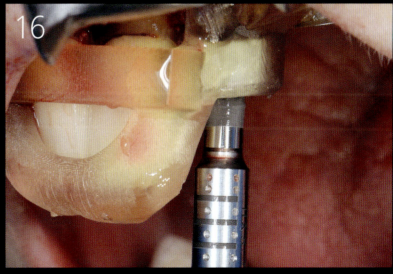

Guided implant placement.

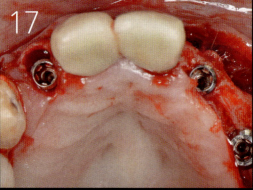

17 Occlusal view of the implants placed before the extraction of teeth 11, 21, and 23 and the fitting of the **immediate** temporary partial denture.

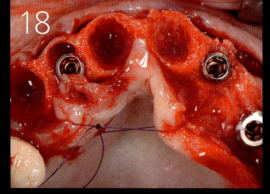

18 Occlusal view after extraction of the condemned guide teeth. The implant in 26 was not visible.

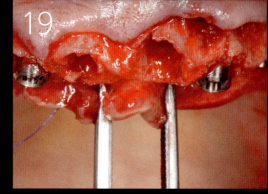

19 Vestibular view of the immediate implants, still with the vertical and palatal positioning increased by 1 mm according to the recommendations in the literature. Note the variations in bone level, a sequela of periodontal disease.

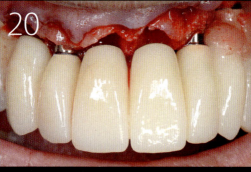

20 Placement of the **instant** temporary partial denture, adapted optimally to NT and RT.

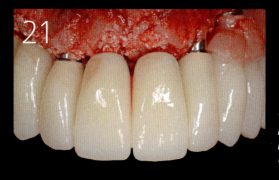

21 GBR compensating for extraction and ridge preservation gaps with DBBM (Bio-Oss with fine particles) incubated in PRGF, phase F2 of plasma in the form of sticky bone.

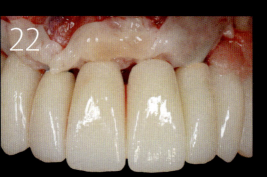

22 Overlay of fibrin membrane from the F1 fraction of plasma.

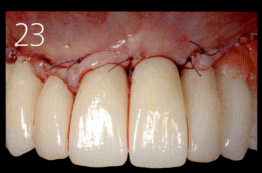

23 Suturing of the flap with ASAF sutures and vertical prosthetic compensation with a false gingiva opposite 24, 25, and 26.

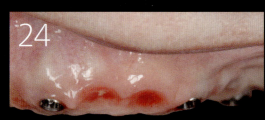

24 Clinical appearance in vestibular view at 3 months. The juxtagingival border of the TLX implant necks is not an esthetic hindrance when viewed from the smile line in relation to the neck line; it was a periodontal asset in the context of the patient's history. Implant osseointegration was validated.

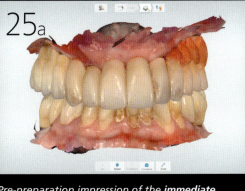

Pre-preparation impression of the **immediate** temporary partial denture, antagonist arch and RIM.

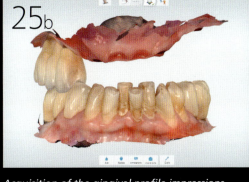

Acquisition of the gingival profile impressions, which were placed in the same occlusion with the antagonist arch.

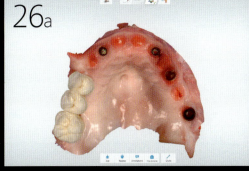

Occlusal view of the optical impression of the gingival profiles. Note the implant beds and pontic beds.

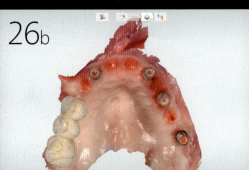

Occlusal view of the TLX scan bodies, the final steps of the digital impressions for the final prosthesis.

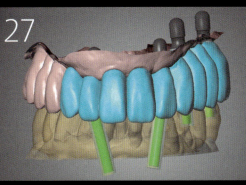

Importation of the pre-preparation impression file into the Dental Wings ecosystem at the Dental Art Technology Laboratory (Richard Demange), overlaid with the STL file of the implant impression.

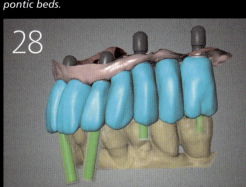

Side view.

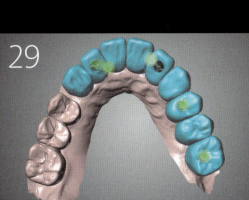

Occlusal view. Note the diastema between the extension in 13 and the partial denture from 14 to 16.

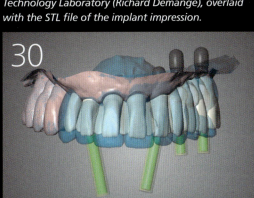

Design of the zirconia framework using a digital homothetic reduction. Note the volumes of 25 and 26, which were slightly more extended at the patient's request to accompany the smile line

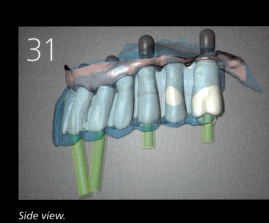

Side view.

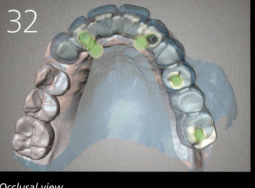
32 Occlusal view.

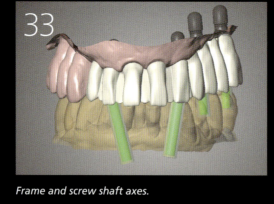
33 Frame and screw shaft axes.

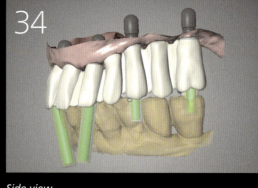
34 Side view.

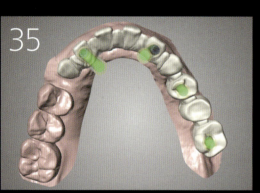
35 Occlusal view.

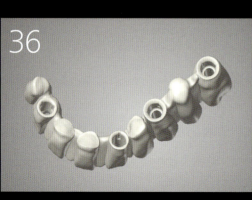
36 STL file of the framework ready to be sent by Richard Demange for machining into Metoxit disks (Createch Medical).

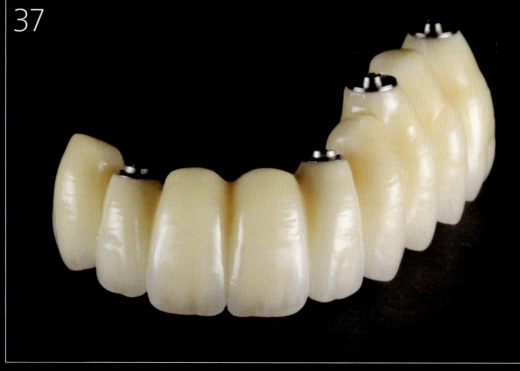
37 The finished partial denture after layering the zirconia framework with CZR Noritake ceramic (Dental Art Technology Laboratory, Richard Demange).

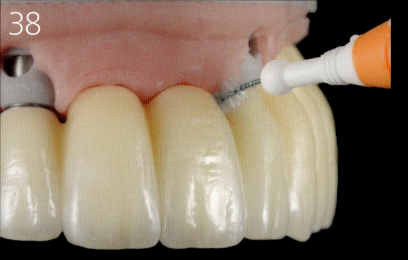

Checking the calibration of interdental brushes. Printed models (Shera).

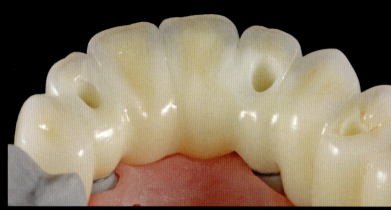

Note the location of the screw wells due to planning that included the prosthetic volume in the positioning criteria.

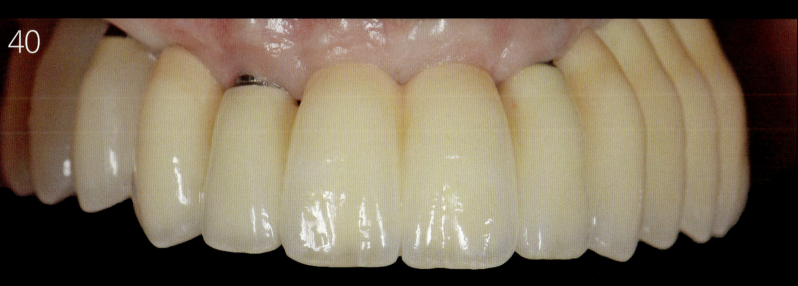

Result in the mouth. The supragingival margins had no esthetic impact but were of real periodontal interest given the patient's history. She is now aware of the need for periodontal maintenance and will follow our instructions.

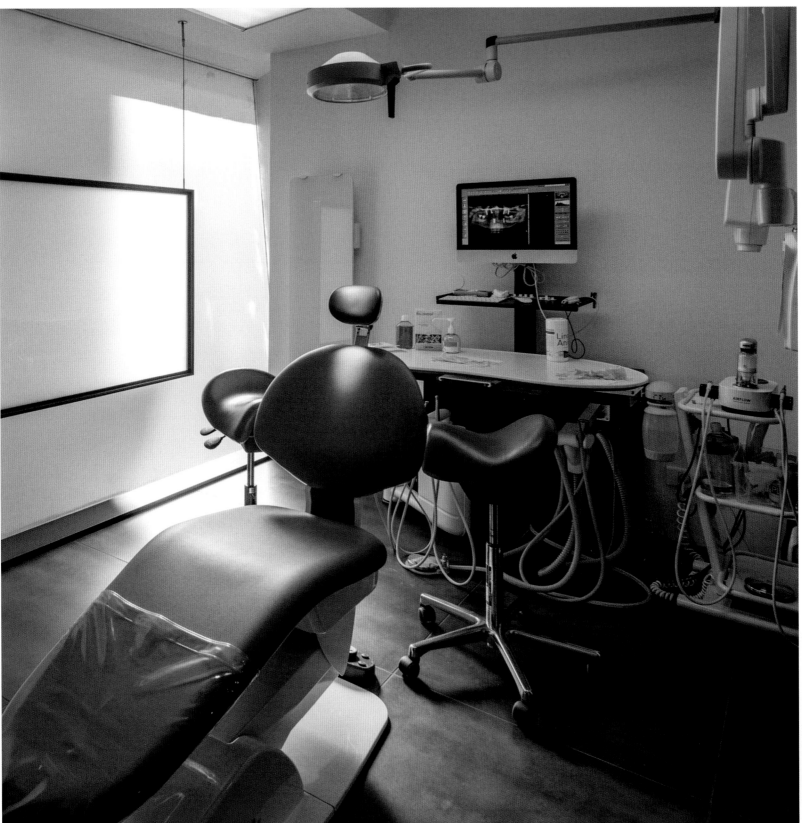

© Vianney Tisseau, 2019.

Plural-unit clinical case 23

62-year-old woman.

Clinical data

- Extraction of teeth 13, 12, and 23 in a context of dental mobility and recurrence of caries lesions the existing six-tooth partial denture.
- Case treated in December 2022.
- Altered bone context with angular losses and different bone levels from 13 to 23.
- Good mucogingival architecture.

Presurgical treatments

- Trios 4 used to take an optical impression and 3Shape X1 used to perform the 3D examination.
- Planning using Implant Studio.
- Placement of Straumann TLX SP NT 3.75 x 12.00 mm implants in 12 and 22 and NT 3.75 x 10.00 mm implants in 13 and 23. The choice of NTs and 3.75 mm diameters was justified by the prosthetic project, which required correction of a midline shift to the left in a constrained space between 14 and 24.
- 3D printing of the guide designed in Implant Studio, printed in the office on a NextDent 5100 printer with NextDent SG resin and polymerized in an LC-3D 3D polymerization unit.
- Straumann T-sockets.
- Temporary partial denture for six screwed-in teeth in 13, 12, 22, and 23, A3 shade, milled in PMMA (Dentitek Laboratory).
- NT Variobase TLX for Bridgework used in 13, 12, 22, and 23, bonded with Multilink Hybrid Abutment HO.

Assessment of the intervention

- Case treated in **three appointments at the office** (impression and 3D examination, surgery, control at 3 months).
- Prosthesis made in the office (Mathias Berger Laboratory).
- The patient came to us as an emergency at the beginning of December 2022 regarding her anterior partial denture that was no longer holding despite repeated sealing. She had already received implants 10 years ago. The roots were mobile in 13, 12, and 23 and the partial denture was on a post, more adapted to the dental support. The difficulty of the case, in addition to the altered bone levels, resided in the significant shift and tilt from the middle to the right in a constrained space between 14 and 24. The patient wished for the immediate implantations associated with the **immediate** restoration to be performed as soon as possible before the holidays.

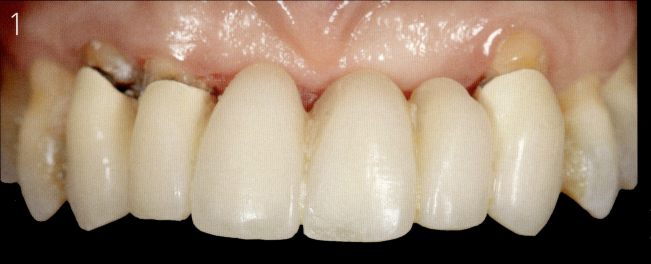

Initial clinical situation with partial denture mobility on the roots.

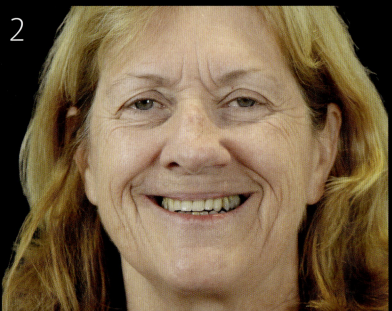

Note the shift and tilt of the interincisal midline in relation to the facial midline. The patient had always noted this problem but had kept the partial denture for more than 15 years; however, she requested that this esthetic aspect be corrected as far as possible.

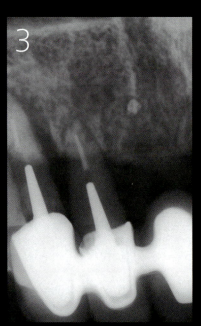

Retroalveolar radiograph of teeth 13 and 12.

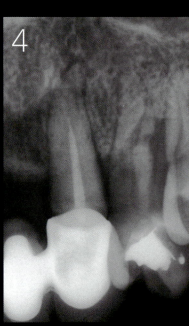

Retroalveolar radiograph in site 23.

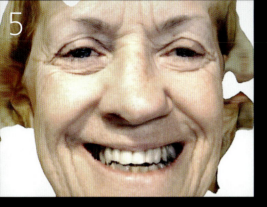

We integrated the esthetic analysis in the RayFace module (Ray Medical), with a 3D facial scanner that made it possible allowing to integrate the STL and DICOM files for esthetic analysis with the spatial references of the different planes and lines of reference in prosthesis and orthodontics. Acquisition stage of the facial scanner.

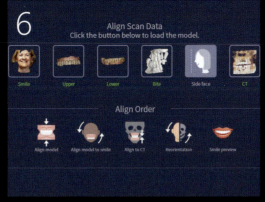

After acquisition and reconstruction of the 3D facial volume, we imported the STL files (acquired using the Trios 4) and DICOM files (acquired using the X1). We could also import a cephalometric radiograph if desired.

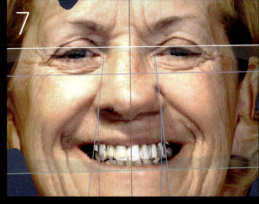

Esthetic project in facial view with the frontal planes of reference. Note the shift to the right, no longer oblique, which still remained, but in a proportion of 2 mm. It was difficult to reduce this shift further to the left as there was limited space between 14 and 24.

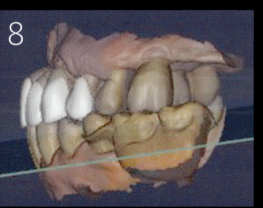

Sagittal view of the montage with the sagittal planes of reference. Note the horizontal bone deficit.

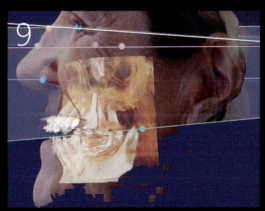

Sagittal view with facial and bone volume.

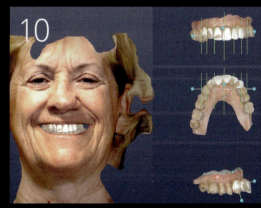

In addition to the design integrating the face, we could work on the volumes in 3D and not only 2D, as in the Smile Design module in Trios.

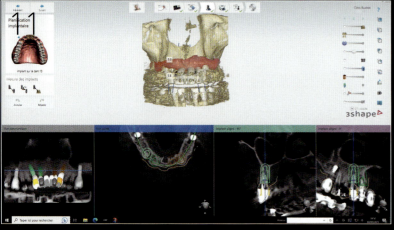

Importation of the file into the 3Shape ecosystem for implant planning in accordance with the prosthetic project.

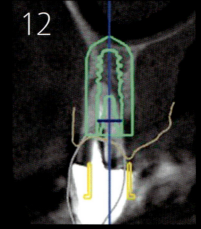

Implant planning in 13. Note the absence of the vestibular bone wall.

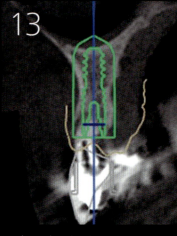

Implant planning in 12. Note the vestibular concavity.

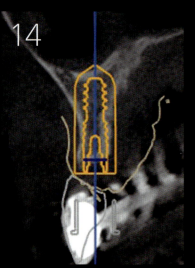

Implant planning in 22. The same vestibular concavity was to be corrected during surgery. Note the orange color of the implant, which means that we had reduced the peripheral spacing envelope of the implant to be able to match the

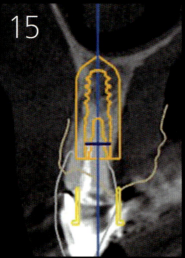

Implant planning in 23. Note the bone compensation work required in the vestibular region.

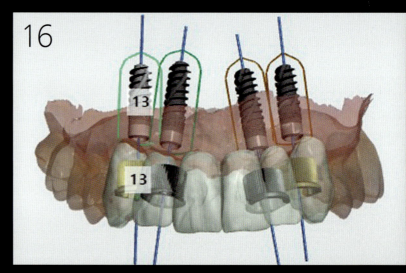

View without the bone filter of the final planning before designing the guide.

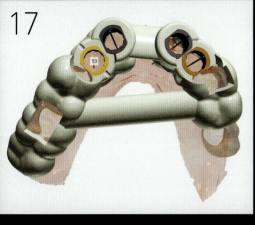

17 Design of the guide with inspection windows, reinforcement bar, and sleeve pockets. Rotational marking is not necessary for partial dentures with a direct connection to the implant.

18 Drilling protocol published by Implant Studio which served as a roadmap during guided surgery.

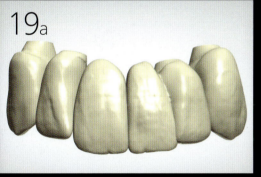

19a STL file of the partial denture designed in Dental System. The rotation of 21 over 11 could have been accentuated to compensate for the width of 21, which was cut to bring the middle back in line with the median axis of the face.

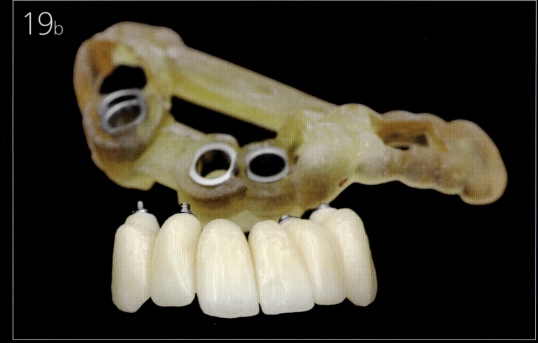

19b Printed guide and milled partial denture. Note the projected emergence profiles to compensate for the horizontal bone deficit. After discussion with the patient, we opted for palatal positioning of the implants with perimplant grafting rather than a pre-implant bone grafting procedure involving wearing a removable prosthesis for at least 6 months.

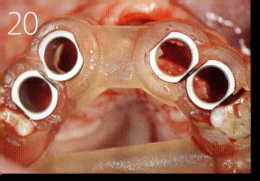

Surgical guide in place after extraction of teeth 13, 12, and 23.

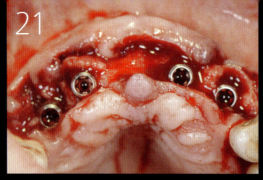

The four NT implants in place in 13, 12, 22, and 23. Note their asymmetric location in relation to the middle of the arch, which is marked by the median raphe.

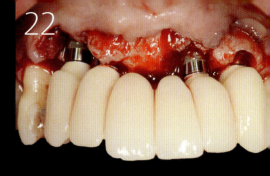

Immediate temporary partial denture in place. Note the bone compensation work by GBR to fill and level the bone defects.

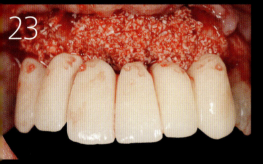

Compensatory GBR with DBBM (Bio-Oss with fine particles) incubated in PRGF fraction F2 of plasma.

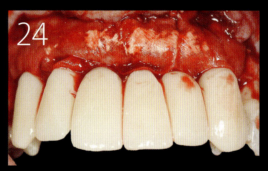

After covering the sticky bone with the fibrin membrane from the F1 fraction of the plasma, a resorbable collagen membrane (Bio-Gide) was placed and stabilized using vestibular pins.

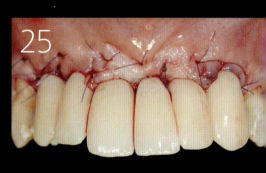

After a half-thickness incision of the vestibular flap was made at the back of the vestibule from 14 to 24 for coronal traction without tension, the flap was sutured using ASAF sutures around 13, 12, 22, and 23 and mattress sutures at 11 and 21.

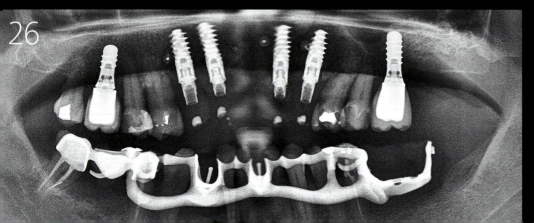

The postoperative control radiograph confirmed optimal seating of the partial denture on the implants.

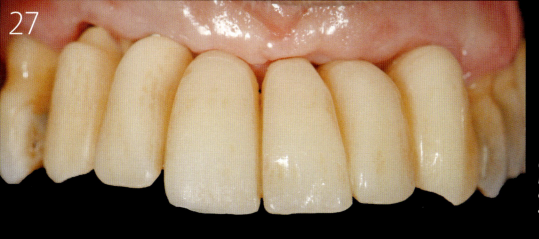

27 Clinical view at 3 months with perfectible hygiene on the part of the patient. The emergence profiles were correct in 23, 22, and 12, but there was a deficit in 13.

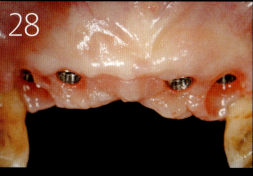

28 Vestibular view after removal of the **immediate** partial denture for implant control. Good leveling of bone defects was achieved with quality implant beds.

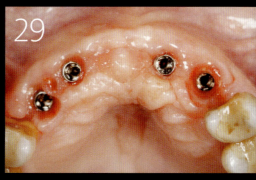

29 Occlusal view of the implant beds. The pontic beds needed to be accentuated.

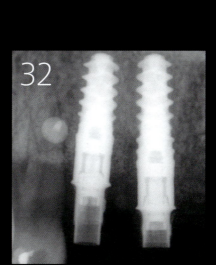

30 We were able to bring the midline back to the median face axis and remove the tilt. The volumes of 11 and 21 still needed to be worked on with animation to improve the esthetic rendering.

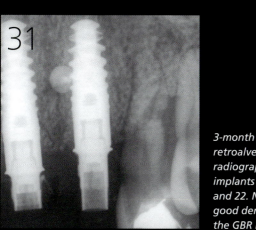

31 3-month retroalveolar radiograph of implants 23 and 22. Note the good density of the GBR material.

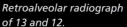

32 Retroalveolar radiograph of 13 and 12.

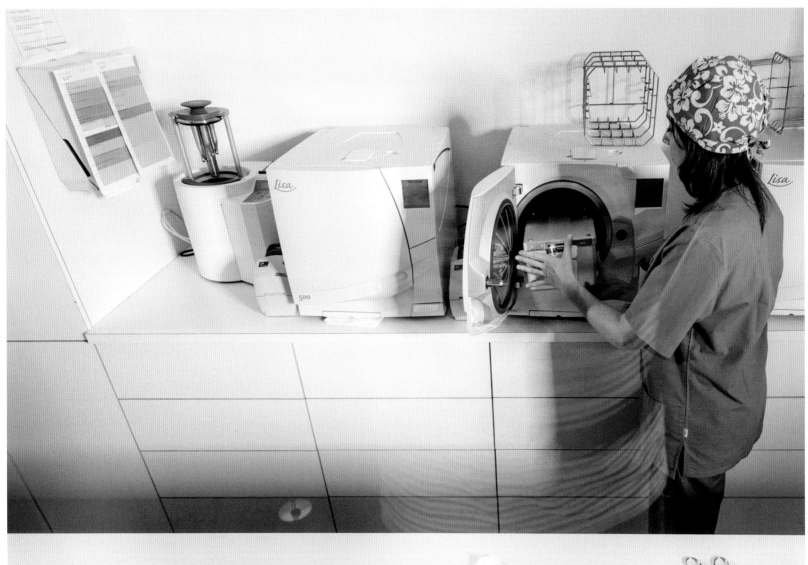
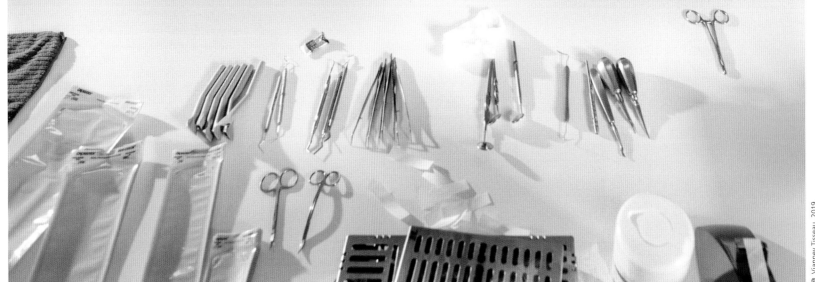

© Vianney Tisseau, 2019.

Plural-unit clinical case 24

70-year-old woman.

Clinical data
- Loss of the partial denture from 33 to 42 supported by 33 and 42, sites of recurring caries lesions and repeated loosening.
- Case treated in March 2021.
- Bone context limited in width.
- Good mucogingival architecture.

Presurgical treatments
- Trios 4 used to take the optical impression and 3Shape X1 used to perform the 3D examination.
- Planning using Implant Studio.
- Placement of Straumann TLX SP RT implant (4.5 x 12.0 mm) in 33 and a NT implant (3.75 x 12.00 mm) in 41. Use of the existing implant in 43.
- 3D printing of the guide designed in Implant Studio, printed in the office on a NextDent 5100 with NextDent SG resin and polymerized in a LC-3D 3D polymerization unit.
- Straumann PEEK sockets for self-locking TLX.
- Temporary partial denture for six teeth, screw-retained in 33 and 41 and attached to a temporary screw-retained abutment for RT in 43 (existing single-tooth BL implant with screw-retained crown in place), A2 shade, milled in PMMA (Dentitek Laboratory).
- NT Variobase TLX for Bridgework used in 41 and RT in 33, bonded with Multilink Hybrid Abutment HO.

Assessment of the intervention
- Case treated in **five appointments at the office** (impression and 3D examination, surgery, control at 3 months and impression, validation index, placement of the prosthesis).
- Prosthesis made in the office (Dental Art Technology Laboratory, Richard Demange).

Additional treatments
- The patient had undergone implant-prosthetic treatment 6 years earlier with lateral and bisinus bone grafting in the maxilla. At 6 months, eight implants were placed in the maxilla (16, 14, 13, 11, 21, 23, 24, and 26) for four partial dentures for three teeth and four implants in the mandible at 34, 36, and 44, 46 for two partial dentures for three teeth. At the time, teeth 33, 43, 32, and 42 were retained. We had to extract tooth 43, which was replaced by an implant 3 years later. The remaining partial denture now had to be extracted. We wanted to rely on the implant in 43 to secure the loading of the two implants by screwing in the **immediate** fixed/removable partial denture in 33 and 41, and securing a temporary screw-in abutment in 43 during surgery. In this context, an implant was positioned in 41, not 42, for a more even implant distribution. This combination of immediate and already osseointegrated implants had been tried two or three times without any convincing success, which made the procedure more complex. In this case, the tooth in 43 was put back in and remained independent of the **immediate** temporary partial denture. We have since been working on a protocol with an impression of the existing implants. This STL file is then integrated into the planning process as an additional file.

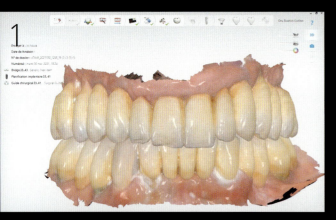

1 Intraoral optical impression of the initial situation (maxillary implant–supported partial dentures after bone grafting and posterior implant–supported restorations). The anterior partial denture from 42 to 33 had just been resealed. Digital data were gathered for **immediate** implantation and restoration.

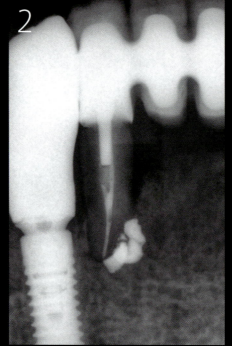

2 Retroalveolar radiograph of 42.

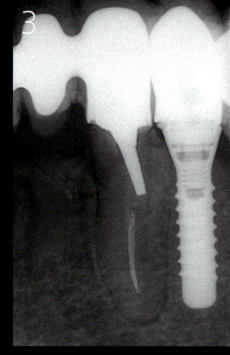

3 Retroalveolar radiograph of 33.

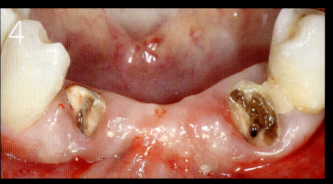

4 Clinical appearance before resurfacing of the partial denture.

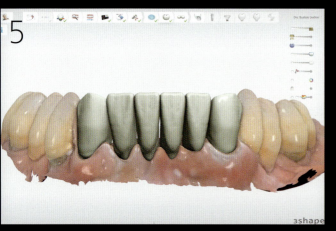

5 Creation of the prosthetic project in Implant Studio.

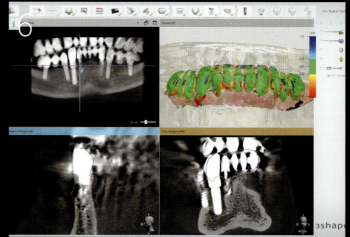

6 Fusion of STL and DICOM files with the colorimetric index. The definition of the DICOM file was good despite the presence of metallic structures (ceramic on a gold alloy frame).

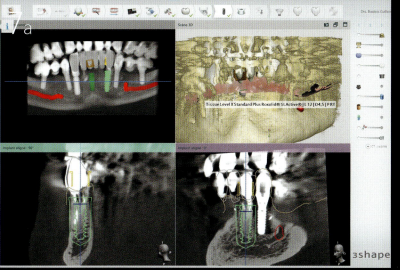

Implant planning in 33.   *Implant planning in 41.*

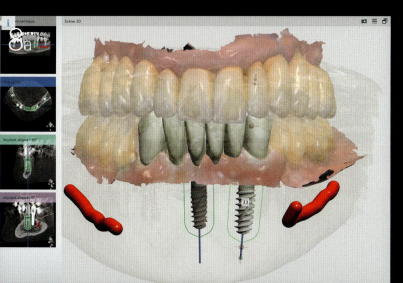

Vestibular view of the relationship of the implants to the prosthetic project.

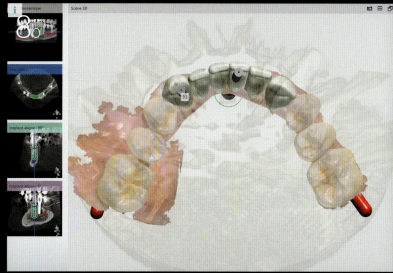

Occlusal view of the same report.

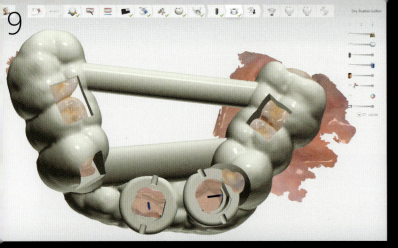

Design of the surgical guide.

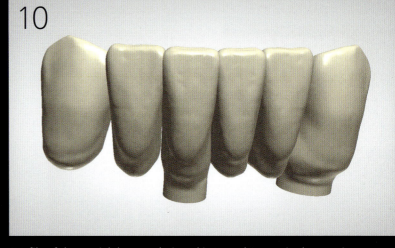

STL file of the partial denture designed in Dental System in the practice.

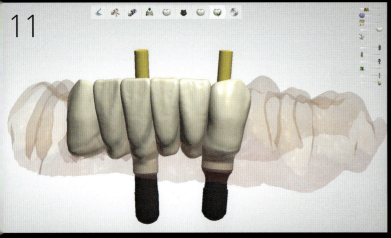

Vestibular view with screw axes.

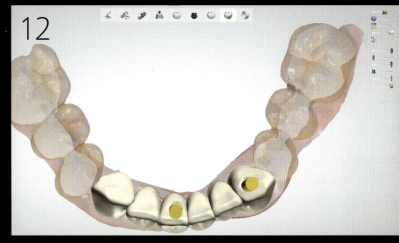

Occlusal view.

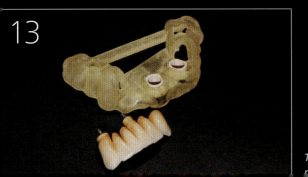

The surgical guide and **immediate** partial denture ready for surgery.

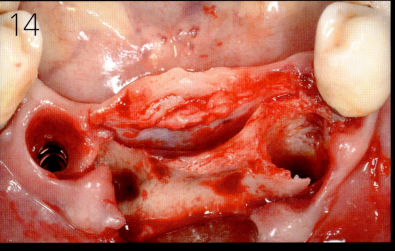

Avulsion of the teeth and removal of the screw-retained implant-supported tooth in 43 at the beginning of surgery.

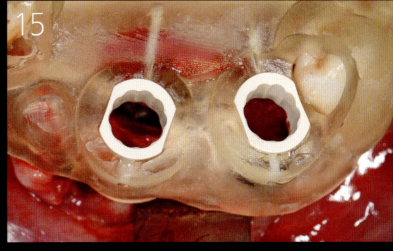

The surgical guide in place with adaptation control windows.

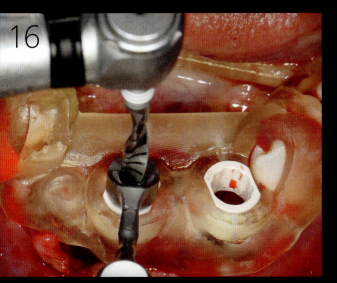

Guided drilling.

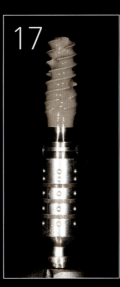

Straumann TLX RT implant, 4.5 x 12 mm.

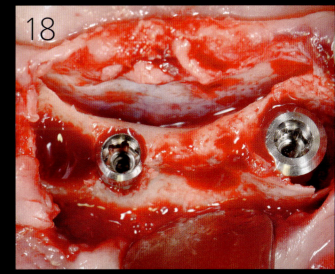

Occlusal view after guided placement of implants 33 and 41 in a vertical subosseous position.

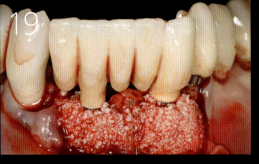

The **immediate** temporary partial denture in place. Tooth 43 had been cut and the screw-retained tooth replaced. Compensatory GBR of the extraction gaps and reinforcement of the ridge volume with DBBM (Bio-Oss with fine particles) incubated in PRGF fraction F2 of plasma.

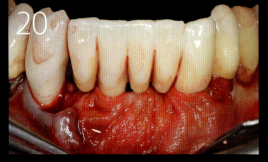

Covering with a resorbable collagen membrane (Bio-Gide).

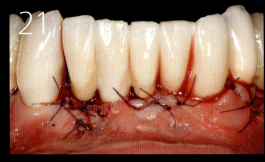

Suturing of the flap around the **immediate** prosthesis.

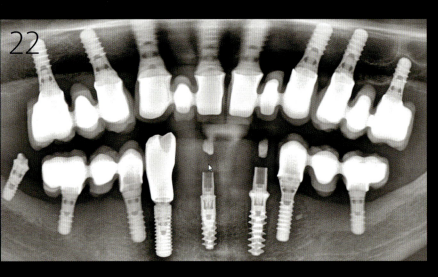

Postoperative panoramic radiograph confirming the fit of the **immediate** partial denture.

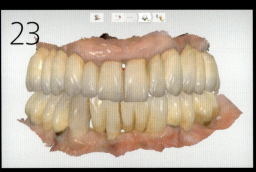

3-month pre-preparation impressions of the provisional partial denture, antagonist arch and occlusion.

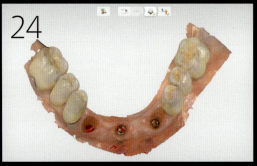

Gingival profile impressions of implants in 33 and 41 and RC in 43.

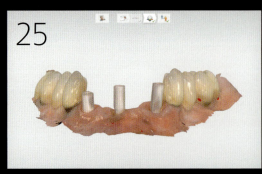

Implant position impressions with TLX scan bodies in 41 and 33 and BL in 43.

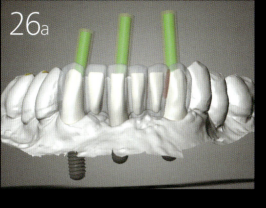
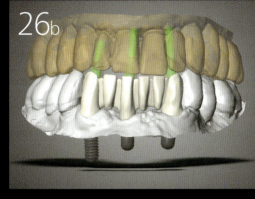

Importation of the overlay files into the Dental Wings ecosystem. (Dental Art Technology Laboratory, Richard Demange) and design of the zirconia framework by homothetic reduction.

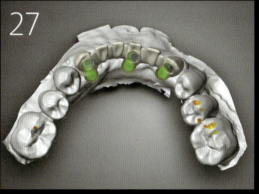

Occlusal view of the framework and screw holes.

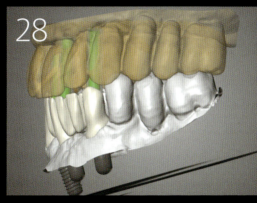

Side view.

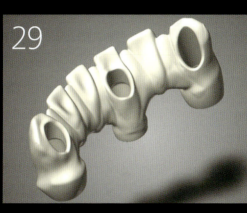

STL file of the zirconia framework ready to be sent to Createch Medical for zirconia machining on a Metoxit disc.

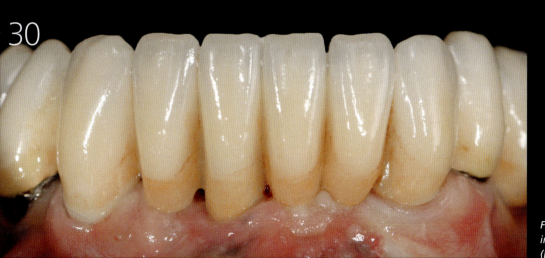

Final outcome with the partial denture in place in 43, 41, and 33. Noritake CZR ceramic (Dental Art Technology, Richard Demange).

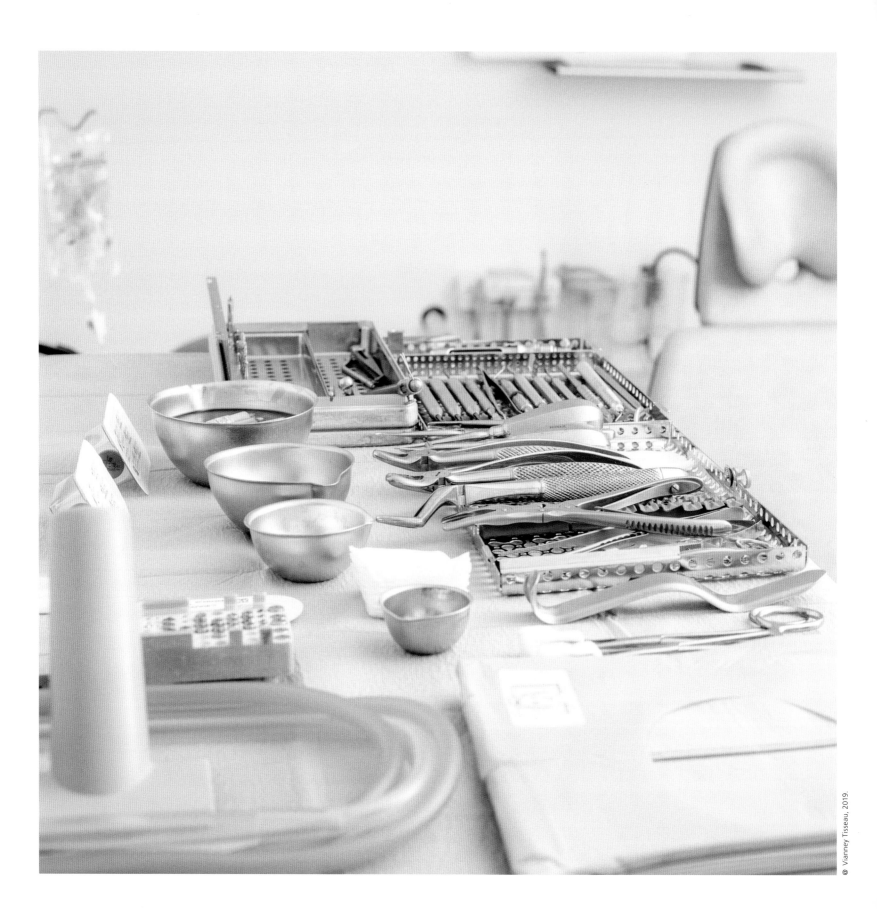

Plural-unit clinical case 25

27-year-old woman.

Clinical data

- Loss of tooth 11 and indication for extraction of 12.
- Case treated in November 2018.
- Vestibular wall present in 12 and 11.
- Altered mucogingival architecture in 11.

Presurgical treatments

- Trios 3 used to take the optical impression and Planmeca ProMax used to perform the 3D examination.
- Planning using Implant Studio.
- Placement of Straumann BL RC implants from 12 to 11.
- 3D printing of the guide designed in Implant Studio (Dentitek Laboratory).
- First-generation Straumann sockets.
- Temporary partial denture for two teeth, screwed in 11 with extension in 12, A3 shade, and milled in PMMA (Dentitek Laboratory).
- Variobase BL RC used for crowns in 11, bonded with Multilink Hybrid Abutment HO.

Assessment of the intervention

- Case treated in **four appointments at the office** (impression and 3D examination, surgery, 3-month check-up, provisionalization in 21 and impression, prosthesis placement).
- Prosthesis made in the office (JC Allègre Laboratory).

Additional treatments

- Tooth 11 was terminally eroded as a result of a trauma during childhood. The presence of a caries lesion in the mandible was treated using composite in 12 with an uncertain durability and which would limit the capacity to recover a non-inflammatory papillary volume in this zone and make a crown with a tight peripheral seal without encroaching on the biological distance. Coronal elongation was not an option in this case. The devitalized tooth 21 also had to be crowned in the final phase.

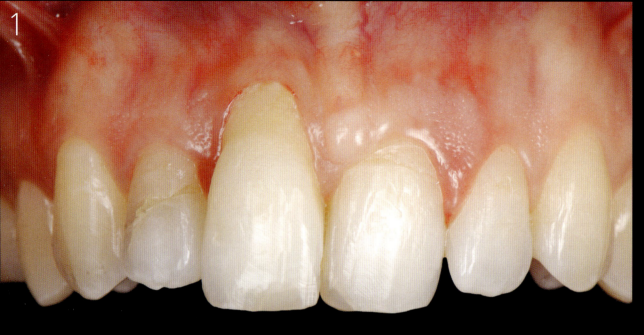

Vestibular view of the initial clinical situation. Note the level of the gingival collar in 11 and the extent of the composite in 12.

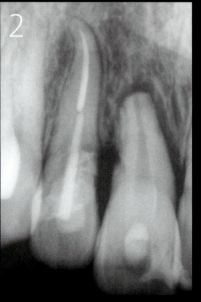

Retroalveolar radiograph showing the need to extract teeth 12 and 11.

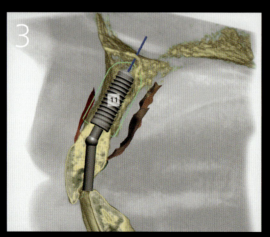

Sagittal section of the plan showing the importance of this step, which made it possible to find the optimal ratio between the bone volume and prosthetic volume, and to plan the GBR or gingival grafts that may have been necessary. It also ensured that the tooth was screwable without weakening the esthetic components of the prosthesis.

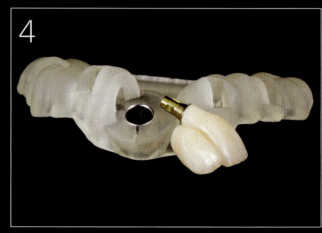

*Surgical guide with rotational registration and an **immediate** temporary partial denture connected to the Variobase RC for crowns.*

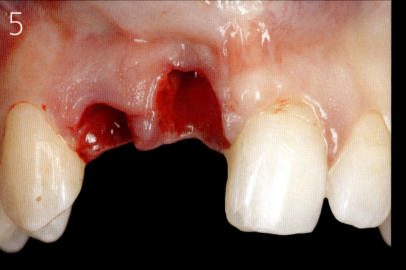

Extraction of the two teeth.

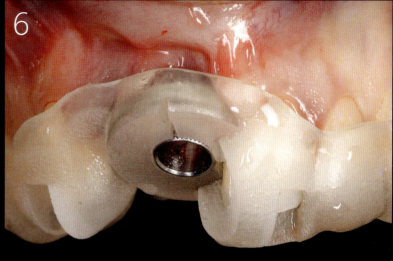

Surgical guide in place with inspection windows for adaptation control.

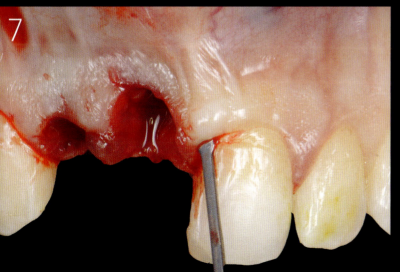

Elevation of a full- and then half-thickness flap by tunneling with a Viper blade (Hu-Friedy, Chicago, IL, USA).

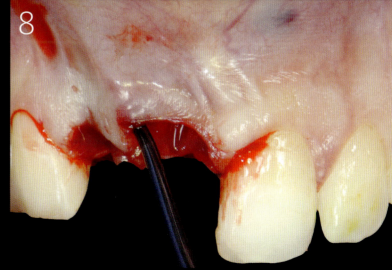

The split-thickness beyond the mucogingival junction that allowed good flap laxity for systematic coronal repositioning in immediate implantation.

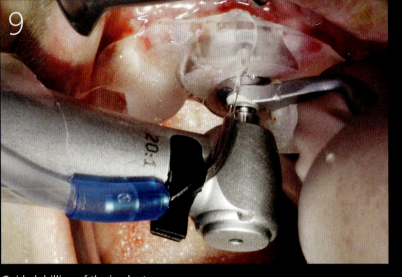

Guided drilling of the implant.

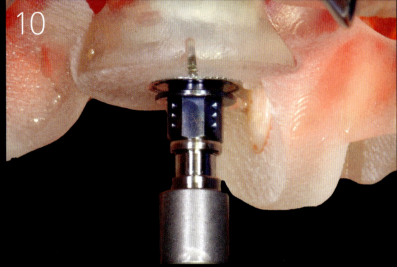

Guided implant placement still with the one-sixth turn offset of the 3Shape ecosystem.

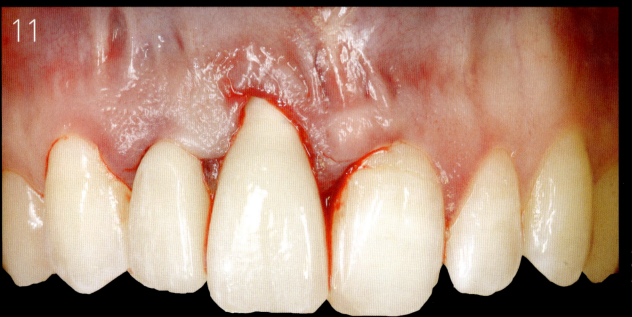

*Fitting of the **immediate** partial denture. Note the precise relationship of the edges.*

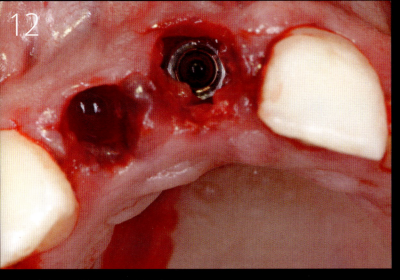

Occlusal view of the implant in place.

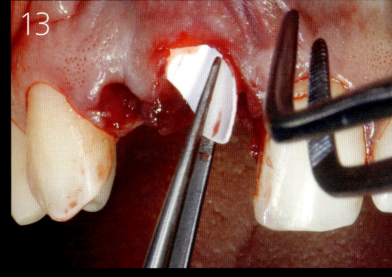

Placement of a collagen membrane under the flap and against the vestibular bone wall to form the future biomaterial (Bio-Gide Perio).

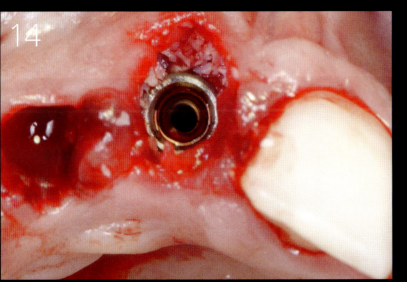

Filling of the extraction gap with DBBM (Bio-Oss with fine particles).

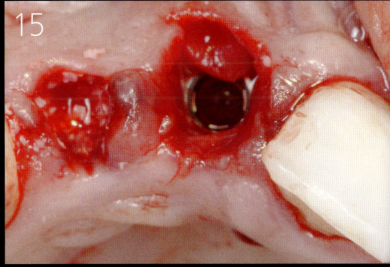

Covering with a collagen membrane.

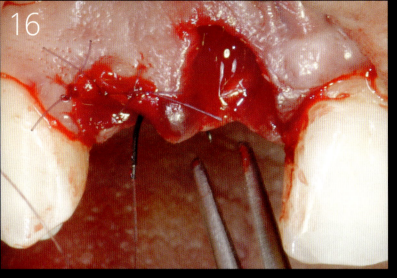

Ridge preservation in 12 with DBBM and closure with a resorbable collagen punch (Mucograft Seal, Geistlich) sutured to the edges of the socket.

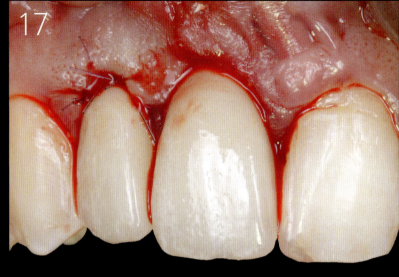

Placement of the **immediate** partial denture.

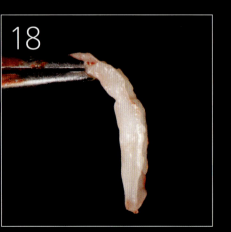

Harvesting of a palatino-conjunctive graft.

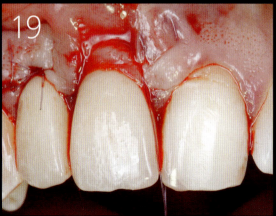

Placement of the connective tissue graft on the vestibular side of 11, stabilized with two simple stitches on the palatal side.

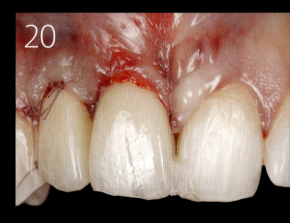

Flap drawn coronally around the **immediate** partial denture, veneered with a hanging suture around 11 and on the contact point between 11 and 21, and bonded with a flowable composite suture.

Chapter 5 - Clinical applications for partially edentulous patients

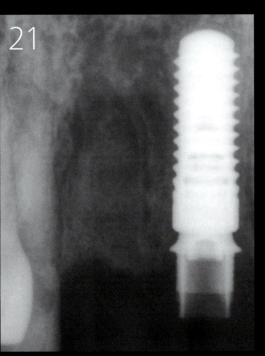

Postoperative retroalveolar radiograph. Note the good density at the level of ridge preservation.

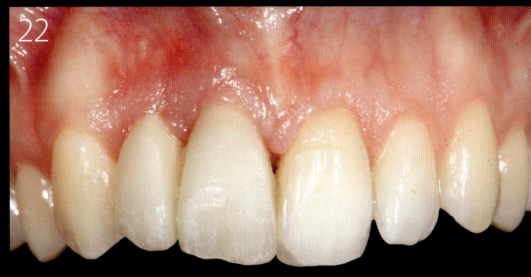

Clinical view of the vestibular region at 3 months. Note the vertical gain of the neck of 11 and the creation of a pseudopapilla between 12 and 11.

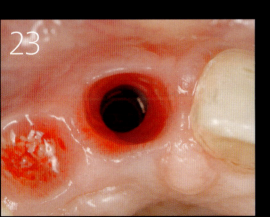

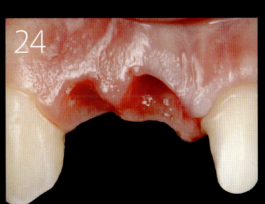

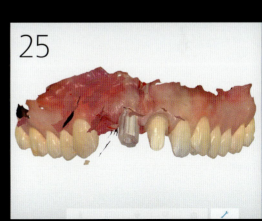

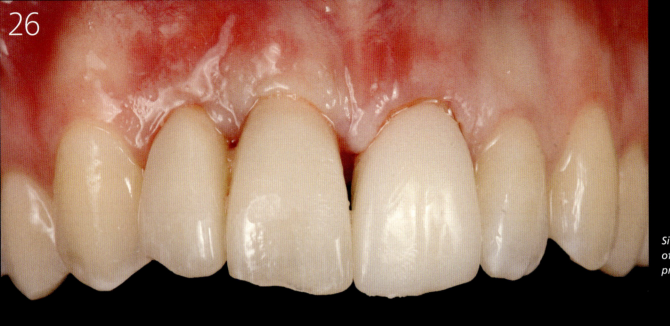

Situation at the end of the session with provisionalization of 21.

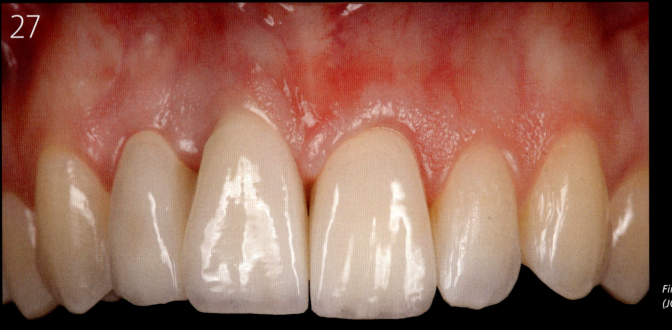

Final prosthetic result (JC Allègre).

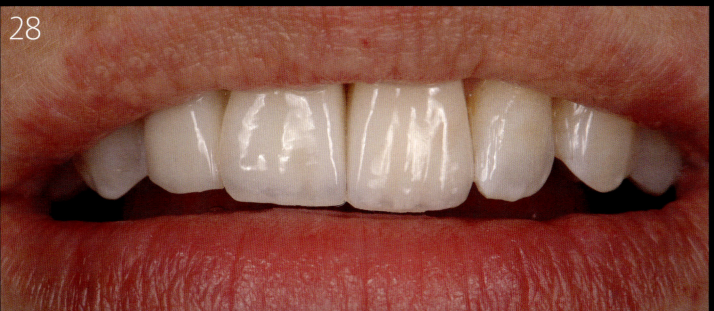

Esthetic integration of the ensemble.

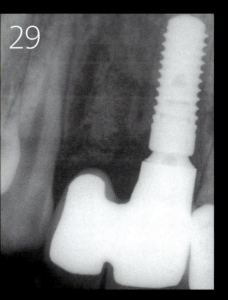

Retroalveolar radiograph.

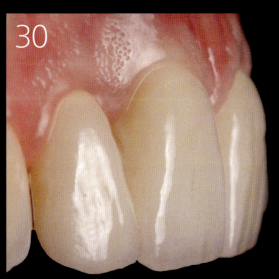

Lateral view showing good periodontal integration, volume management, and gingival health. Note the quality of the pontic emergence profile.

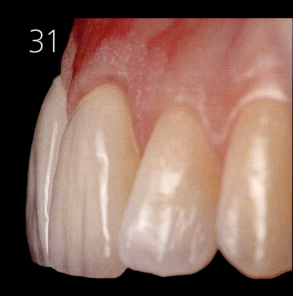

View of the opposite side.

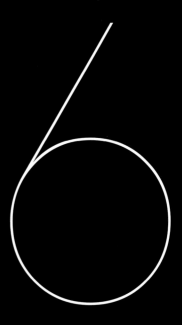

Full-arch clinical applications

| Toothed unimaxillary
Full-arch clinical cases 26 to 37 .... 273 |
| Edentulous unimaxillary
Full-arch clinical cases 38 and 39 .... 393 |
| Maxillomandibular
Full-arch clinical cases 40 and 41 .... 417 |

The impossible always retreats when you walk towards it.

Antoine de Saint-Exupéry

Let's take a look at the most controversial clinical application since we started communicating about full digital flow. The road to the **immediate full** partial denture is a succession of steps and exchanges. As with any clinical procedure, the Quokka "full arch" involves a learning curve of successes, failures, analysis and understanding.

In January 2016, when we began immediate implantation and loading, single cases and small plural cases (two implants, three teeth) were very quickly validated with a provisional prosthesis connected to the titanium bases before surgery, in a purely digital environment, without going through a physical model. At the time, we were convinced that the same approach was impossible for a full-arch rehabilitation. Digital flow was a powerful prosthetic planning tool, a relevant implant planning tool and a comfortable aid for immediate loading during surgery. It enabled us to bond provisional abutments to the hollowed-out partial denture. Thanks to the precision of drilling and guided implant placement, adjustments were limited during surgery, enabling us to suture the flaps to the prosthesis in place.

The idea of a full provisional partial denture connection was always a tempting technical projection in a protocol that had already standardized a qualitative implant-prosthetic approach. Reflection and exchange convinced us to try this connection before surgery, in order to remain in a 100% digital environment. We began with a simple all-on-four maxillary case in November 2019. The result was a partial failure. Partial, because the patient still had a partial denture placed at the end of the surgery. At this stage, we could have given up. We analyzed and identified possible bias factors in the digital and clinical chains of the protocol.

Since 2020, we've been using a standardized total digital flow approach for complete rehabilitations. The large number of cases we have dealt with and the protocol training we have received at CampusHB have enabled us to refine and secure this approach, which is now part of our daily clinical routine. Our case studies and the practical work carried out by participants during the teaching sessions enable us to confirm that the level of technical precision of the tools available with the Straumann guided surgery kit, Trios, Implant Studio, CodiagnostiX on TL, BL, TLX and BLX is sufficient and necessary to enable the partial denture to be connected to the titanium bases prior to surgery. Any failure – and there are some, as in any treatment procedure – would be due to a bias in use. The cases to follow illustrate this evolution. However, in our daily practice, our patients are able to receive an **immediate** partial denture during surgery, with the management of possible failures but always allowing suturing around the partial denture in place during surgery under local anesthesia.

The debate should no longer be "to believe or not to believe", but "to understand, train and practice". The outlook for the future is clear: the final prosthesis must be fitted during surgery. We're working on it. We have gained in humility and will no longer allow ourselves to think that this procedure is impossible.

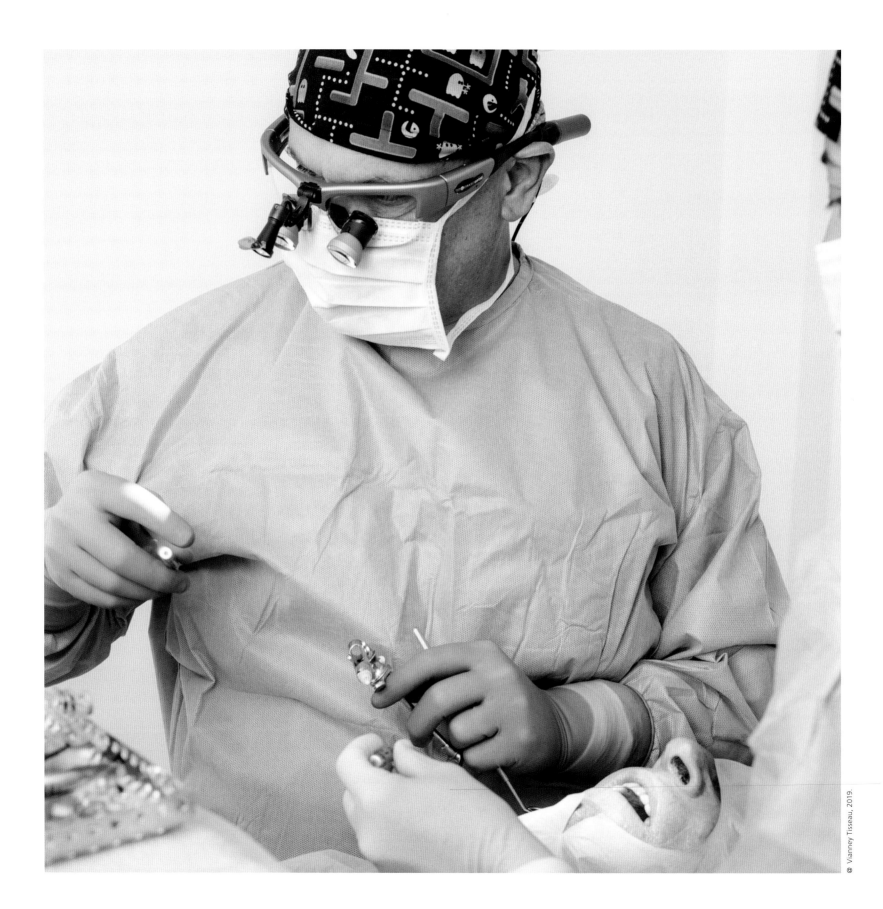

© Vianney Tisseau, 2019.

Full-arch clinical case 26

51-year-old woman.

Clinical data

- Desire to remove the partial removable appliance from the maxilla as a priority, and from the mandible, if possible. The patient had been edentulous for 30 years (since the age of 20).
- Case treated in March 2016 (bone graft).
- Bone reconstruction necessary in pre-implantation.
- Good mucogingival architecture.

Presurgical treatments

- Optical impression taken using a Trios 3 (3Shape, Copenhagen, Denmark) and 3D examination performed using a Planmeca ProMax (Helsinki, Finland).
- Planning using Implant Studio (3Shape) 6 months after bone grafting.
- Straumann TL SP RN 8-mm in 15, RN 12-mm in 13 and 23, RN 10-mm in 25, and NC 12-mm in 12 and 22.
- 3D printing of the guide designed in Implant Studio (Dentitek Laboratory).
- First-generation Straumann socket.
- Temporary partial denture milled in PMMA (Ivotion Dent Multi, Ivoclar) (Dentitek Laboratory).
- A model was printed to prepare the temporary screw-retained abutments for RN and NC. These abutments were set in occlusal height and covered with an opaquer. The partial denture was recessed around the abutments with an additional 1 mm of peripheral space (Dentitek Laboratory).
- The partial denture was bonded to the abutments during surgery with Structur resin (Voco, Cuxhaven, Germany) after application of a primer (Telio Activator, Ivoclar, Schaan, Liechtenstein).

Assessment of the intervention

- Case treated in the office in **nine appointments** (DSD and digital impression, esthetic mock-up, esthetic and functional validation partial denture, pre-implant bone grafting, radiopaque partial denture and implant planning, immediate loading surgery, implant impression, impression validation, CAD/CAM model, placement of final ceramic partial denture).
- Prosthesis made in the office (JC Allègre Laboratory).
- This was the approach with a partial denture conversion as we practiced it between early 2016 and late 2019. This is a pre-implant grafting case with removal of the removable partial denture and placement of a fixed provisional before pre-implant surgery, following the esthetic analysis. This allowed the patient to be comfortable and achieve an esthetically pleasing result in accordance with the expected final goal. The partial denture was used as a therapeutic guide throughout treatment and during pre-implant bone grafting.

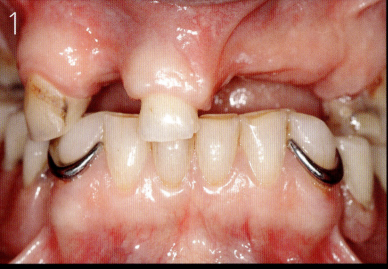

Initial frontal situation without the maxillary removable partial denture (RPD). Note the mandibular removable partial denture and the abrasion of the occlusal surfaces of the maxillary anterior teeth related to anterior overload, but without anterior rotation of the mandible. The articular and muscular functionality was good. There was no joint noise, the Farrar diagram was balanced, and there was no muscle pain on palpation. The midlines were aligned.

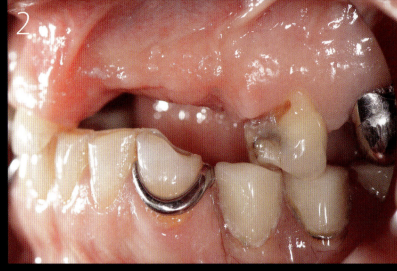

Left-side view.

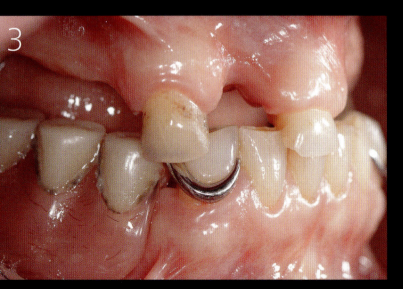

Right-side view.

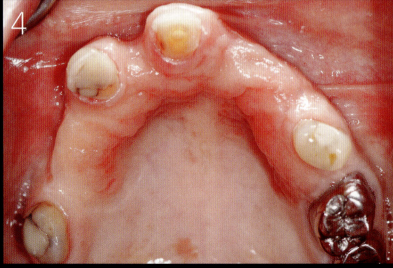

Occlusal view clearly showing the bone resorption. This can be classified as a complex case with pre-implant bone grafting.

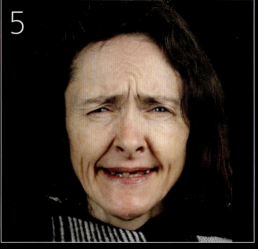

Frontal facial photograph.

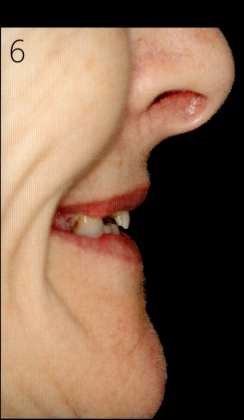

Profile photograph. Note the opening of

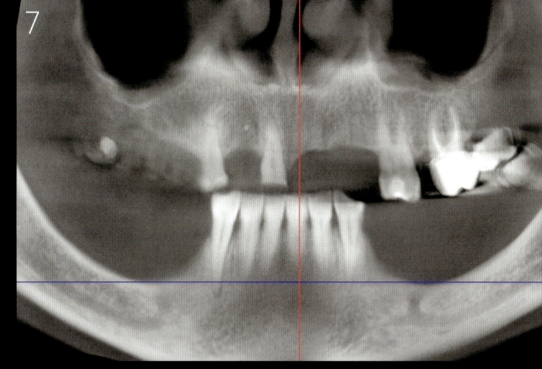

Panoramic view of the CBCT examination. The vertical bone volume was correct in the maxilla; thus, we essentially had a horizontal volume problem. Note the posterior vertical loss in the mandible. Since vertical grafts are the riskiest (from the perspective of success rates), one solution would be to perform an all-on-four procedure to eliminate the removable partial denture. The patient was understandably traumatized due to the extractions she had undergone at a young age and wanted to keep her anterior teeth. We therefore performed a new removable partial denture while waiting for possible posterior mandibular bone grafts.

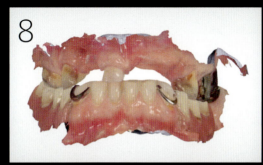

Optical impression taken with a Trios 3 for esthetic analysis.

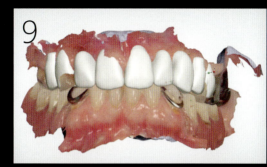

In parallel to the Smile Design performed in the Trios workflow and sent to the Dentitek Laboratory to prepare a model for the fitting of a mask in the mouth, we performed a quick setup in Implant Studio to evaluate the volume of bone graft

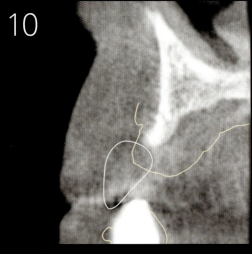

Prosthetic plan, gingival volume, and bone volume correlated in Implant Studio.

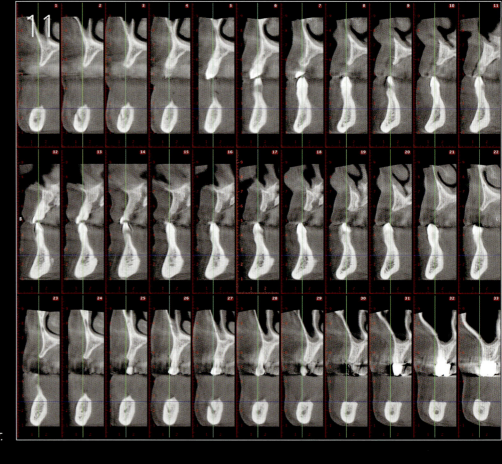

Digital view of the sagittal sections of the CBCT.

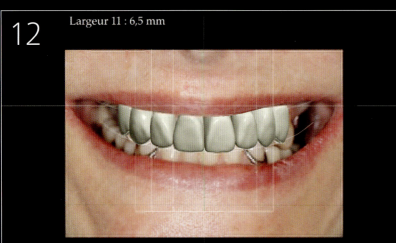

RealView view of the esthetic assembly in the Trios 3.

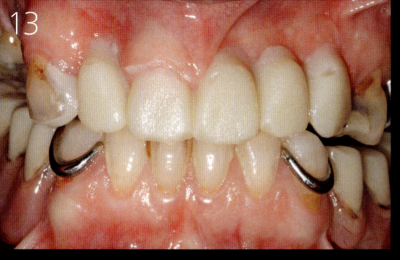

13 Resin mask made in the mouth from the silicone key during the second esthetic analysis session.

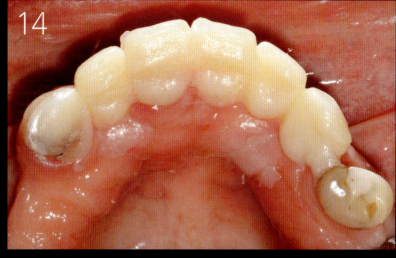

14 Occlusal view.

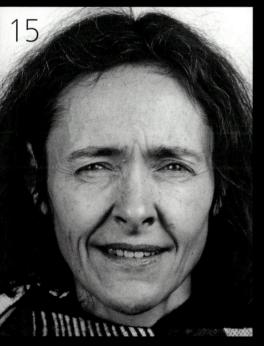

15 Photograph showing the mask in the mouth. Note the rejuvenation of the smile and the good integration of the proposed volume. The good relationship between the vestibular incisal edge and the lower lip was confirmed with the phoneme /f/ (dry line and wet line).

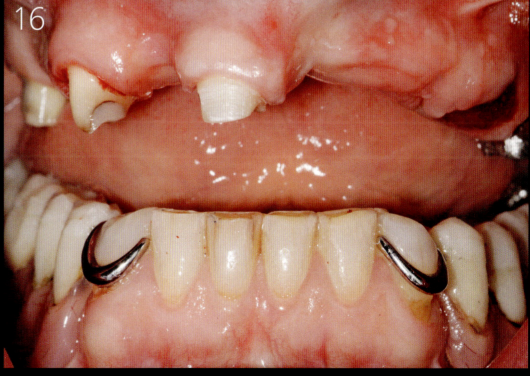

16 Clinical view after tooth preparation for placement of the esthetic and functional validation temporary partial denture for the esthetic analysis. The rotated tooth 25 was extracted to simplify the placement of the temporary partial denture.

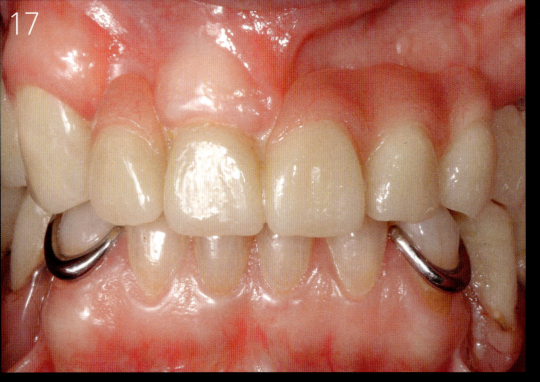

17 Esthetic validation temporary partial denture in place. Note the compensatory pink false gingiva and horizontal bone loss.

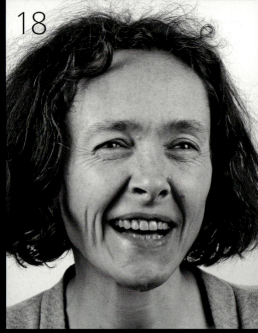

18 Integration of the temporary partial denture into the smile. Note the change in the facial appearance, with which the patient was extremely satisfied, and she very quickly regained fixed teeth and confidence in the rest of the treatment.

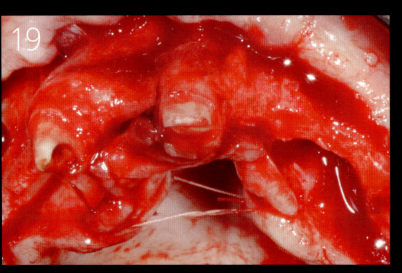

19 With the prosthetic project validated, we proceeded to the reconstruction phase. Full-thickness flaps were elevated to perform the lateral apposition bone graft.

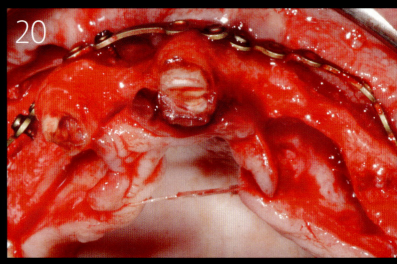

20 Placement of the osteosynthesis plates, which determined the volume of the formwork in accordance with the prosthetic volume.

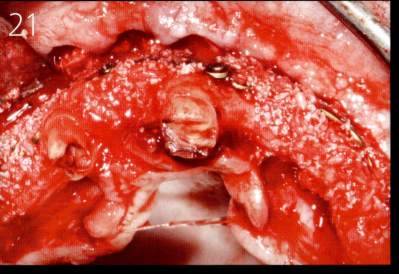

21 Filling of the spaces thus determined with a composite graft. This graft was composed of 50% autogenous cortical bone chips taken from the external oblique line and DBBM (Bio-Oss with fine particles, Gestlich, Wolhusen, Switzerland).

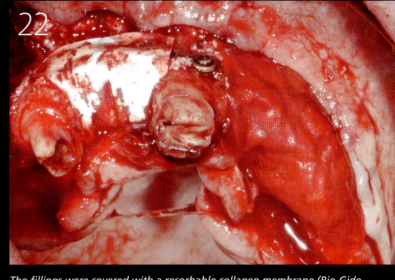

22 The fillings were covered with a resorbable collagen membrane (Bio-Gide, Geistlich).

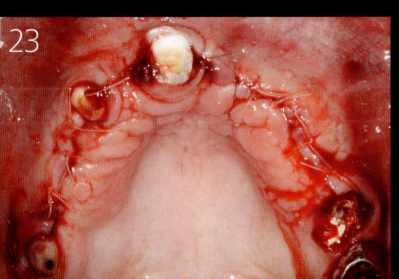

23 After the half-thickness incision of the vestibular flap, coronal traction and a single suture without tension were performed.

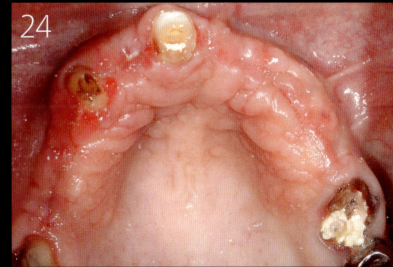

24 Removal of the provisional partial denture at 6 months to check the bone graft planning.

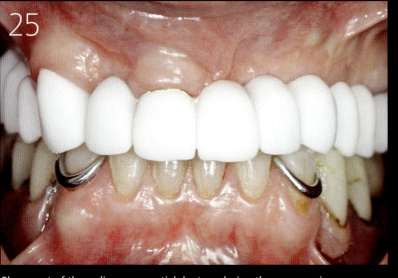

25 Placement of the radiopaque partial denture during the same session, a copy of the esthetic and functional validation partial denture. An intraoral impression was taken using a Trios 3, then a CBCT examination was performed.

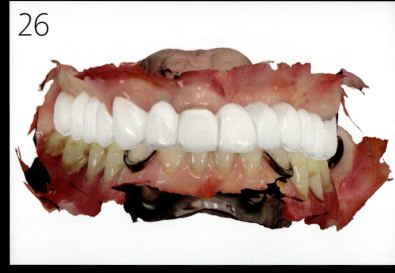

26 Digital impression of both arches in occlusion in the 3Shape ecosystem.

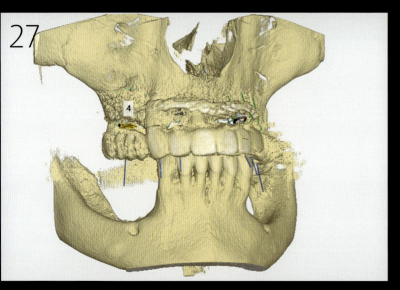

27 DICOM file of the CBCT scan imported into Implant Studio.

28 Merging of the intraoral STL file and the bone DICOM file.

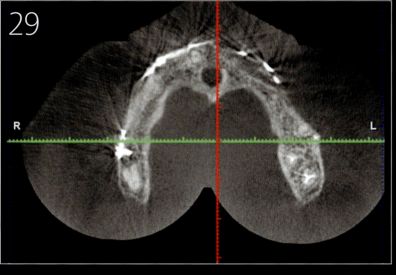

29 Axial view. Note the microplates that delineate the vestibular bone wall.

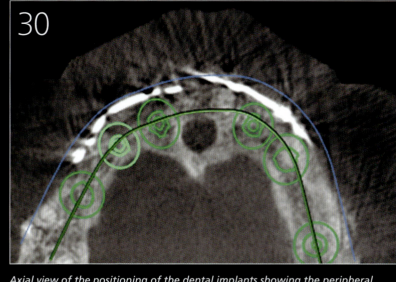

30 Axial view of the positioning of the dental implants showing the peripheral bone volume in accordance with biologic laws.

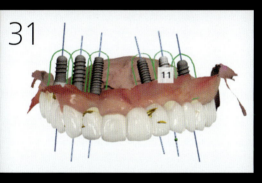

31 3D planning view without the bone filter. This made it possible to appreciate the relationship between the implant axes and the prosthesis and gingiva.

32 Comparison of the implant axes and the prosthetic volume.

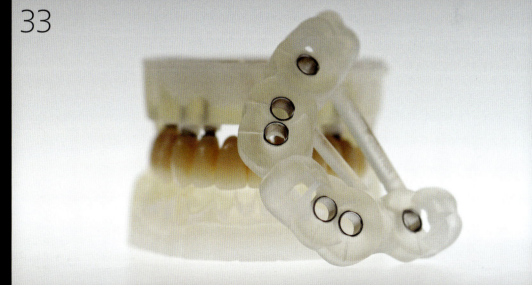

33 First-generation Quokka full-arch protocol. Printing of a resin model was necessary to prepare the provisional abutments and hollow out the milled immediate loading partial denture for bonding in the mouth. The surgical guide was printed with the bonded sockets.

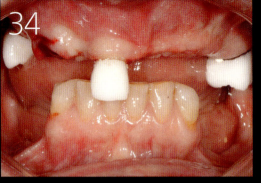

Implant surgery phase with teeth as supports for the surgical guide.

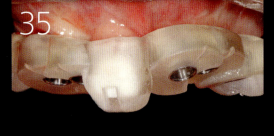

Surgical guide in the mouth with inspection windows.

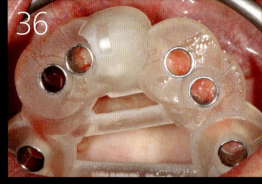

Occlusal view of the surgical guide in place.

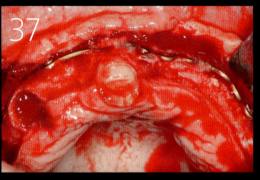

Elevation of full-thickness flaps. Note the presence of the microplates in the vestibular region, which were removed before implant drilling, and the horizontal bone gain and extraction of the implant in site 13.

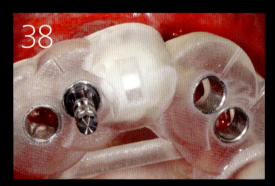

Guided placement of a first-generation Straumann RN implant.

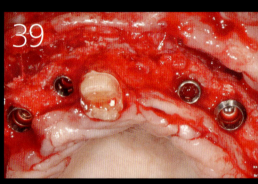

Axial view of the implants placed after removal of the guide and before teeth extraction.

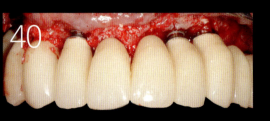

Immediate loading temporary partial denture connected to the temporary abutments and screwed in during surgery before suturing.

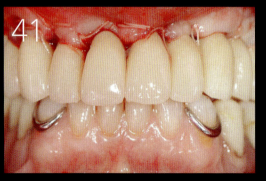

Suture around and guided by the partial denture. Note the precision of the volumes and occlusion from the digital plan.

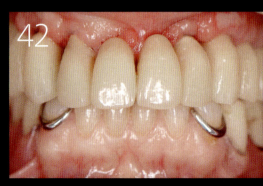

3-month view of the clinical situation. Note the more heterogeneous resin in the bonding areas.

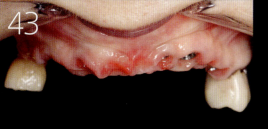
Vestibular view of the clinical situation after removal of the temporary partial denture.

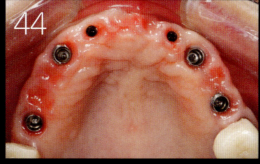
Occlusal view of the clinical situation after removal of the temporary partial denture.

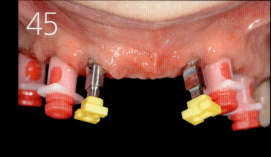
Implant impressions with closed tray transfers.

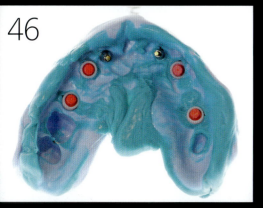
View of the silicone double-mix impression (Aquasil, Dentsply Sirona, Charlotte, NC, USA).

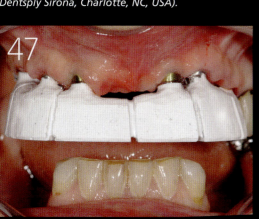
Plaster key to validate the impression.

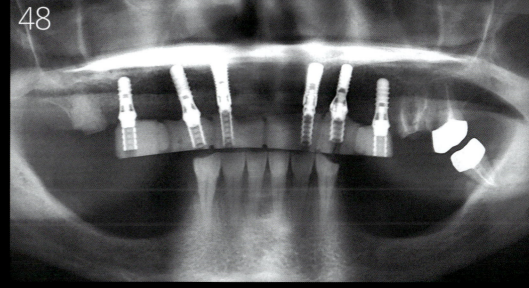
Panoramic radiograph to check the adaptation of the plaster index. A transfer of the occlusion chairside with the articulator and the silicone index of the partial denture was performed in the same session.

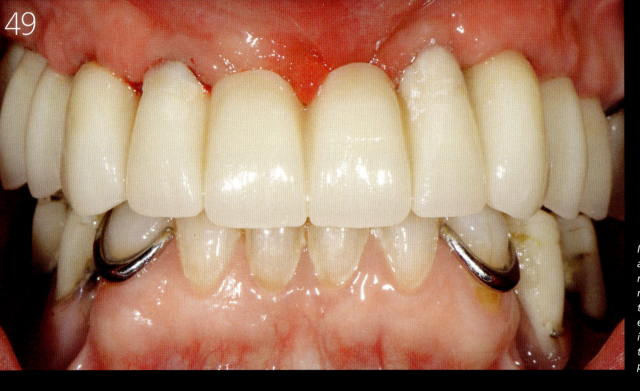

49 In a fourth prosthetic appointment, a provisional model, known as a CAD/CAM model, was tried in the mouth to confirm the occlusion and esthetic volumes, particularly in the emergence profiles. Note the reworking of the emergence profiles in 12 and 22.

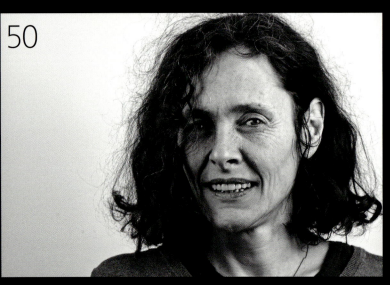

50 Photograph of the face with the model in place to validate the expected result with the patient. Note the quality of the upper lip support, the result of the prosthetic assembly, and the bone graft.

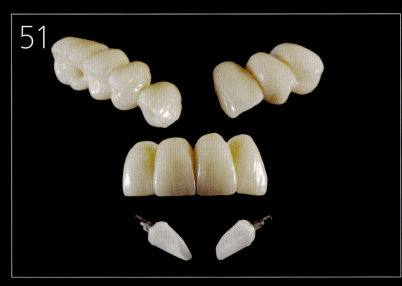

51 Final prosthesis before placement. The rehabilitation was in three parts: two posterior screw-retained sectors and an anterior sector of four teeth, cemented on two zirconia false stumps.

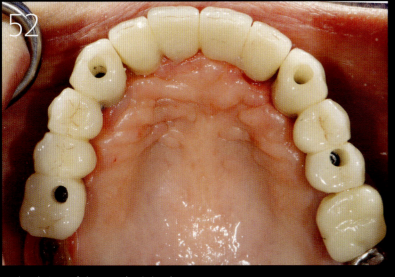
Occlusal view of the prosthesis in place.

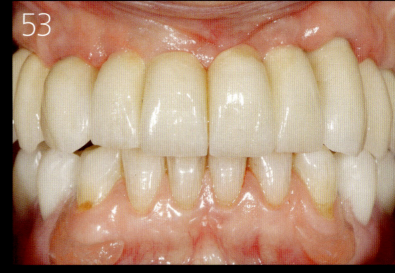
Buccal view of the final result.

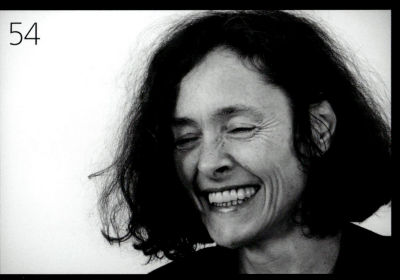
Esthetic integration of the prosthesis during smiling.

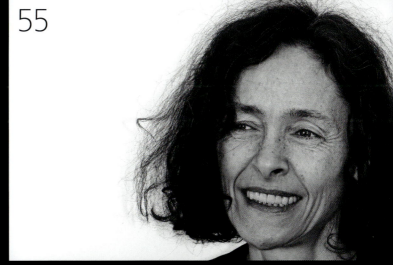
Frontal view. Two esthetic analysis appointments, one bone grafting appointment, one planning appointment, one implant surgery appointment, and four prosthetic appointments were required to complete this case over 12 months.

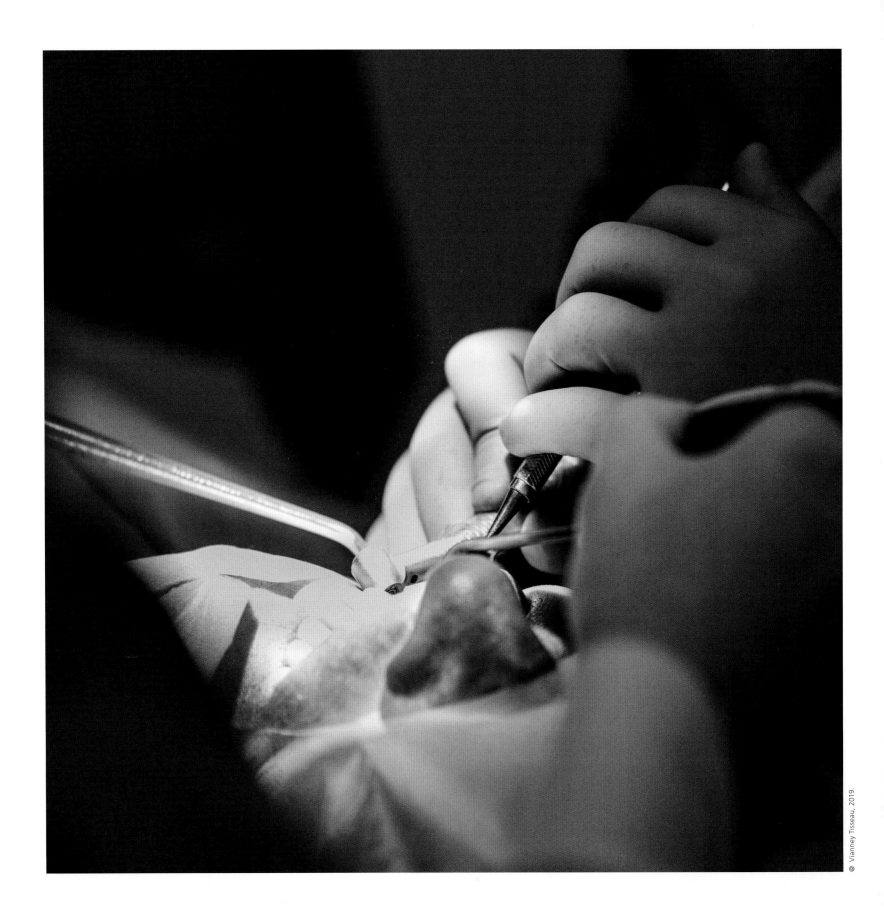

© Vianney Tisseau, 2019.

Full-arch clinical case 27

59-year-old man.

Clinical data

- The patient presented for a fixed implant supported maxillary rehabilitation in place of the hopeless full teeth supported restorations.
- Case treated in October 2020.
- Heterogeneous vertical bone loss.
- Heterogeneous mucogingival architecture in a context of a very low smile line.

Presurgical treatments

- Trios 4 used to take an optical impression and 3Shape X1 used to perform a 3D examination.
- Planning using Implant Studio.
- Placement of Straumann TL RN 8-mm implants in 16, 24, and 25, RN 10-mm in 14 and RN 12-mm in 12 and 22.
- 3D printing of the guide designed in Implant Studio (Dentitek Laboratory).
- First-generation Straumann TL sockets.
- Temporary partial denture milled in PMMA (Ivotion Dent Multi, Ivoclar) (Dentitek Laboratory) on a shade A3 base.

Assessment of the intervention

- Case treated in the office in **seven appointments** (esthetic analysis, validation fixed/removable partial denture, radiopaque fixed/removable partial denture, implant surgery, impression preparation, validation of the impression and CAD/CAM model, placement of the final prosthesis).
- Prosthesis made in the office.

Additional treatments

- Both arches were condemned to complete extraction. The patient wished to delay treatment of the mandible for financial reasons. His compliance with hygiene was excellent since we took over his care. He knew that the same treatment would have to be performed on the mandible in 2 years' time, with the possibility of earlier **immediate loading** if the situation deteriorated. A nocturnal muscle deprogramming splint was placed at the end of treatment and quarterly periodontal maintenance was performed. The Class II division 2 intermaxillary relationship complicated the treatment. A prosthesis with a polyetheretherketone (PEEK) framework and resin teeth was chosen due to its more tolerant mechanical behavior in this mechanical context.

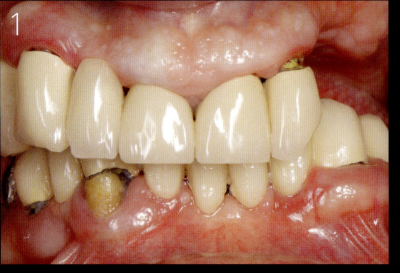

Initial clinical view. The mandibular full bridge also ideally needed to be removed. The patient wished to keep it for financial reasons and was aware of its fragility and the need to rehabilitate it quickly.

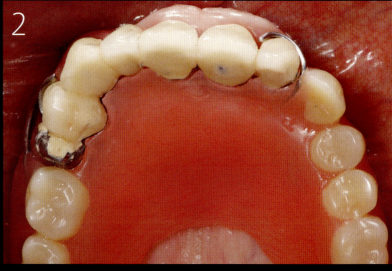

Occlusal view with the removable appliance. The patient could no longer tolerate the presence of the RPD and, despite the deleterious condition of the mandibular denture, wanted to start with the maxilla.

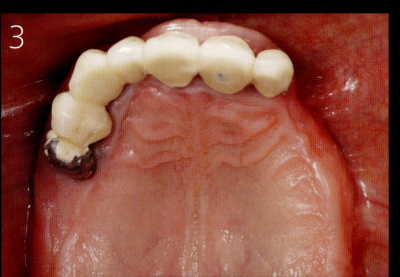

Occlusal view without the RPD. Note the bone resorption asymmetries.

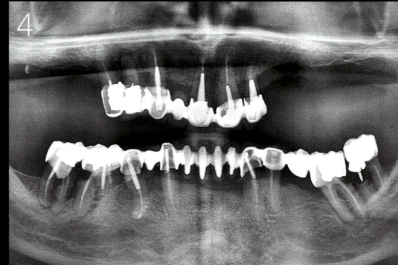

Panoramic radiograph of the initial situation. The multiple carious recessions under the mandibular denture limited our ability to place a provisional partial denture in the mandible while waiting for the maxillary part to be made. Indeed, the dental abutments were too fragile to allow a reliable provisional partial denture over 1 or 2 years.

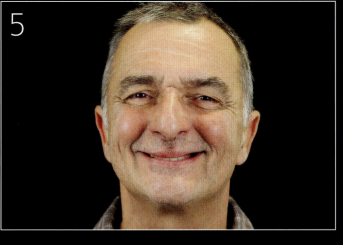

Facial photograph for esthetic analysis with the smile.

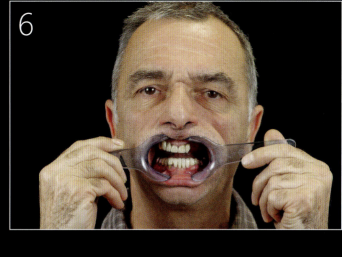

Facial photograph with a retractor to be superimposed on the photograph of the smile.

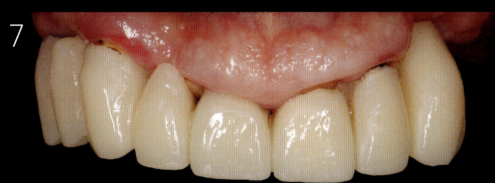

Provisional partial denture for esthetic and functional validation based on the esthetic and occlusal analyses. The mandibular occlusal plane, although not ideal, allowed us to create a balanced maxllary denture.

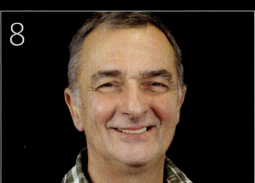

Facial image showing the integration of the esthetic project.

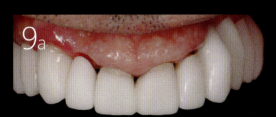

Radiopaque partial denture in place a while after the esthetic and functional validation partial denture placement session to give the patient time to perceive the esthetic setup and functionality of the proposed partial denture. During this session, we took an intraoral digital impression of the radiopaque partial denture in place and performed

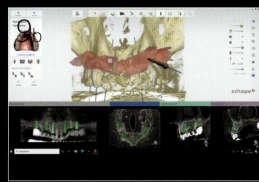

Planning carried out in Implant Studio after merging the STL and DICOM files.

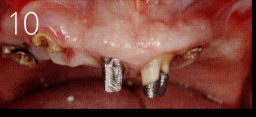

The temporary partial denture was removed at the beginning of surgery to accommodate the radiopaque teeth, which support the surgical guide. In this case, a radiopaque partial denture was necessary because the residual tooth surfaces were too limited in volume to allow proper surfacing during planning.

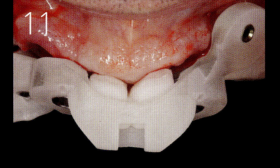

Fitting of the surgical guide. Note the key on the left side to compensate for the lack of tooth support.

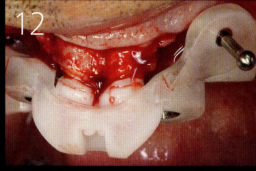

Surgical guide locked after vestibular flap removal.

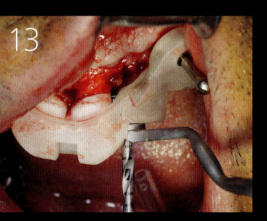

Guided drilling for the Straumann TL RN 12-mm implant in 22.

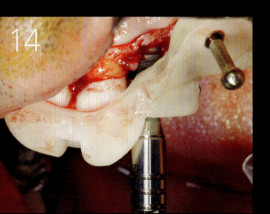

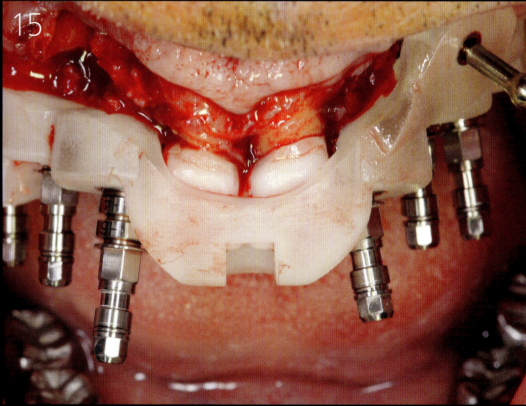

The six guided implants (first-generation, delivered with the guided gripper screwed onto the implant once in place) according to the drilling and vertical positioning protocol delivered by the planning software.

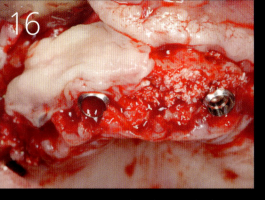

Compensatory GBR around implants and ridge preservation on non-implant extraction sockets with DBBM (Bio-Oss with fine particles, Geistlich) incubated in the F2 fraction of plasma rich in growth factors (PRGF) (Endoret, BTI).

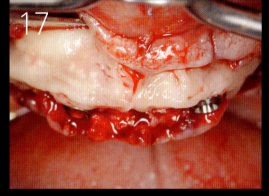

The GBR material was covered with the fibrin membrane from the F1 fraction of the plasma.

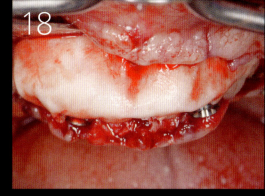

A resorbable collagen membrane (Bio-Gide, Geistlich) was used according to the biologic rules of GBR.

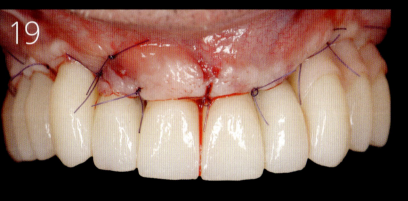

The **immediate** provisional partial denture in place with ASAF sutures guided by the prosthesis. The 8-mm RN 16 implant was not loaded due to a lack of primary stability. We drove it in with two additional turns to increase its anchorage and placed a cover screw. The occlusion was unloaded in the area of 15 and 16.

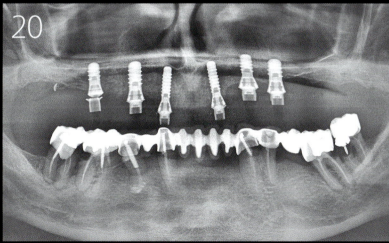

Postoperative panoramic radiograph.

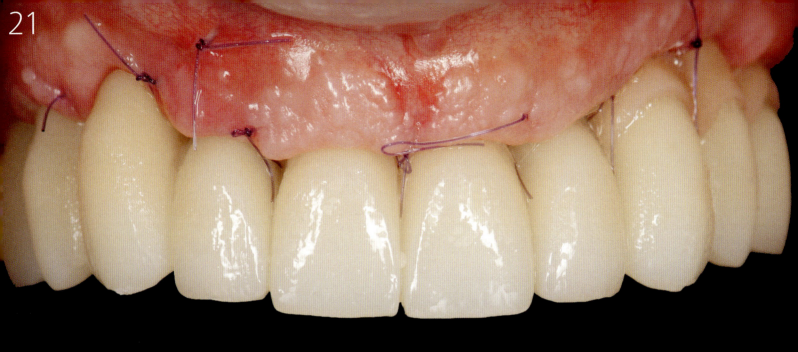

21 Clinical view at 8 days.

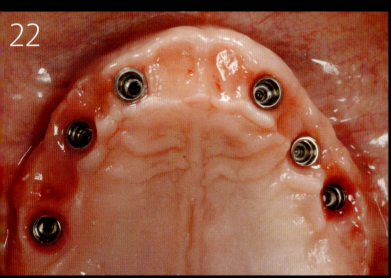

22 Occlusal view at 3 months when the partial denture was removed for impressions. Note the correction of the arch asymmetry, to be compared with Fig 27-3.

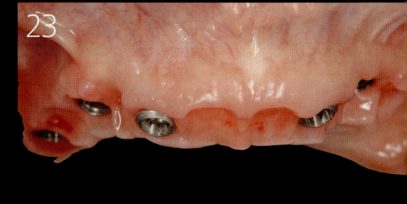

23 Vestibular view.

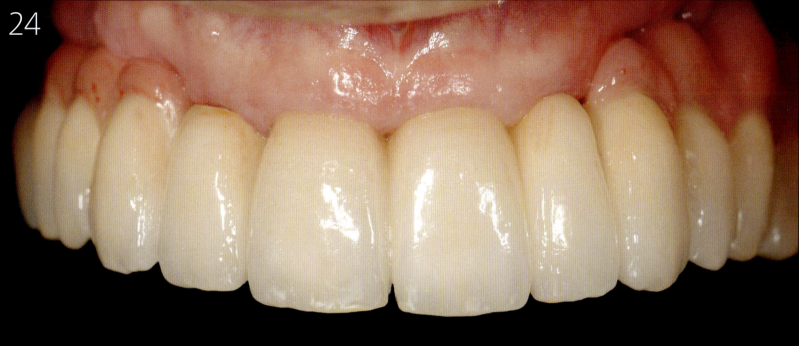

Final partial denture in place.

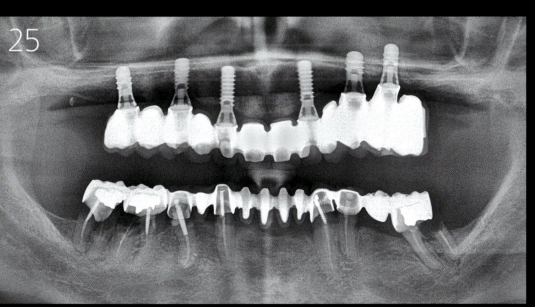

Panoramic radiograph of the final partial denture in place.

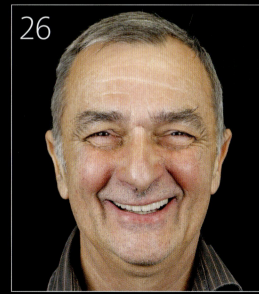

Facial image showing the esthetic integration of the rehabilitation.

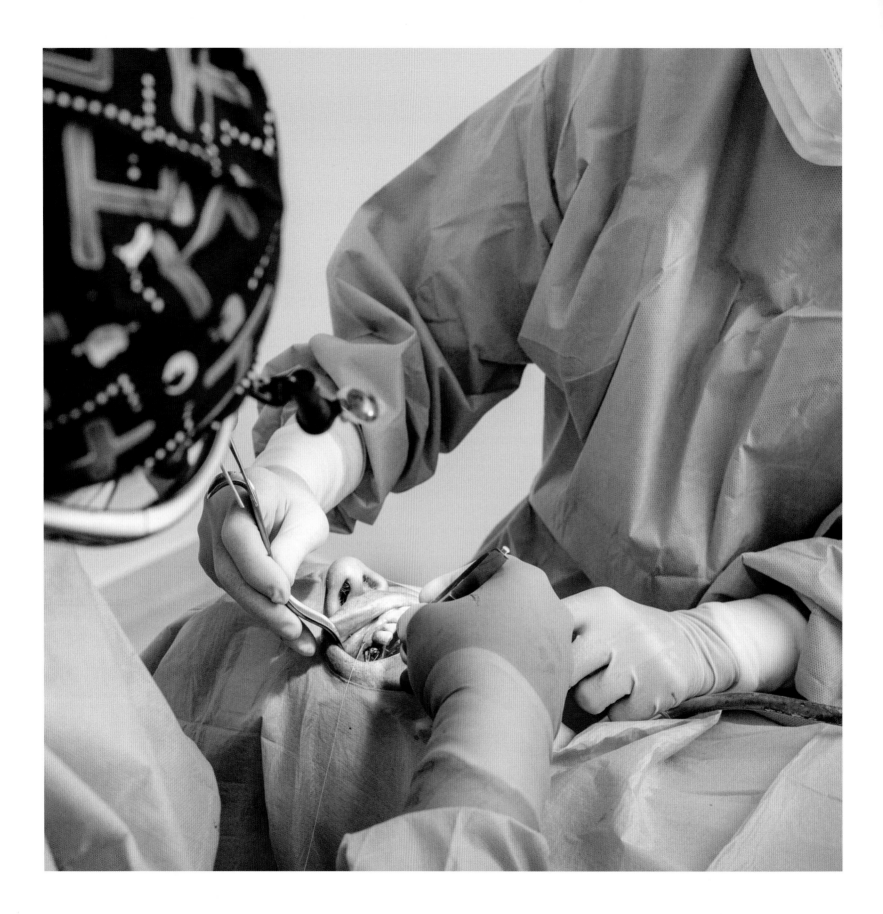

Full-arch clinical case 28

66-year-old man.

Clinical data

- The patient wanted to remove the removable partial appliance in the maxilla due to the increasing mobility of incisors. He did not want a temporary removable appliance.
- Case treated in November 2020.
- Heterogeneous vertical bone loss.
- Correct mucogingival architecture. Hygiene to be modified.

Presurgical treatments

- An optical impression was taken using a Trios 4 and the 3D examination was performed using a 3Shape X1.
- Planning using Implant Studio.
- Placement of Straumann TL SP RN 12-mm implants in 14, 12, and 22, and RN 10-mm implant in 24.
- 3D printing of the guide designed in Implant Studio (Dentitek Laboratory).
- Straumann T-socket.
- Temporary partial denture milled in PMMA (Ivotion Dent Multi) (Dentitek Laboratory) on a shade A3 base.

Assessment of the intervention

- Case treated in the office in **five appointments** (esthetic analysis, implant surgery, implant impression preparation, validation of the impression, placement of the final prosthesis).
- Prosthesis made in the office (JC Allègre Laboratory).
- The patient had no specific esthetic requests. He wished to get rid of his loose teeth and his mobile appliance if a simple and quick solution was possible. He did not want a solution that involved bone grafting and general anesthesia, as proposed by a colleague, despite his fears about dental care; his fears about general anesthesia and grafts was too great. The one-step approach with **immediate loading** appealed to him due to its speed and the comfort between steps, which met his functional and tranquility requirements. To reduce the cost we proposed four implants for ten teeth with a digital wax-up as a prosthetic project, without a validation partial denture, allowing for prosthesis-guided planning. The final prosthesis was planned in resin with a false gingiva, mounted on a PEEK framework.

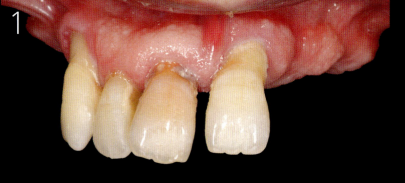

Frontal clinical view displaying very poor dental hygiene.

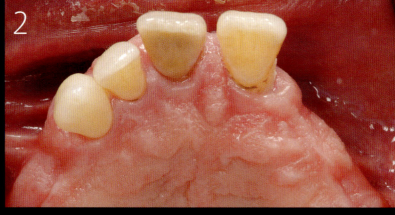

Occlusal view showing the migration of the central incisors.

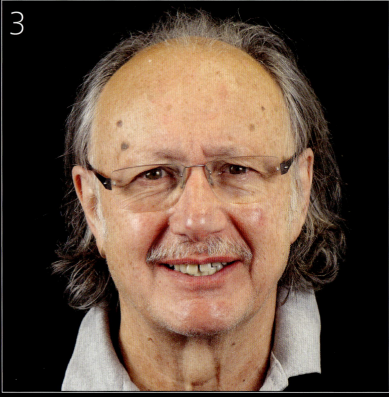

Frontal facial photograph.

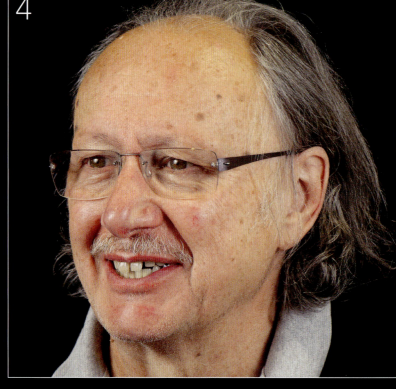

Facial photograph.

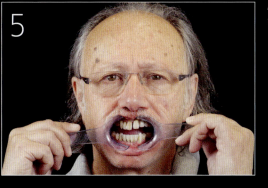

Photograph with retractor for the Smile Design Trios 4.

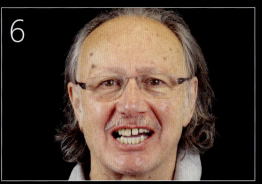

Photograph of the (moderate) smile for the Smile Design Trios 4.

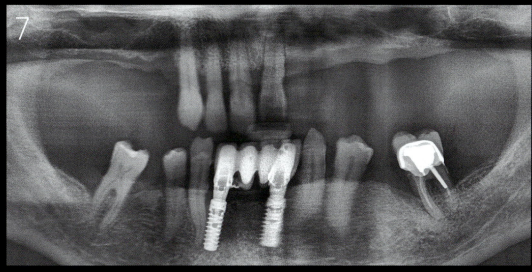

Panoramic radiograph. Note the serum tartar in 43 treated during periodontal maintenance.

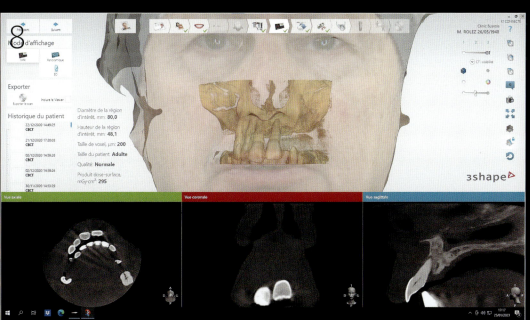

CBCT acquisition with the 3Shape X1 with the possibility of a facial scan.

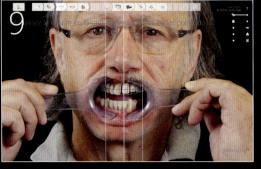

Esthetic analysis in the Trios 4 flow.

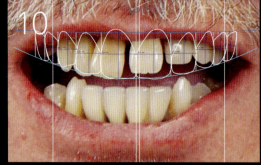

Enlarged view of the 2D esthetic project with size ratios. Note the shift in the midlines, related to the heterogeneity of the rehabilitations over time. The mandibular canine tips were abraded to harmonize the mandibular plane.

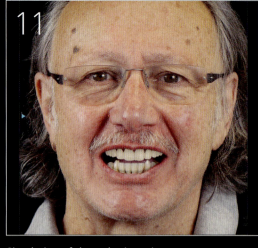

Simulation of the esthetic project.

Digital wax-up in an STL file (3Shape DCM file) made in Dental System and imported into Implant Studio.

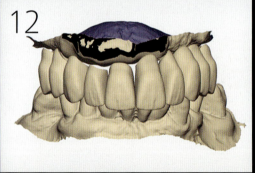

Occlusal view of the overlay between the existing

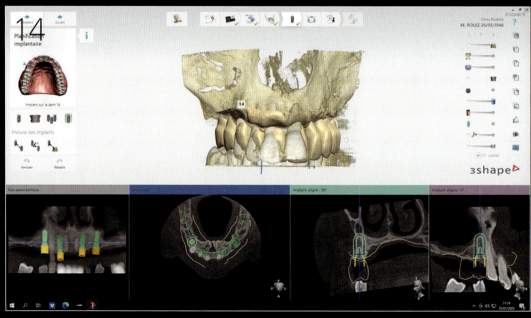

View of the planning window in Implant Studio.

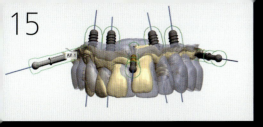

Frontal view of the final plan without the bone filter with the guide stabilization pins and the four RN implants.

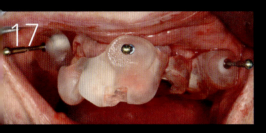

The second appointment was the implant surgery session. The guide was in place, supported at 13, 11, and 21, and keyed at three points.

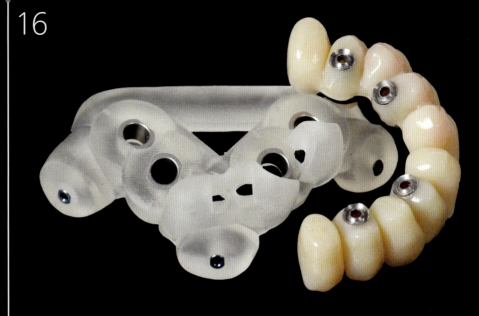

Radiographic guide and *immediate* temporary complete denture (Dentitek Laboratory).

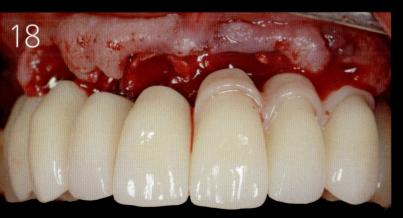

immediate partial denture in place during surgery before GBR and suturing.

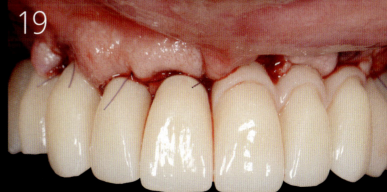

Use of interrupted sutures. The cervical margin line was not exposed and the final prosthesis were made with artificial gingiva.

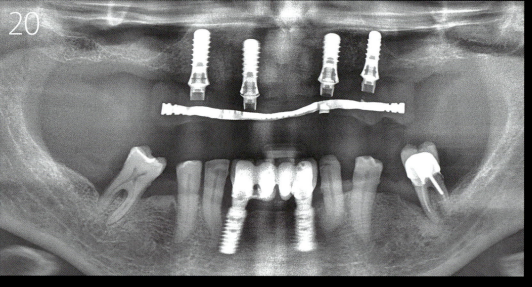

20 Postoperative panoramic radiograph. The result was quite satisfactory. The offset in 12 had no clinical consequence or significance compared to the comfort and benefits offered by **immediate loading**. Tightening was performed on all four implants.

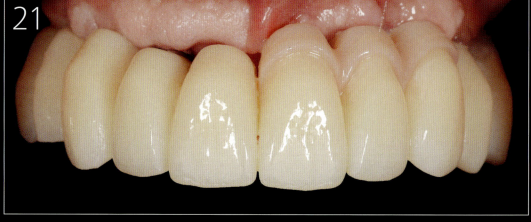

21 Clinical view at 3 months. Fortunately, the patient was well aware that good hygiene was essential to ensure durability of the implants. Note the gingival collapses due to a more limited compensatory GBR because of the objective of a final resin prosthesis with artificial gingiva.

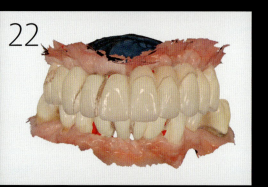

22 Trios 4 optical impression of the full-arch denture with the pre-preparation scan, occlusion, and antagonist, allowing the laboratory to transfer all the information needed to produce the final prosthesis. These impressions were taken during the third appointment at 3 months after implant surgery, after the implant osseointegration had been checked.

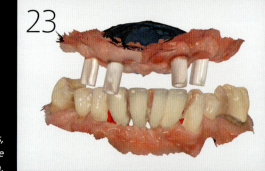

23 Scan of the implants with scan bodies, superimposed onto the scan of the emergence profiles in the patient's occlusion.

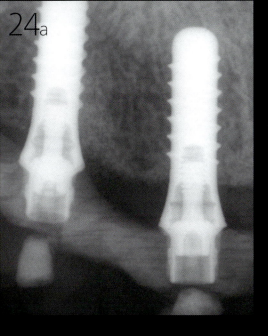
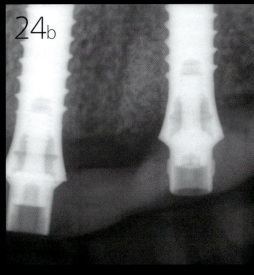

Retroalveolar radiograph in 14 and 12 of the plaster key during the fourth appointment dedicated to validation of the impression and retroalveolar radiograph in 22 and 24.

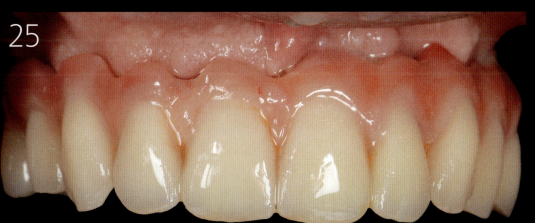

Final resin partial denture for 10 teeth on a PEEK framework with resin mounting of teeth and false gingiva. Note the openings for the interdental brushes. Placement was completed in the fifth treatment session. The patient did not experience any phases where his functional and esthetic comfort was altered; he gained in comfort, esthetics, and functionality with each session.

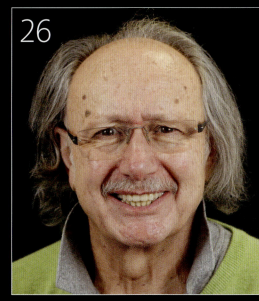

Final result integrated into the face.

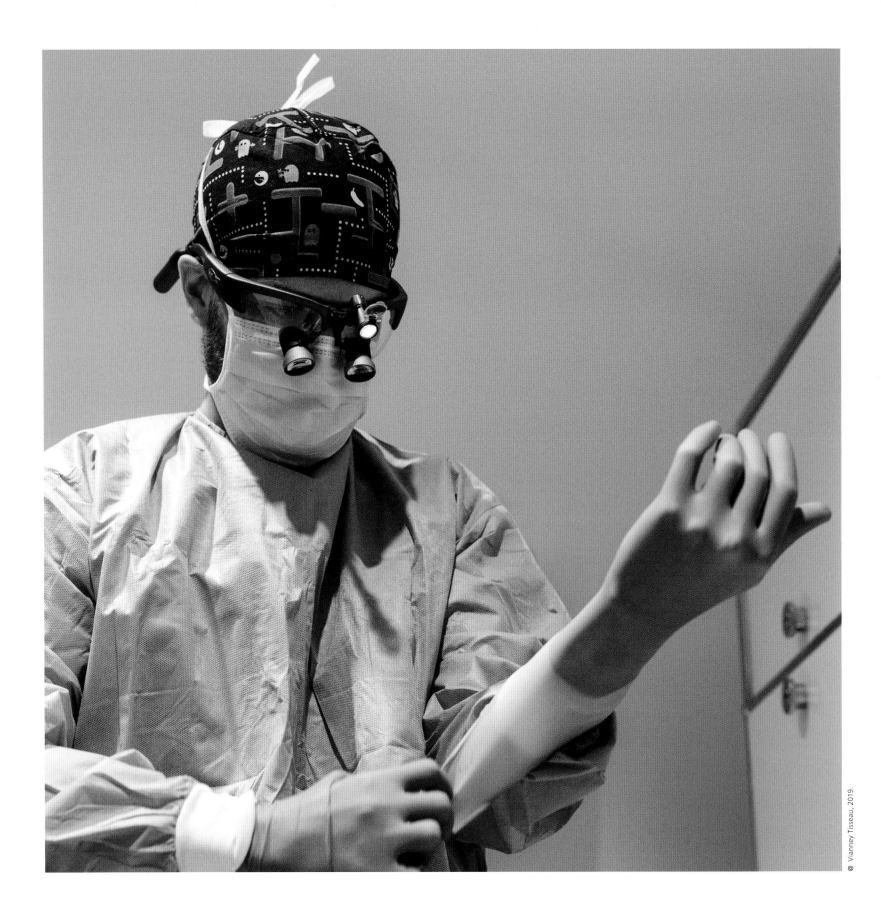

© Vianney Tisseau, 2019.

Full-arch clinical case 29

61-year-old woman.

Clinical data

- The patient was referred to our practice by her daughter who wished to take over her care before her retirement. The case was treated during a live surgery in CampusHB training session.
- Case treated in March 2021.
- Good mucogingival architecture.

Presurgical treatments

- Optical impression taken using a Trios 4 and 3D examination performed using a 3Shape X1.
- Planning using Implant Studio.
- Placement of a Straumann TL SP RN 3.3 x 8.0 mm implant in 15 and 25, and RN 3.3 x 10.0 mm in 14, 12, 22, and 24.
- 3D printing of the guide designed in Implant Studio (Dentitek Laboratory).
- Second-generation Straumann T-socket.
- Temporary partial denture milled in PMMA (Ivotion Dent Multi) (Dentitek Laboratory).

Assessment of the intervention

- Case treated in the office in **six appointments** (esthetic analysis, validation fixed/removable partial denture and radiopaque fixed/removable partial denture, implant surgery, control and impression, validation of the impression, placement of the final prosthesis).
- Final prosthesis made in the office (JC Allègre Laboratory).
- The patient wished to regain masticatory efficiency and a harmonious smile. We began with maxillary **immediate loading** in March 2021. In May 2021, we placed three Straumann SP TL RN 6-mm implants in 45 and 46 and one Straumann SP TL RN 8-mm implant in 36. The final maxillary ceramic partial denture and mandibular ceramic crowns were placed in September 2021 and treatment was completed in early November 2021.

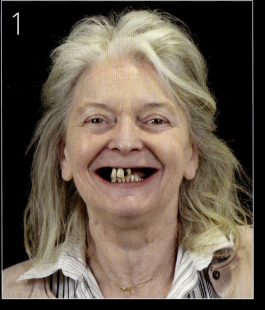

Frontal facial photograph.

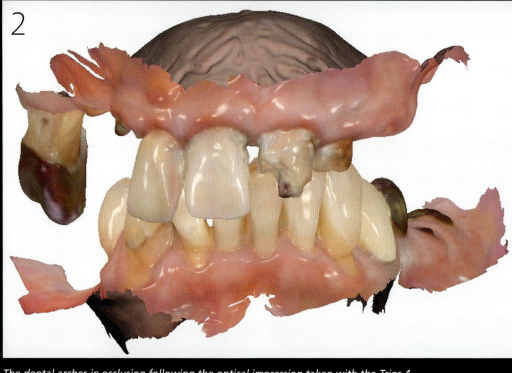

The dental arches in occlusion following the optical impression taken with the Trios 4.

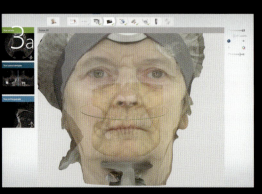

Frontal view of the CBCT scan matching with a facial scan of the patient (3Shape X1).

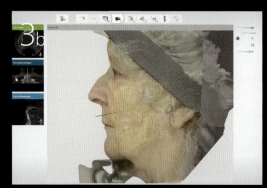

Side view of the CBCT scan matched with the facial scan of the patient (3Shape X1). The aim was to analyze the support of the upper lip via the line of Ricketts (the line passing through the tip of the nose and chin). This esthetic line of Ricketts made it possible to determine the advancement or retreat of the prosthetic project on the frontal plane to obtain better lip support if necessary. There was no need to modify the anteroposterior positioning of the prosthetic project.

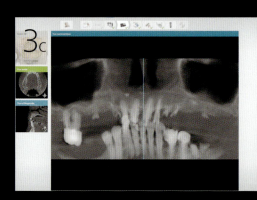

CBCT panoramic mode visualization.

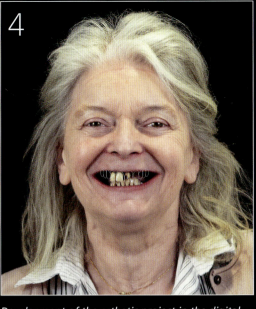

Development of the esthetic project in the digital Smile Design tool by 3Shape.

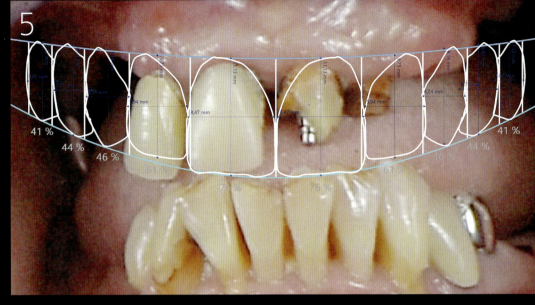

Creation of the new tooth contours corresponding to the prosthetic project. A reference measurement was imported into the Smile Design software to measure the changes to be made in relation to the original clinical situation. This allowed the dental technician to design the esthetic and functional validation partial denture based on the clinical situation and the esthetic simulation.

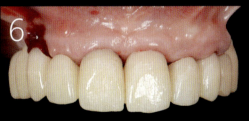

Esthetic and functional validation provisional partial denture placement of 15 to 25 after first-line extraction of teeth 13, 24, and 27; however, the provisional partial denture rested on teeth 12 to 22 and on the root-form teeth in 15 and 23. These two root-form teeth, which were ultimately to be extracted, were important to keep at this stage to provide sufficient anchorage for the temporary partial denture (Dentitek Laboratory).

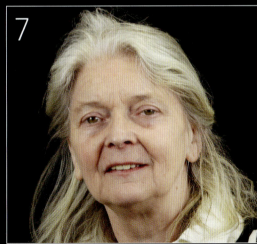

Frontal photograph of the patient's face at rest with the esthetic and functional validation partial denture.

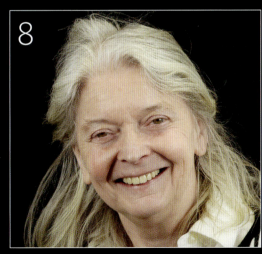

Frontal view of the patient's face and smile with the esthetic and functional validation partial denture. Its design fit very well with the patient's face and smile, with the free edges following the lower lip in a harmonious way.

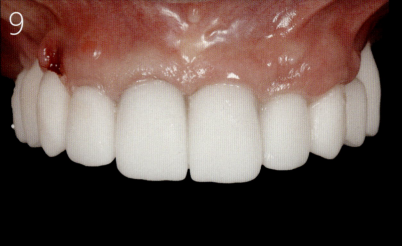

Frontal view of the radiopaque partial denture in place, a duplicate of the esthetic and functional validation partial denture.

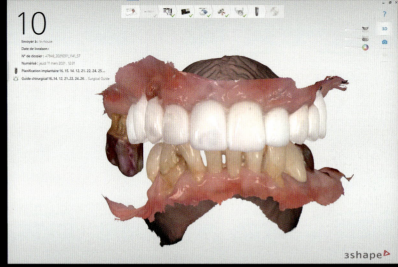

Gathering of the necessary elements for implant planning with the radiopaque partial denture (STL file of the digital impression).

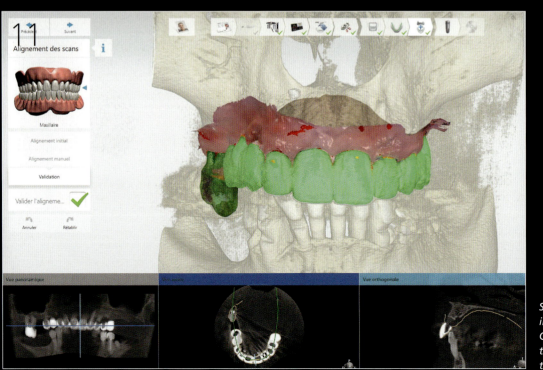

Surfacing between the STL file of the digital impression and the DICOM file of the CBCT scan. Good surfacing quality is essential to be able to accurately transpose the digital implant position to the implant position during surgery.

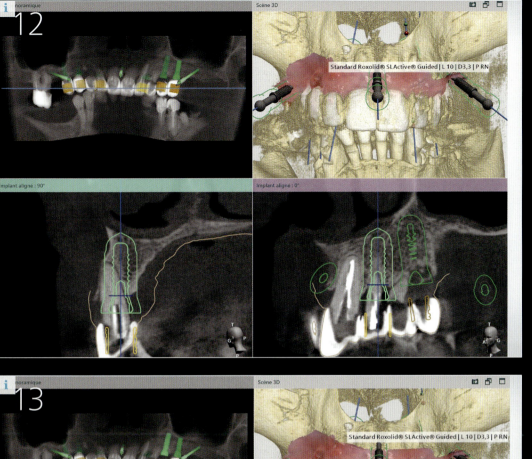

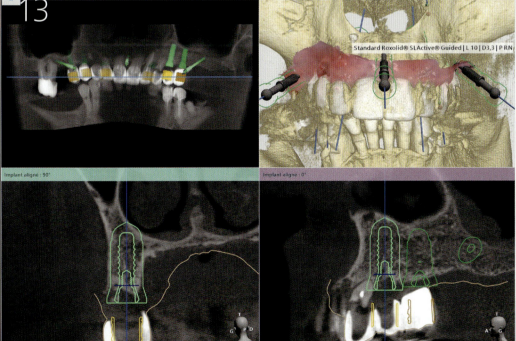

Planning for the implant to be placed in site 22 (Straumman TL RN 3.3 x 10.0 mm) in Implant Studio. Note the proximity of a proximal mesial bone peak to the implant neck.

Planning for the implant to be placed in site 24 (Straumman TL RN 3.3 x 10.0 mm) in Implant Studio.

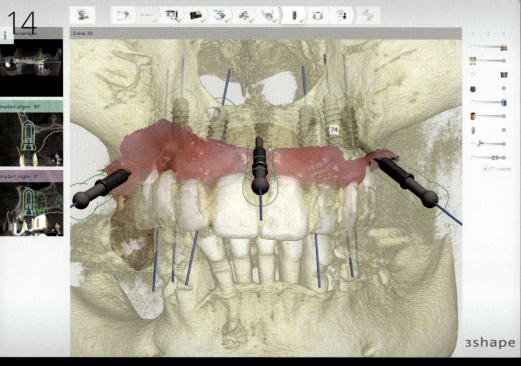

Visualization of the planning of the holding pins for the future surgical guide.

Visualization of implant planning based on the prosthetic plan. The implant angulation was in accordance with the prosthetic plan, without the use of angled prosthetic abutments.

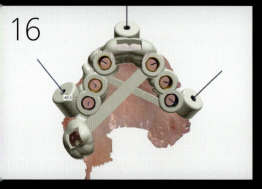

Visualization of the design for the surgical guide with its retaining wedges. The lack of posterior dental support necessitated the use of retaining pins to ensure the stability of the surgical guide during drilling.

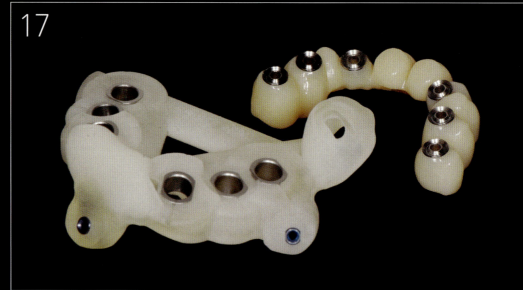

The complete temporary partial denture with **instant loading** and surgical guide before surgery.

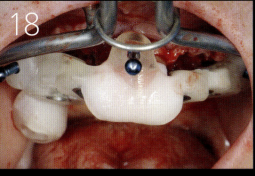

Frontal view of the keyed surgical guide in the mouth.

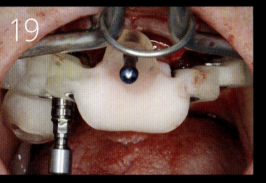

Guided implant placement in site 12 (Straumann TL RN 3.3 x 10.0 mm).

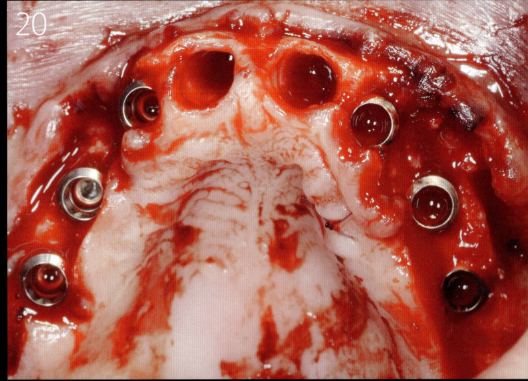

Occlusal view of the six implants placed after extraction of the guide teeth.

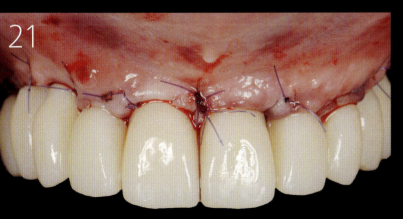

Frontal view of the provisional instant loading partial denture screwed onto the six implants, with ASAF 6/0 monofilament sutures guided by the prosthesis (Dentitek Laboratory).

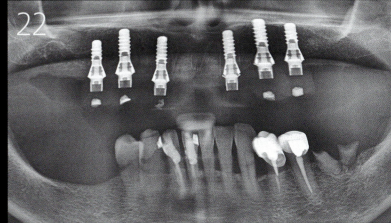

Postoperative panoramic radiograph. Note the slight misfit of the partial denture on the implant in site 22 due to the distal offset of the implant neck because of the bone peak present.

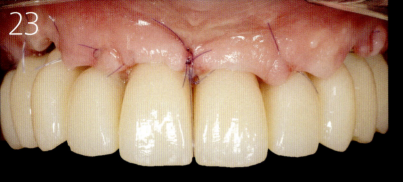

Clinical view at 8 days.

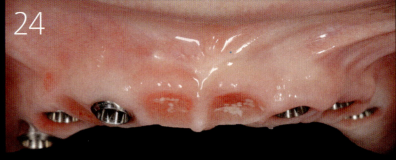

Vestibular view of gingival healing after removal of the instant loading partial denture.

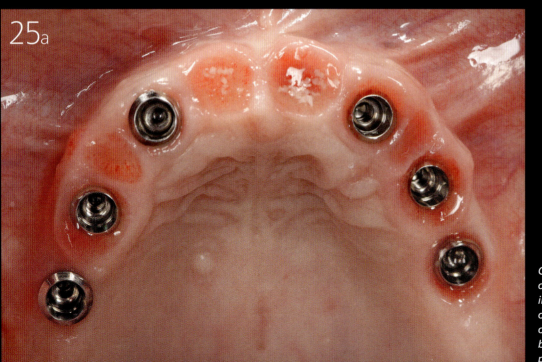

Occlusal view of gingival healing after removal of the instant loading partial denture. Note the implant beds and pontic beds with their absence of inflammation; also note the good preservation of the maxillary bone crest and the good vestibular bone and gingival volumes in the implant and pontic areas.

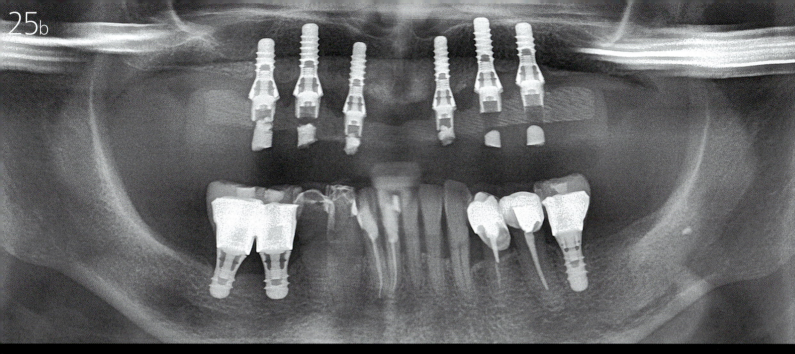

25b Panoramic radiograph of the finalized clinical situation with the six maxillary implants and the mandibular implants placed after instant loading surgery.

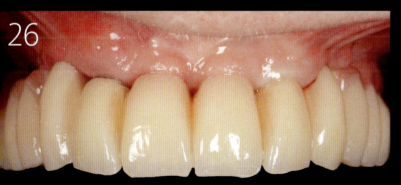

26 Frontal view of the clinical situation at 3 months. The final ceramic partial denture with a zirconia framework was made in the JC Allègre Laboratory. Note the macrofeatures added to the prosthetic project to make the final restoration more personal, while keeping the dental volumes that were validated by the patient beforehand.

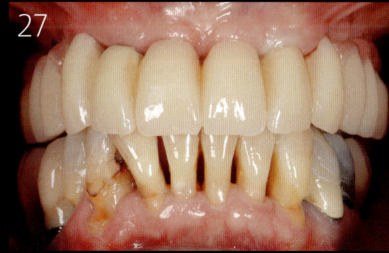

27 Frontal view of the final maxillary partial denture in occlusion. 3 months after the instant loading surgery, three mandibular implants were placed (Straumann TL SP RN 6-mm implants in 45 and 46 and Straumann TL SP RN 8-mm implants). The final maxillary partial denture and mandibular implant crowns were made at the same time in the JC Allègre Laboratory.

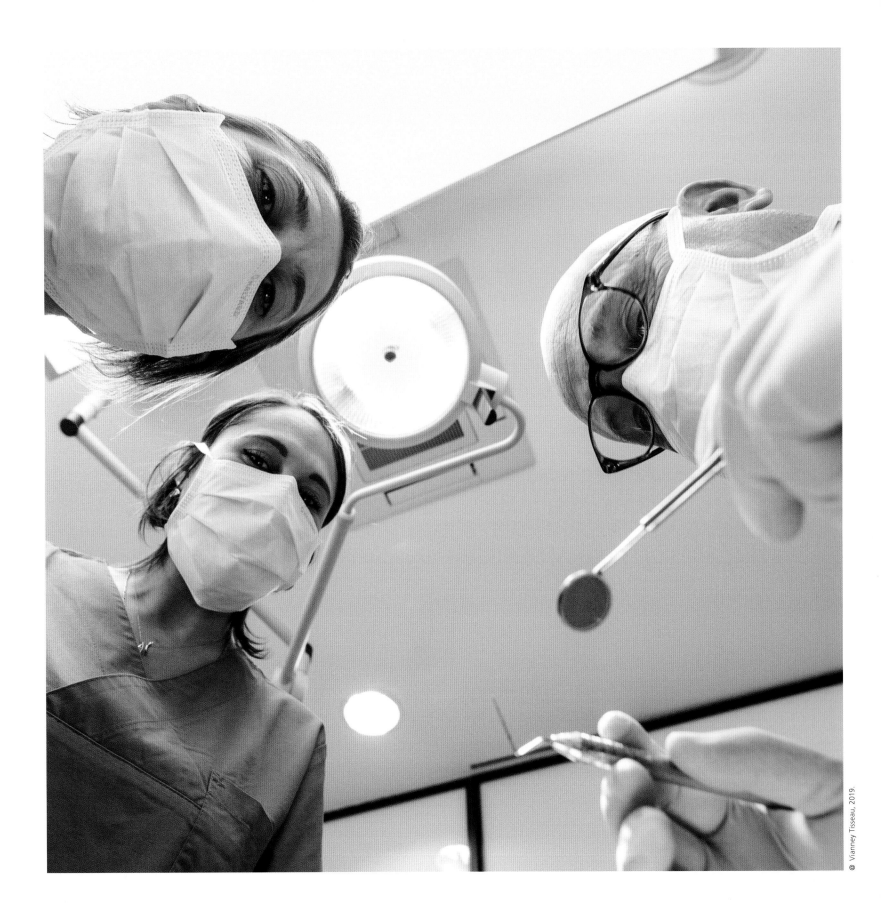

© Vianney Tisseau, 2019.

Full-arch clinical case 30

67-year-old woman.

Clinical data

- The patient had been monitored in the office since 2004 and had experienced frequent episodes of crown loosening in 11 in 2019 and 2020. Tooth 11 was devitalized and crowned and had a low root post height compared to the height of the clinical crown. The prognosis for this tooth was uncertain, so the patient wanted a global esthetic solution. Indeed, she was very concerned about her maxillary incisors due to the fact that their proportions were not balanced.
- Case treated in December 2020.
- Complex mucogingival architecture with the presence of existing implants (in the area of teeth 17, 15, 22, 25, and 27) and old dental crowns. Lack of alignment of the collars.

Presurgical treatments

- Optical impression taken using a Trios 4 and 3D examination performed using a 3Shape X1.
- Planning using Implant Studio.
- Placement of Straumann TL SP RN 3.3 x 10.0 mm implant in 12 and 24, and RN 3.3 x 12.0 mm implant in 14.
- 3D printing of the guide designed in Implant Studio (Dentitek Laboratory).
- Straumann T-socket.
- Temporary partial denture milled in PMMA (Ivotion Dent Multi, Ivoclar) (Dentitek Laboratory).

Assessment of the intervention

- Case treated in the office in **six appointments** (esthetic analysis, validation and radiopaque partial dentures, implant surgery, control and impression, validation of the impression, placement of the final prosthesis).
- Final prosthesis made in the office (JC Allègre Laboratory).
- The patient wished to shorten the free edge of her incisors which were too long, appeared too thin, and interfered with her lower lip. In addition, she expressed her esthetic discomfort with her smile, having discovered the non-alignment of the necks of her teeth and the excessive length of her incisors when smiling. To respect the patient's wishes, the implant prosthesis had to include a part of false gingiva to balance the gingiva–crown ratio.
- The patient wore the esthetic and functional validation partial denture for 3 months prior to the immediate loading surgery so she could become accustomed to her new tooth volumes.
- The final partial denture was made of ceramic with a zirconia framework. A brush calibration session was scheduled with the patient so that she could clean the junction between the prosthetic false gingiva and her gingiva.

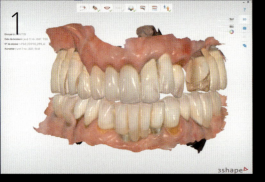

Digital impression of the initial clinical situation. The patient had Straumann TL implants in zones 17, 15, 25, and 27, and a Straumann Narrow Neck (NN) implant with external hex in 22. The implant in site 22, with its highly apical prosthetic platform, determined the vertical positioning of future implants to facilitate accessibility for hygiene maintenance and obtain a more harmonious visual appearance.

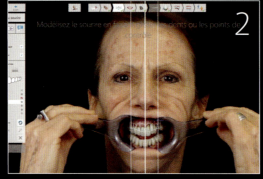

Frontal view of the digital smile design in the 3Shape workflow. In this situation, this tool was used to diagnose the future apical limit of the implant prosthesis; indeed, the neck of the digital dental contours indicates the future limit of the implant platforms, and thus the future limit between the prosthetic false gingiva and the patient's gingiva. For this boundary to be invisible, it must be at least 3 mm below the lip when smiling. The apical limit of the prosthetic project must be aligned with the prosthetic platform of the implant in 22.

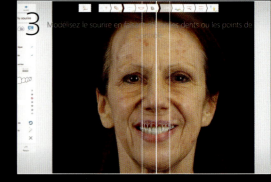

Indication of the boundary of the future prosthetic false gingiva during smiling. This boundary was covered by the patient's upper lip when smiling; the implant treatment plan was therefore validated and feasible. Note the interference of her current teeth with the lower lip.

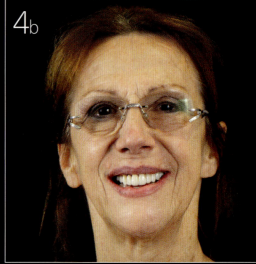

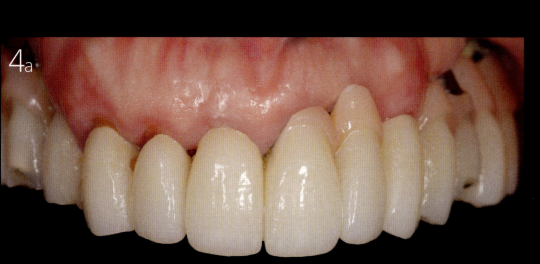

Frontal view of the esthetic and functional validation provisional partial denture screwed onto the existing posterior implants and relined onto the existing anterior teeth. The length of the free edges of the anterior teeth was reduced and the height–width ratio of the crowns was decreased. False gingiva was made on teeth 21 and 22 so the patient could validate the gingiva–crown ratio of the prosthetic project.

Frontal view of the patient's face with the esthetic and functional validation partial denture. The patient wished to further reduce the height–width ratio of her teeth significantly. The reduction in height of the clinical crown was in favor of the false gingiva. The width and anteroposterior positioning of the crowns were validated by the patient. Note the good relationship of the free edges with the patient's lower lip (Dentitek Laboratory).

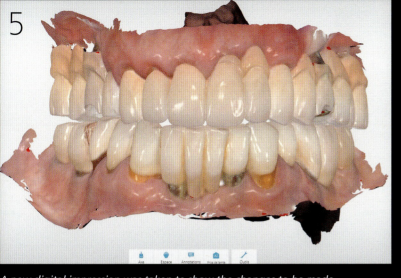

A new digital impression was taken to show the changes to be made in the laboratory.

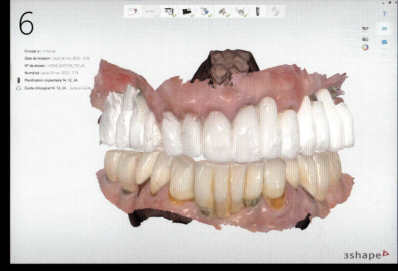

Digital impression of the radiopaque partial denture, a duplicate of the esthetic and functional validation partial denture. At this stage, changes in the height–width ratio of the clinical crowns would not affect the implant planning.

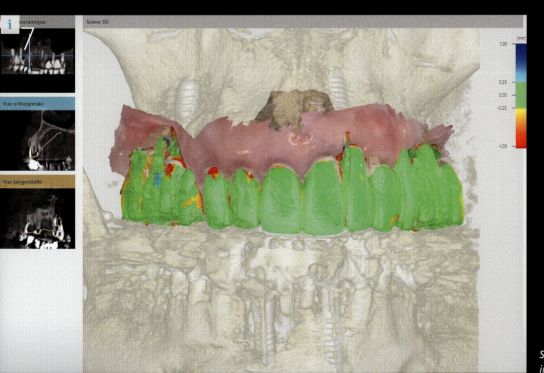

Surfacing between the STL file of the digital impression and the DICOM file of the CBCT scan.

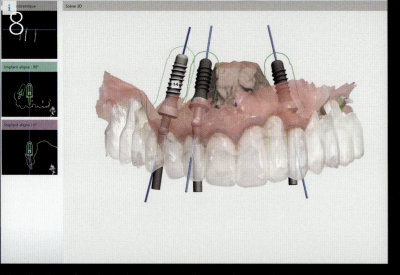

Visualization of implant planning according to the prosthetic project.

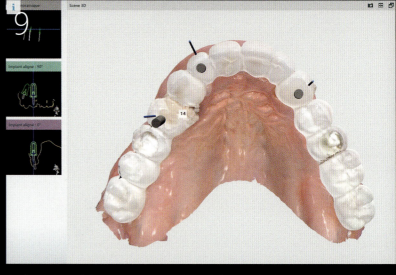

Occlusal view of the emergence profiles of the prosthetic screw shafts in accordance with the prosthetic project.

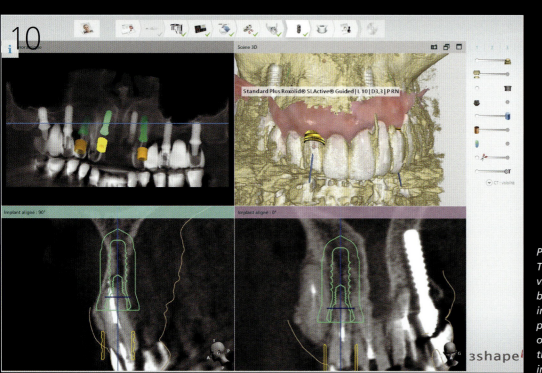

Planning for the implant in zone 12 (Straumann TL RN 3.3 x 10.0 mm) in Implant Studio. Note the visualization of the amount of bone resection to be applied after extraction of tooth 12 and before implant insertion (sagittal section window), and the placement of temporary screw-retained abutments on the implants already in place in 15 and 25, and the retention of Synocta abutments on the implants in 17 and 27 (panoramic window).

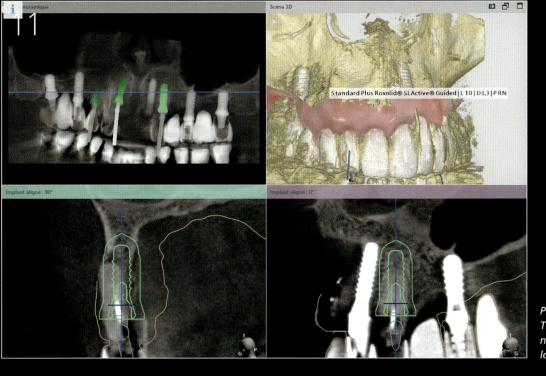

Planning for the implant in zone 23 (Straumann TL RN 3.3 x 10.0 mm) in Implant Studio. Note the need to perform peri-implant GBR during instant loading surgery to correct the vestibular bone defect.

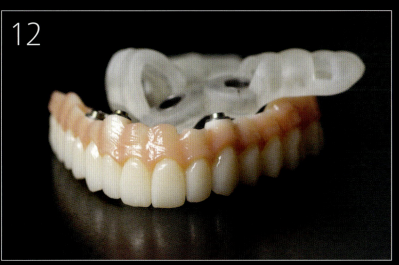

Visualization of the surgical guide with the **immediate loading** partial denture. The gingiva–crown ratio was changed to false gingiva to reduce the length of the clinical crowns, as requested by the patient. The posterior implants, present in the mouth and osseointegrated, were attached to the prosthesis with temporary abutments and brief relining with autopolymerizing resin.

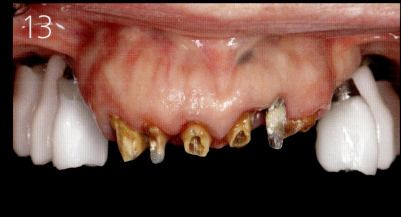

Frontal view of the clinical situation before placement of the surgical guide. The radiopaque partial denture was cut to allow placement of the surgical guide teeth (teeth 15 to 17 and 25 to 27). These teeth supporting the partial denture were placed on the implant abutments.

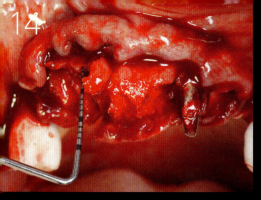

14 Frontal view of the bone situation after the vestibular flap had been removed and the anterior teeth extracted. The measurement of the periodontal millimeter probe indicated the amount of bone resection to be performed to align the apical limit of the future prosthetic soft tissue with the implant platforms.

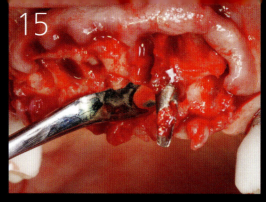

15 Frontal view of the bone situation after anterior bone resection. Note the alignment of the bone level with the implant platform in site 22.

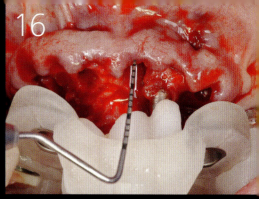

16 Frontal view of the surgical guide and its good adaptation on the supporting teeth. Visualization with the periodontal millimeter probe of the new bone level in relation to the neck of tooth 21, with distance corresponding to the height of the prosthetic false gingiva (photograph taken not perpendicular to the periodontal probe, 7 mm measurement).

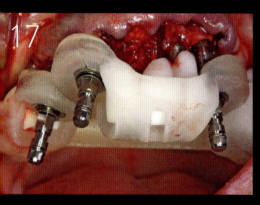

17 Frontal view of the implant grippers guided through the surgical guide. The vertical embedding of the implants (first-generation, delivered with the guided gripper screwed on the implant in place) was determined by the planning software (here, H6).

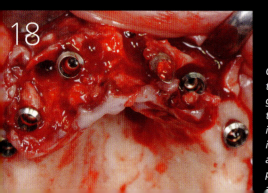

18 Occlusal view of the three newly placed guided implants. Note the distal offloading incisions away from the implants in zones 15 and 25 to preserve the peri-implant circular attachment.

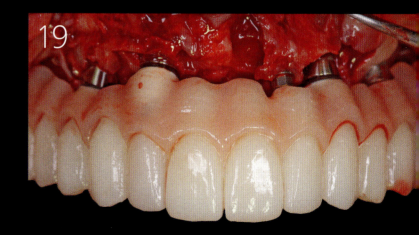

19 Try-in and screwing in of the connected instant loading provisional partial denture on the three newly placed implants and securing of the partial denture to the posterior implant abutments with autopolymerizing resin. Note the presence of fibrous tissue at the implant body in 22 that made it difficult to lift the buccal flap.

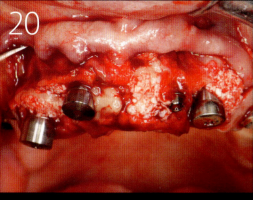

Compensatory GBR around the implants and ridge preservation on the non-implant extraction sockets with DBBM (Bio-Oss with fine particles) incubated in the patient's plasma F2 fraction (PRGF). Note the tear in the vestibular alveolar mucosa opposite tooth 22.

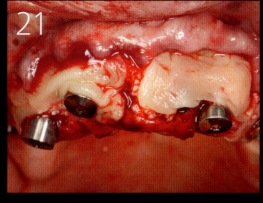

Placement of F1 fibrin membranes from the patient's plasma and covering of the GBR material.

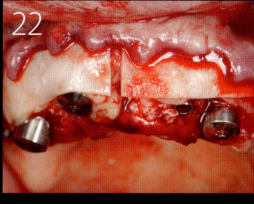

A resorbable collagen membrane (Bio-Gide) was used according to the biologic rules of GBR.

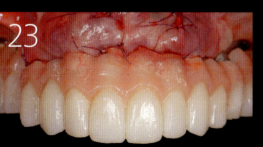

Frontal view of the postoperative situation with the immediate loaded temporary partial denture in place. Apical repositioning sutures were placed from 13 to 23. In this situation, the sutures were made before the partial denture was inserted.

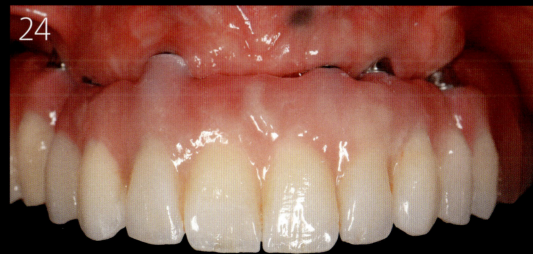

Frontal view of the clinical situation at 6 months, final ceramic partial denture with a zirconia framework made in the office (JC Allègre Laboratory).

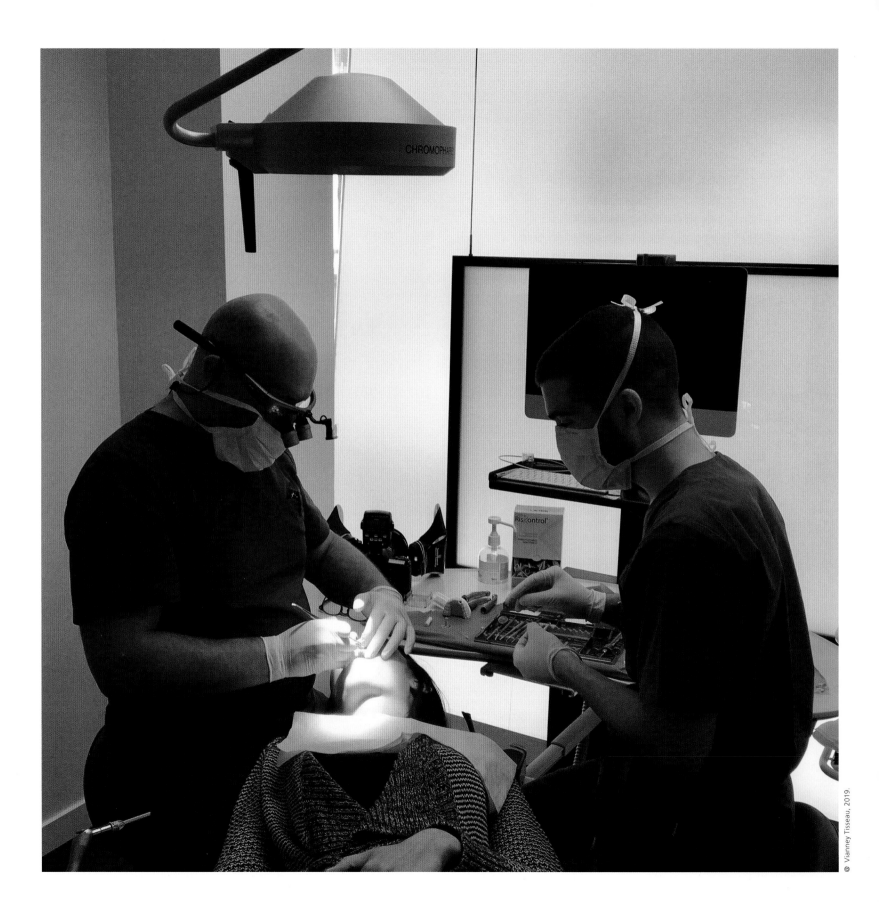

© Vianney Tisseau, 2019.

Full-arch clinical case 31

56-year-old man.

Clinical data

- Presented for a fixed implant supported maxillary rehabilitation in place of the condemned full dentoportal partial denture.
- Case treated in February 2022.
- Heterogeneous vertical bone loss.
- Complex heterogeneous mucogingival architecture in the context of a gingival smile.

Presurgical treatments

- Trios 4 used to take optical impression and 3D examination performed using a 3Shape X1.
- Planning using Implant Studio.
- Placement of 3.75 x 10.00 mm Straumann TLX RT implants in 14 and 24, 4.5 x 10.0 mm in 26, 3.75 x 8.00 mm in 16, NT 3.75 x 12.00 mm in 22, and 3.75 x 10.00 mm in 12.
- 3D printing of the guide designed in Implant Studio (Dentitek Laboratory).
- Straumann TLX self-locking PEEK sockets.
- Temporary partial denture milled in PMMA (Ivotion Dent Multi) (Dentitek Laboratory) on an A3 shade base.

Assessment of the intervention

- Case treated in the office in **seven appointments** (esthetic analysis, validation partial denture, radiopaque partial denture, implant surgery, implant impression preparation, validation of the impression and CAD/CAM model, placement of the final prosthesis).
- Prosthesis made in the office (Dental Art Technology Laboratory, Richard Demange).

Additional treatments

- Both arches were condemned to complete extraction. The patient wished to delay extraction of the mandible for financial reasons. His compliance with hygiene was optimal since we took over his care. He knew that the same treatment would have to be performed on the mandible in the next 2 years, with the possibility of earlier **immediate loading** if the situation deteriorated. A nocturnal muscle deprogramming splint was placed at the end of treatment and quarterly periodontal maintenance was delivered.

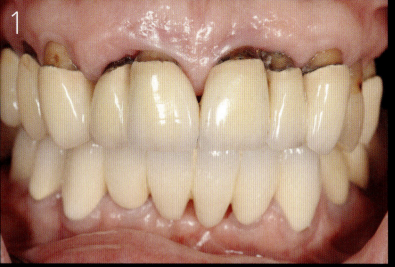

Frontal view of the occlusion.

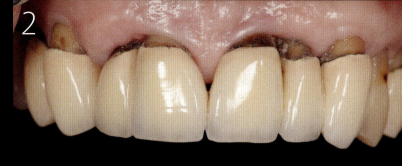

View of the maxilla.

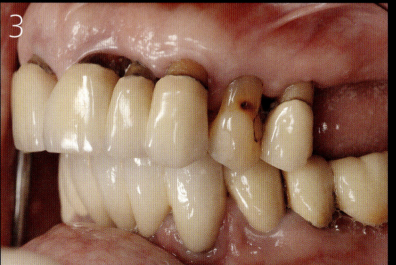

Occlusion, left lateral view.

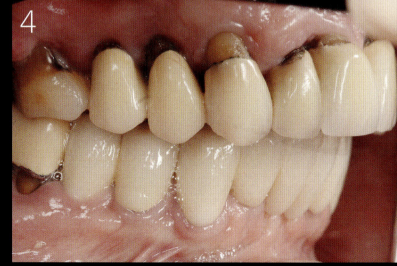

Occlusion, right lateral view.

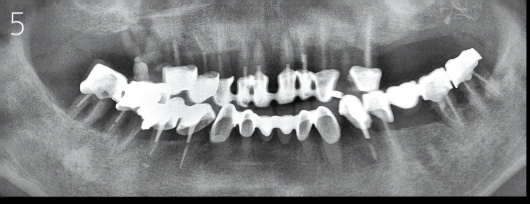

Panoramic radiograph of the initial clinical situation.

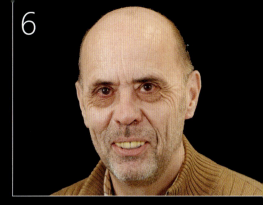

Frontal facial photograph of the patient.

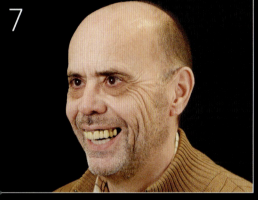

Facial photograph, three-quarter view.

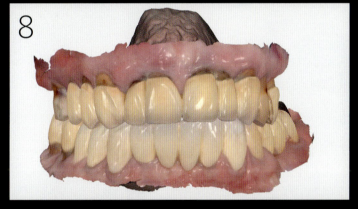

The dental arches in occlusion following the optical impression taken with the Trios 4.

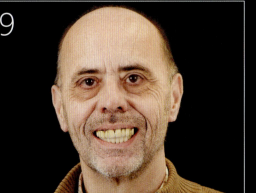

Facial photograph of the patient smiling when recording elements for the esthetic analysis during the first treatment appointment.

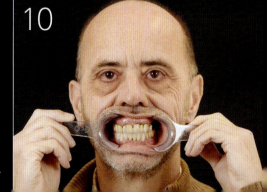

Facial photograph of the patient with retractors for esthetic analysis.

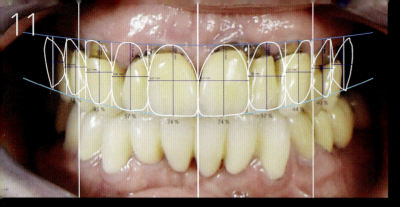

Development of the esthetic project in the 3Shape flow.

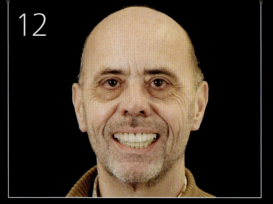

The finished esthetic project in RealView mode.

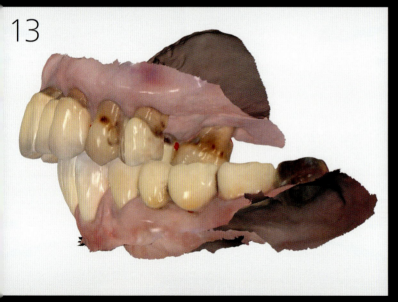

The optical impression in addition to the esthetic analysis on which the esthetic and functional validation partial denture was to be made, in accordance with the esthetic simulation performed in the 3Shape flow. The partial denture was designed in Dental System after importing the photos from Smile Design and the optical impressions (Dentitek Laboratory).

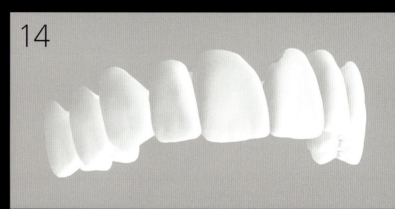

STL file of the esthetic and functional validation temporary partial denture in vestibular view.

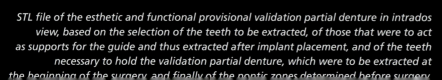

STL file of the esthetic and functional provisional validation partial denture in intrados view, based on the selection of the teeth to be extracted, of those that were to act as supports for the guide and thus extracted after implant placement, and of the teeth necessary to hold the validation partial denture, which were to be extracted at the beginning of the surgery, and finally of the pontic zones determined before surgery.

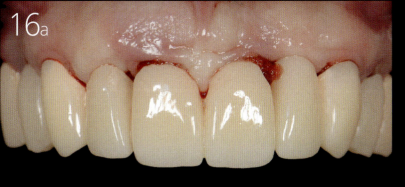 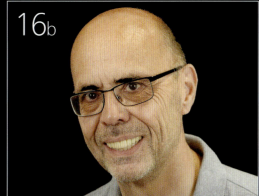

Placement of the esthetic and functional validation temporary partial denture with first-line extractions. The central and lateral incisors were extracted to improve the mucogingival level differences via gingival healing. Facial view with the validation partial denture in the mouth for evaluation of the integration of the esthetic result.

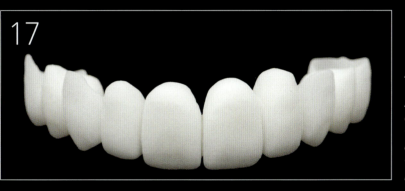

After the patient validated the esthetic setup, a copy of the esthetic and functional validation partial denture was milled in radiopaque resin. A follow-up appointment was scheduled to place this radiopaque partial denture to gather the information required for implant planning, namely the optical impression and the 3D examination. The optical impressions of the extrados and intrados of the provisional partial denture for esthetic validation were taken at the end of the session in order to machine the radiopaque partial denture without the need for relining in the next session.

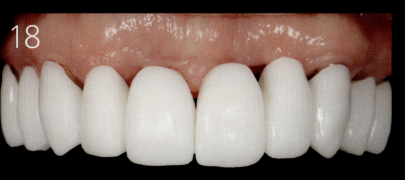

The radiopaque partial denture in place for the planning session.

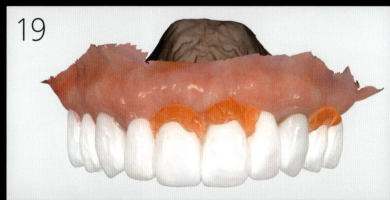

Optical impression of the radiopaque partial denture in place. Note the wax filling of the gaps to simplify the cutting of the teeth. The latest Trios update negates the need to seal these gaps.

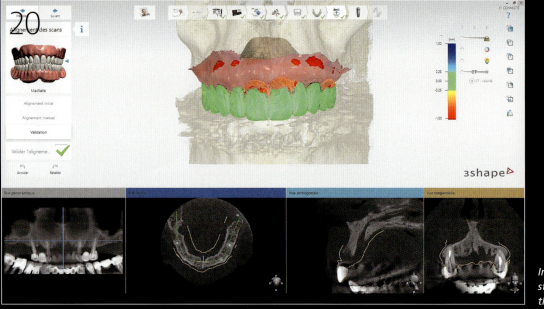

Implant Studio software window in the surfacing step between the STL optical impression file and the DICOM file of the CBCT acquisition.

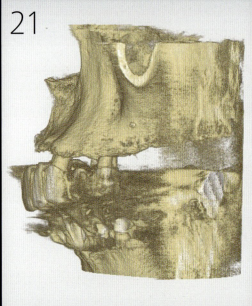

Profile view of the DICOM file showing the relationship between the prosthetic project and

CBCT panoramic view showing the supporting teeth for the temporary partial denture.

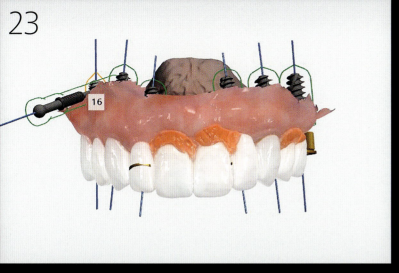

Planning overview with the STL file, without the DICOM file.

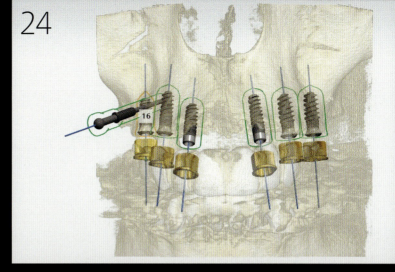

Planning overview in the bone volume, without the intraoral STL volume. The socket heights were finalized: H4 posterior and H6 anterior were defined.

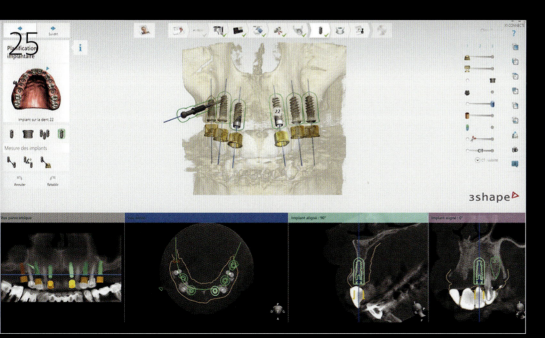

Planning also determined the surgical requirements during implantation. In site 22, note the need for corrective GBR of the vestibular concavity.

STL file for the instant loading partial denture. It was milled in a PMMA disk before being connected to the titanium bases (Dentitek Laboratory).

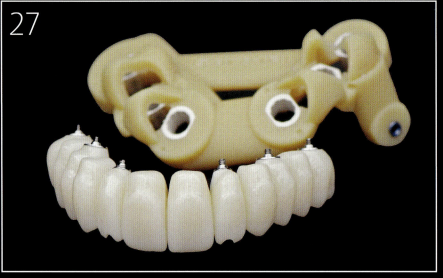

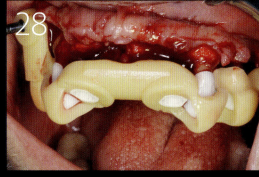

Surgical guide in place on the supporting teeth and keyed on the right side.

Temporary complete denture with instant loading and surgical guide ready for surgery.

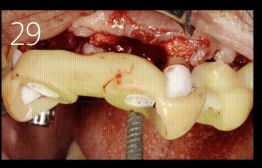

After guided drilling, guided placement of the 3.75 x 10.00 mm TLX NT implant in 22.

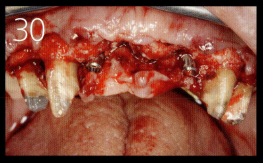

Vestibular view of the implants placed before extraction of the guide teeth.

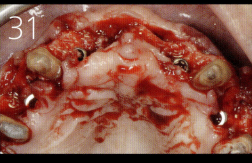

Occlusal view of the implants placed before extraction of the guide teeth.

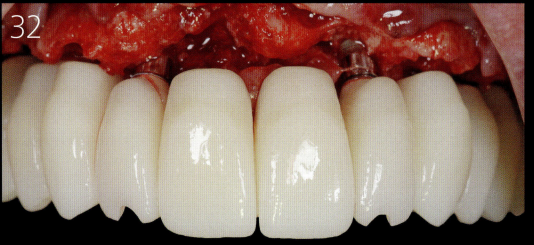

The instant loading partial denture in place on the implants during surgery. Note the emergence of the screw shaft on the incisal edges in 12 and 22, related to the fact that there was no Variobase SA (angled screw shaft) for partial denture work.

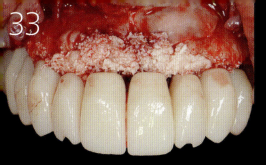

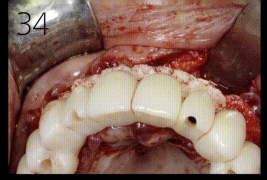

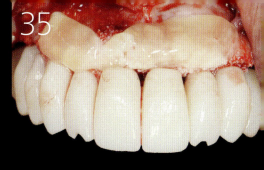

Vestibular view of the compensatory prosthesis-guided GBR, associated with the preserved ridges of the extraction sockets that will be pontic areas with DBBM (Bio-Oss with fine particles) incubated in the plasma F2 fraction (PRGF).

Occlusal view of the compensatory GBR guided by the prosthesis.

Covering of the deproteinized bovine bone mineral (DBBM) with a fibrin membrane from the F1 plasma fraction.

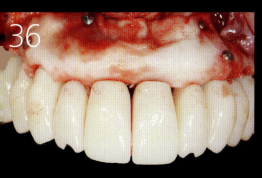

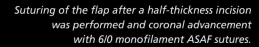

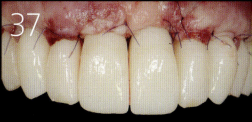

Covering with a resorbable collagen membrane (Bio-Gide) stabilized using impacted pins.

Suturing of the flap after a half-thickness incision was performed and coronal advancement with 6/0 monofilament ASAF sutures.

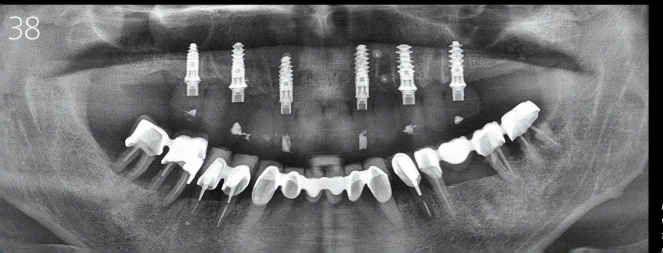

Postoperative panoramic view confirming the optimal fit of the instant temporary partial denture.

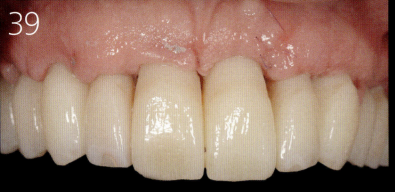

Clinical view at 8 days. Note the good tissue reaction.

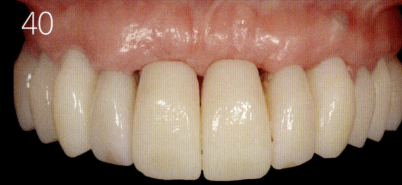

Clinical view at 3 months. Note the lack of pseudopapillae between the central and lateral incisors that would have to be worked on with the supports of the final prosthesis.

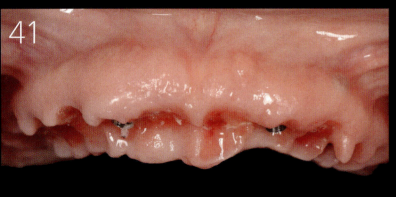

Vestibular view of gingival healing after removal of the immediate loading partial denture.

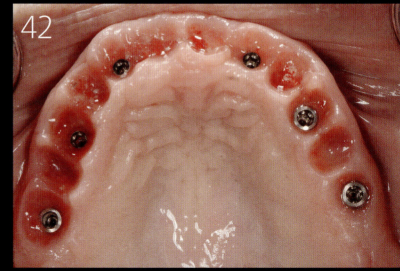

Occlusal view of gingival healing after removal of the immediate loading partial denture. Note the implant and pontic beds.

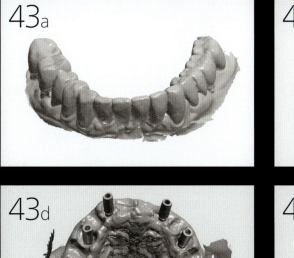
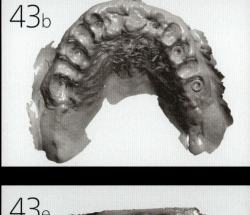
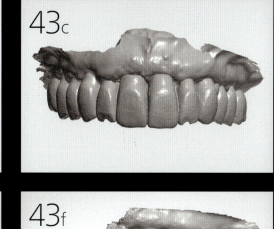
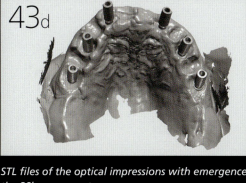
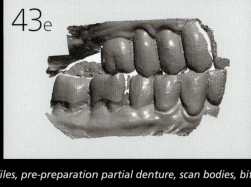
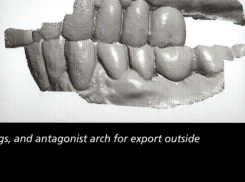

STL files of the optical impressions with emergence profiles, pre-preparation partial denture, scan bodies, bitewings, and antagonist arch for export outside the 3Shape ecosystem.

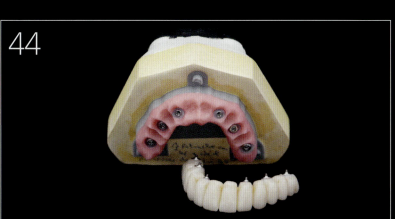

A CAD/CAM model was used to correct the esthetic details identified. This model was placed on the same day as the plaster key fitting for validation of the impression and volumes. The model was scanned in duplicate to allow

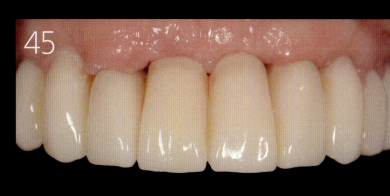

The model in place. Note the flattening of the vestibular surfaces.

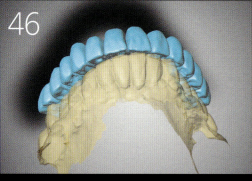

Window in Dental Wings laboratory software with the final prosthetic volume modeled (Dental Art Technology Laboratory).

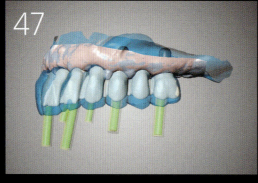

Lateral view of the homothetic reduction of the framework (Dental Art Technology Laboratory).

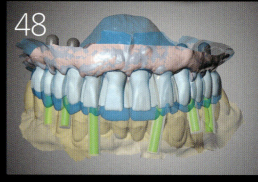

Vestibular view of the homothetic reduction of the framework (Dental Art Technology Laboratory).

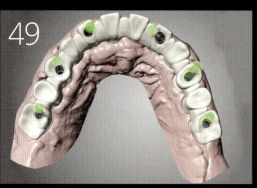

Occlusal view of the framework with the screw axes (Dental Art Technology Laboratory).

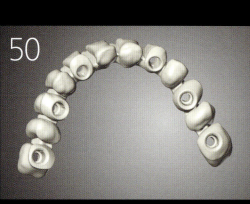

STL file of the completed framework, ready to be sent for machining in zirconia in Metoxit discs (Createch Medical) (Dental Art Technology Laboratory).

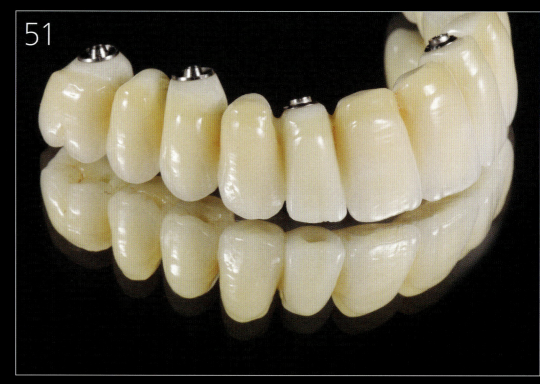

Mounting the ceramic (CZR; Noritake, Nagoya, Japan) on the zirconia framework. Note that this is the first step involving physical work on the model since the start of treatment (Dental Art Technology Laboratory).

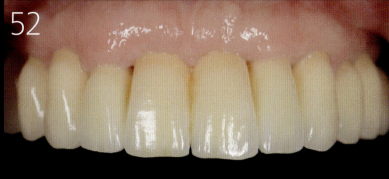

52 The final screw-retained partial denture.

53 Panoramic radiograph of the final partial denture in place.

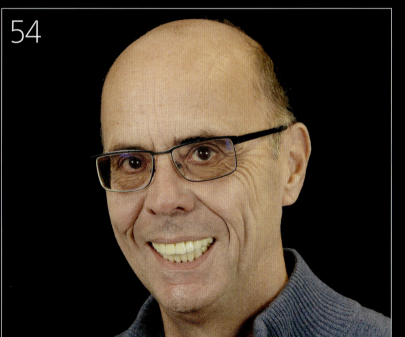

54 Esthetic integration of the final prosthesis in the face.

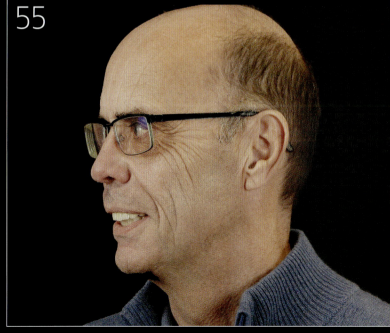

55 Integration into the patient's profile.

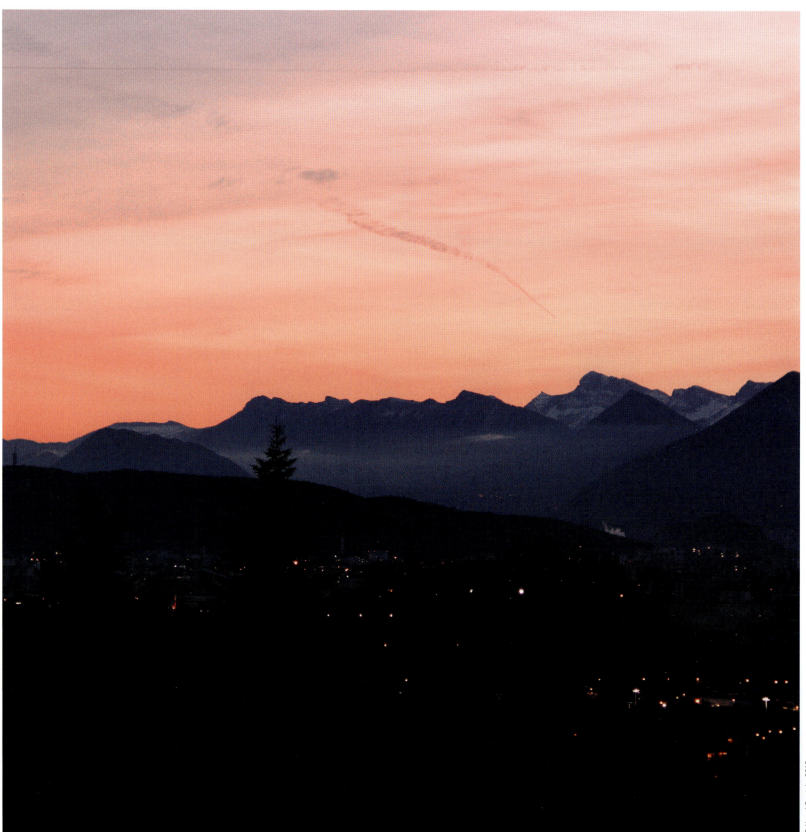

© Hervé Buatois, 2018.

Full-arch clinical case 32

56-year-old woman.

Clinical data

- Referred for a fixed implant supported maxillary rehabilitation in place of a full teeth supported denture.
- Case treated in May 2022.
- Favorable bone context.
- Favorable mucogingival architecture.

Presurgical treatments

- Optical impression taken using a Trios 4 and 3D examination performed using a 3Shape X1.
- Planning using Implant Studio.
- Placement of Straumann 3.75 x 12.00 mm TLX NT implants in 12 and 22, RT 4.5 x 12.0 mm in 14, and RT 4.5 x 8.0 mm in 16, 26, and 24.
- 3D printing of the guide designed in Implant Studio (Dentitek Laboratory).
- Straumann TLX self-locking PEEK sockets.
- Temporary partial denture milled in PMMA (Ivotion Dent Multi) (Dentitek Laboratory) on an A2 shade base.

Assessment of the intervention

- Case treated in the office in **six appointments** (esthetic analysis, validation and radiopaque partial denture, implant surgery, control and impression, validation of the impression, placement of the final prosthesis).
- Prosthesis made in the office (Mathias Berger Laboratory).
- The patient attended the practice because she was considering a complete implant-supported maxillary rehabilitation. In addition to the missing molars, we had caries recurrence under the existing partial denture. This partial denture was already a third generation with history of recurring caries lesions. The radiographic and clinical examinations confirmed these findings. Teeth 15, 11, 21, and 22 would be conservable and eligible for new prostheses with a sufficient seal. Strategically, and after discussion with the patient, we opted for a complete implant-prosthetic rehabilitation using six implants to replace twelve teeth.

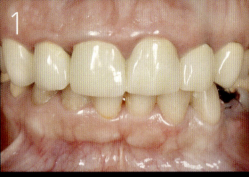
Frontal clinical view.

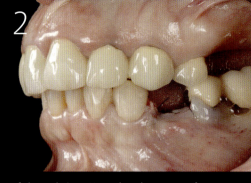
Left lateral view. Note the placement of a Straumann TLX implant in 34.

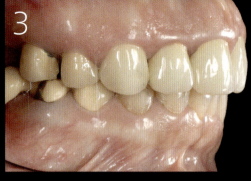
Right-side view.

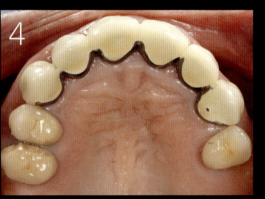
Occlusal view.

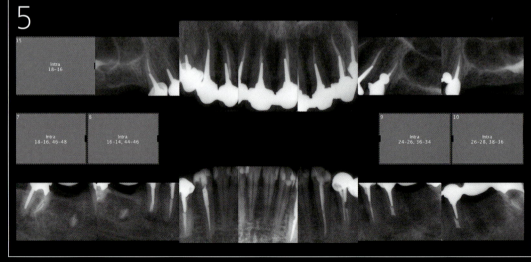
Retroalveolar long cone assessment to evaluate the intrinsic value of each maxillary tooth and understand the recurrent loosening of 14 and 15.

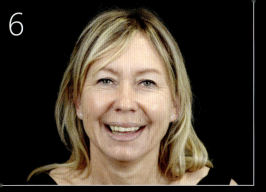

Frontal view for esthetic analysis.

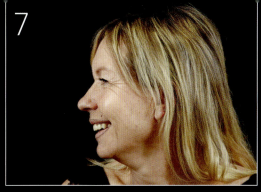

Profile view to complement the esthetic analysis views to judge the tooth–lip ratio.

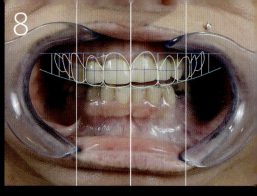

Development of the esthetic assembly in the Smile Design module in Trios 4.

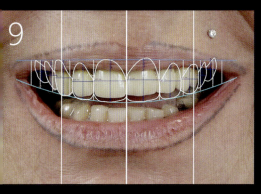

Final view of the assembly with length–width ratios.

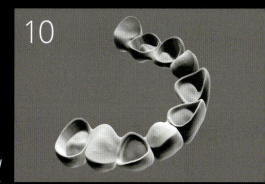

STL file of the esthetic and functionally validated partial denture.

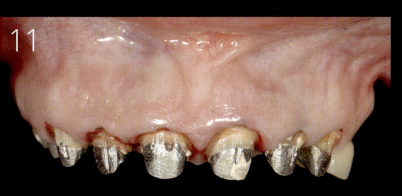

Situation after cutting and removing the existing partial denture.

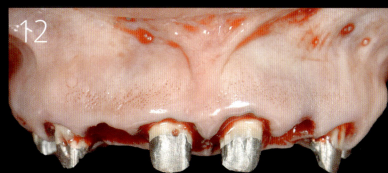

Situation after extraction of teeth 14, 12, 22, and 25.

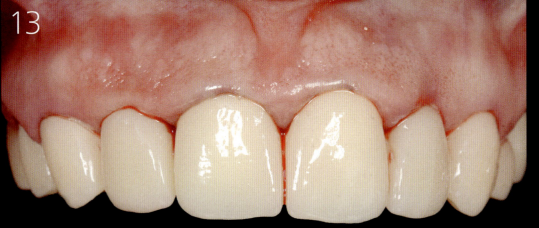
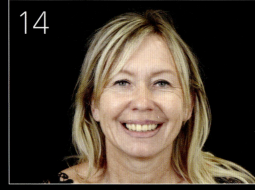

Temporary partial denture in place at the end of the session after relining and polishing.

Facial view a few days after the session to evaluate the esthetic integration of the project. Note the slight tilt in the midlines due to teeth 11 and 21 shifted to the right, which would be corrected later on.

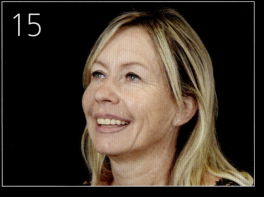
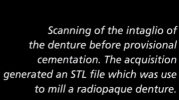
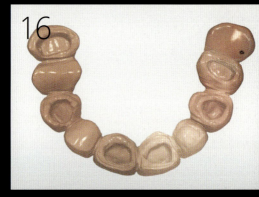

Three-quarter view to evaluate the integration of the partial denture with the smile.

Scanning of the intaglio of the denture before provisional cementation. The acquisition generated an STL file which was use to mill a radiopaque denture.

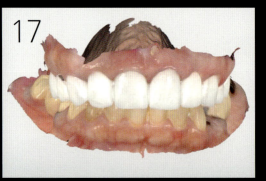
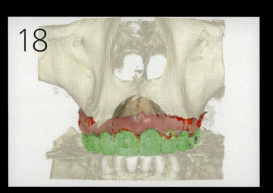
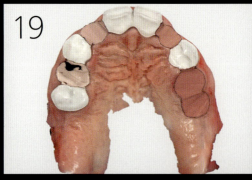

Intraoral digital impression of the radiopaque denture in place and the antagonist arch in occlusion for implant planning.

Matching step between the STL file and the CBCT DICOM file. Note the colorimetric index to control the accuracy of the matching process.

Occlusal view of the impression after virtual extraction of the teeth used for the surgical guide.

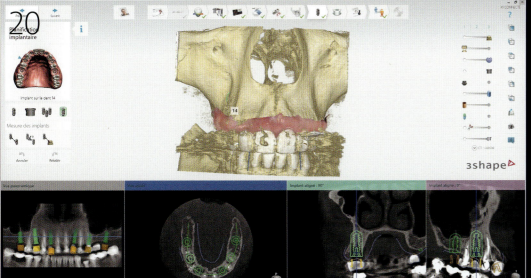

Implant planning in Implant Studio.

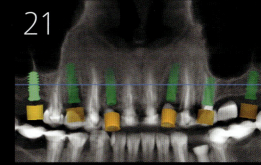

Panoramic view of the planning for six implants.

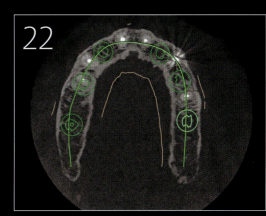

Planning view on an axial section.

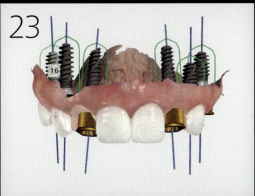

Planning view without the bone filter of the six implants and their relationship to the gingiva and the prosthetic project.

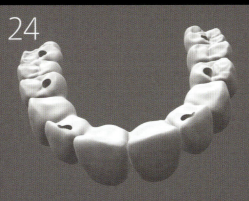

*STL file of the provisional **immediate loading** denture, prepared in Dental System after exporting the planning files (Dentitek Laboratory).*

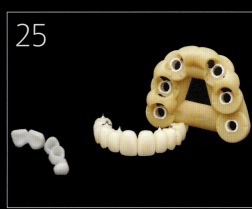

Instant loading partial denture, surgical guide, and radiopaque guide teeth before surgery.

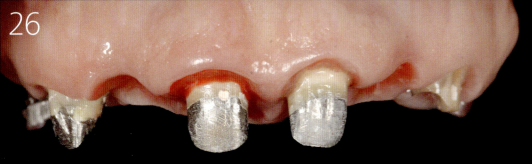

Removal of the temporary partial denture on the day of surgery.

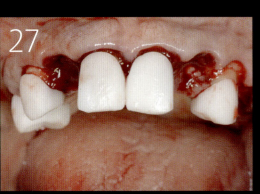

Placement of the radiopaque guide teeth after the sulcal incisions and flap preparation.

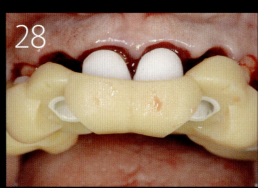

Surgical guide in place for guided drilling.

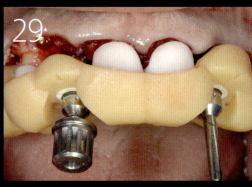

Guided placement of implants, either manually or on a contra-angle.

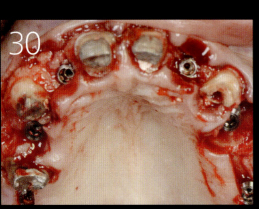

Occlusal view of the six implants placed before extraction of the guide teeth.

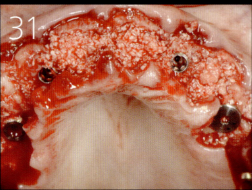

Compensatory GBR of extraction gaps around implants and ridge preservation in pontic alveoli with DBBM (Bio-Oss with fine particles) incubated in the F2 plasma fraction (PRGF). Note that the implant in 24 was not to be loaded due to a lack of primary stability in a large socket. A 2-mm healing

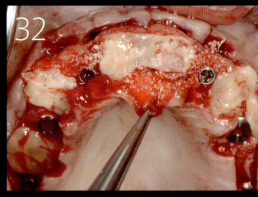

Covering of the fillings with a fibrin membrane from the F1 plasma fraction.

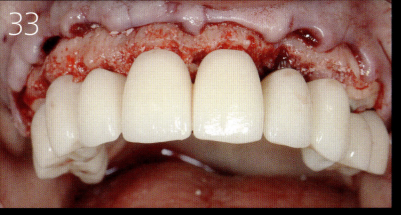

Immediate loading partial denture in place, screwed onto the implants. Note the good relationship with the bone volumes.

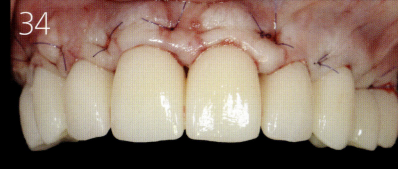

Suturing of prosthesis-guided flaps using ASAF sutures.

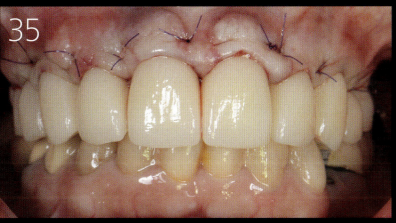

Occlusal view of the temporary partial denture at the end of surgery.

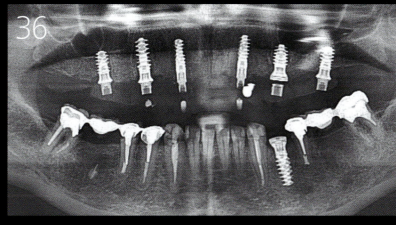

Postoperative panoramic radiograph.

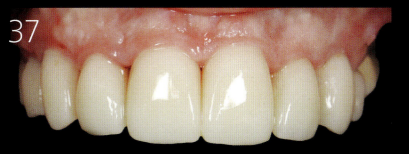

Clinical view 3 months postoperatively showing optimal gingival integration of the temporary partial denture.

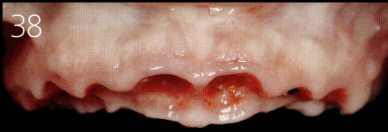

Vestibular view of the healing situation of the gingiva after removal of the partial denture.

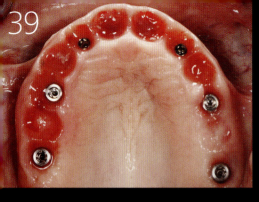

39

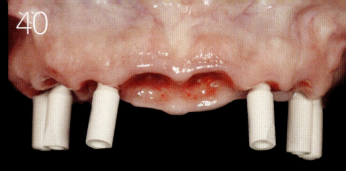

40

Occlusal view. Note the quality of the implant emergence profiles and pontic beds.

Impression scan bodies in place.

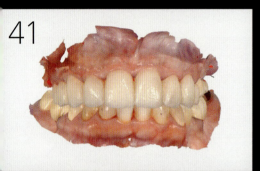

41

Acquisition file with the Trios 4 of the provisional bridge in pre-preparation file in occlusion with the antagonist arch.

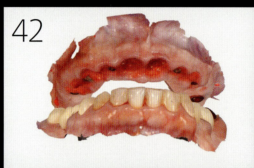

42

Acquisition file of the emergence profiles of the maxilla automatically in occlusion with the antagonist arch.

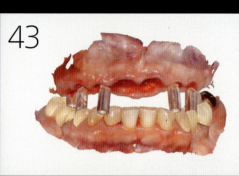

43

Acquisition file of the scan bodies automatically in occlusion with the antagonist arch.

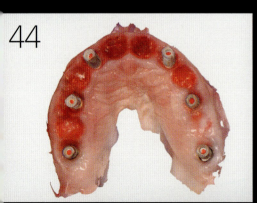

44

Occlusal view of the acquisition file of the scan bodies.

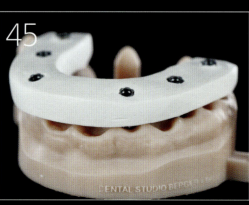

45

Plaster key for validation of the impression (Berger Laboratory).

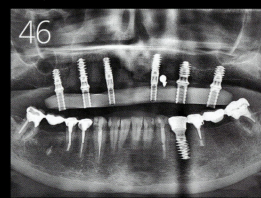

46

Panoramic radiograph of the plaster key in place, allowing validation of the optical impression.

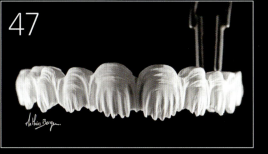

Zirconia framework milled on a Katana Zirconia HTML Plus disc (Kuraray Noritake, Tokyo, Japan) before sintering (Berger Laboratory).

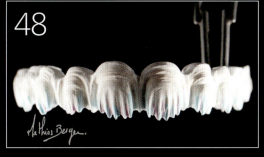

Framework stained before sintering to improve its appearance in support of the ceramic layering (Berger Laboratory).

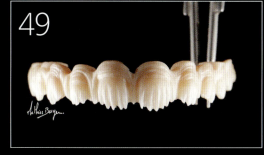

Rendering of the sintered framework after application of staining (Berger Laboratory).

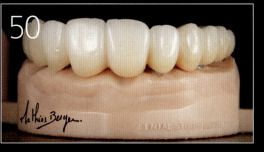

Layered ceramic partial denture on a zirconia framework in its final stage in the laboratory (CZR ceramic) (Berger Laboratory).

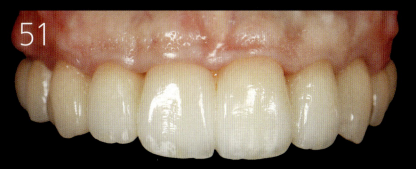

Final partial denture in the mouth on the day of placement.

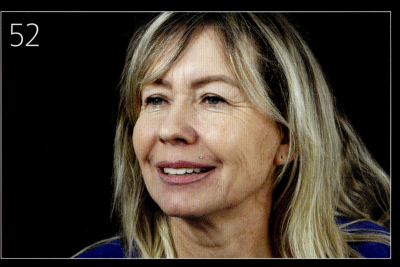

Three-quarter view of the face showing the integration of the prosthesis.

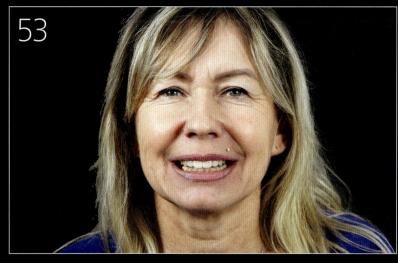

Frontal facial photograph showing the integration of the prosthesis.

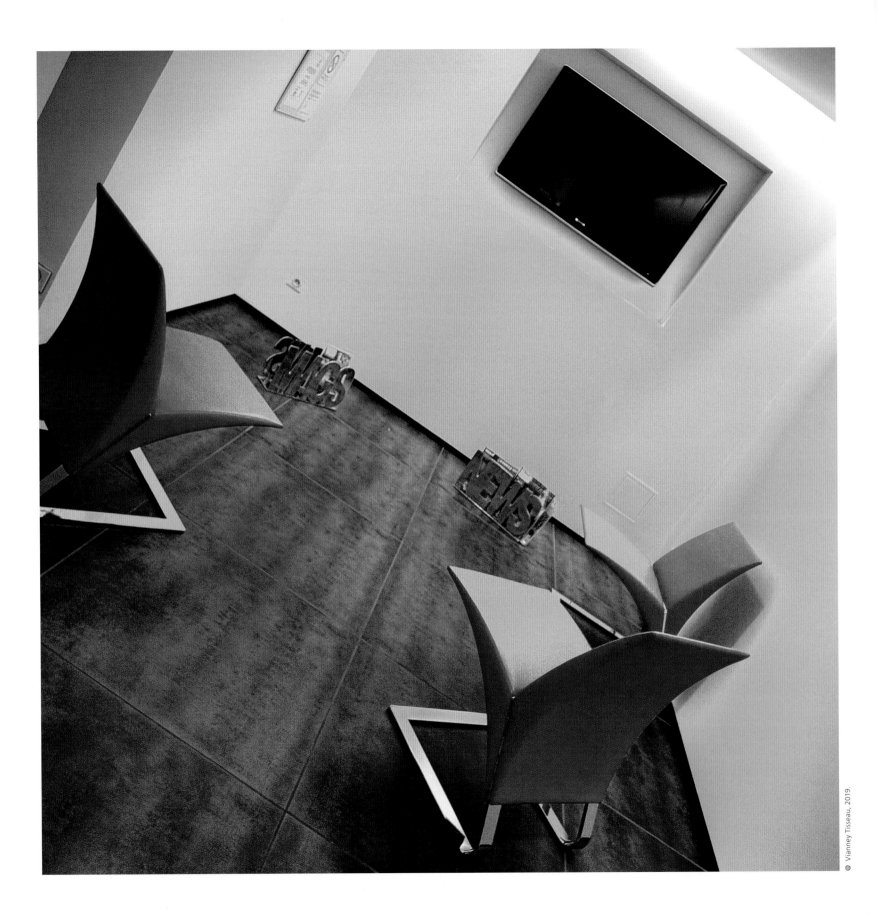

© Vianney Tisseau, 2019.

Full-arch clinical case 33

31-year-old woman.

Clinical data

- After facing some difficult personal events, this patient wished to take care of herself and her health. She wanted to restore functional and efficient chewing and rehabilitate her smile.
- The first consultation at the office took place in October 2021.
- No vertical bone loss observed.
- Correct mucogingival architecture. Hygiene to be modified.

Presurgical treatments

- Optical impression taken using a Trios 4 (3Shape, Copenhagen, Denmark) and 3D examination performed using a 3Shape X1.
- Planning using Implant Studio (3Shape).
- Placement of Straumann TLX SP NT implants (Basel, Switzerland) in 12 and 22, and RT in 16, 14, 24, and 26.
- 3D printing of the guide designed in Implant Studio (Dentitek Laboratory).
- Straumann T-socket, self-locking.
- Temporary partial denture milled in polymethylmetylacrylate (PMMA) (Ivotion Dent Multi, Ivoclar VIvadent, Schaan, Liechentenstein) (Dentitek Laboratory) on a shade A3 base.

Assessment of the intervention

- Case treated in the office in **three appointments** (esthetic analysis, placement of a temporary partial denture for esthetic and functional validation, implant surgery). The appointments to check the provisional partial denture for esthetic and functional validation and the implant osseointegration were not counted.

Additional treatments

- The patient wanted complete removable maxillary and mandibular appliances. Due to her young age and difficult personal history, we persuaded her to have a fixed implant-prosthetic rehabilitation. Treatment was performed during a CampusHB training course, with the placement of six implants and an **immediate loading** partial denture for 12 teeth in September 2022.
- The patient wanted to keep the immediate loaded temporary maxillary partial denture for as long as possible before the final ceramic partial denture was fabricated. She wished to treat the mandible first for financial reasons. Mandibular treatment in progress at the office involving removal of carious lesions, devitalization of tooth 31, and placing 34 to 44 under a partial denture.

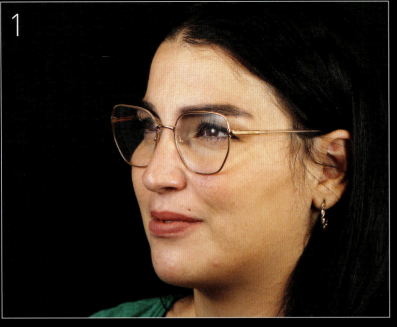

Three-quarter view of the patient's face at rest.

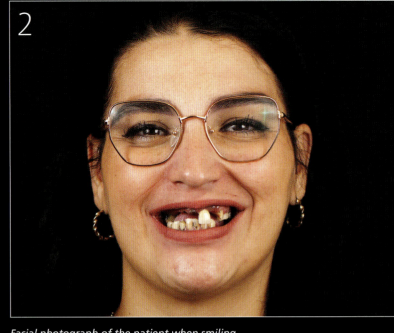

Facial photograph of the patient when smiling.

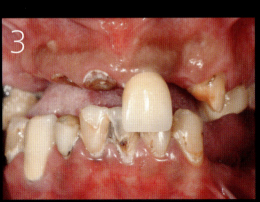

Front view of the initial clinical situation with both arches in occlusion.

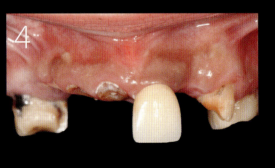

Frontal view of the maxilla.

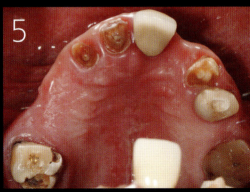

Occlusal view of the maxilla. Note the vestibular bone concavity in the area of 22, which needed to be treated to restore a favorable gingival architecture compatible with easy brushing.

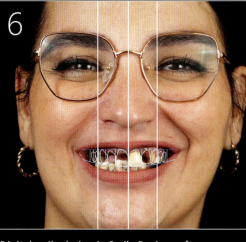

Digital smile design in Smile Design software (3Shape, Copenhagen, Denmark) with a photograph of the patient's smile in frontal view. The digital dental contours correspond to the prosthetic design. The analysis of the digital smile design was used to validate the position and volume of the dental crown in 21.

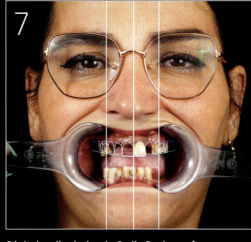

Digital smile design in Smile Design software with a photograph of the patient with a retractor in frontal view. Tooth 21 was used as a reference for the new smile design.

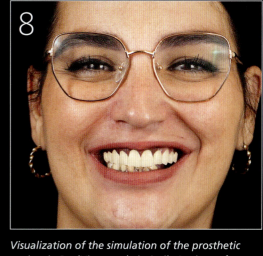

Visualization of the simulation of the prosthetic project in RealView mode in Smile Design software. The patient validated the esthetic setup.

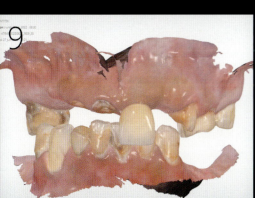

The patient's digital impressions with the arches in occlusion. The digital impressions and the design of the patient's smile were sent to the prosthetic laboratory to create the temporary partial denture for esthetic and functional validation (Dentitek Laboratory).

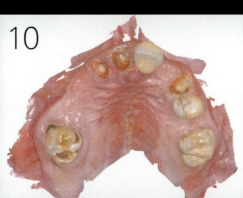

Visualization of the maxillary digital impression corresponding to the initial situation. The digital impressions were taken with a Trios 4 optical camera (3Shape).

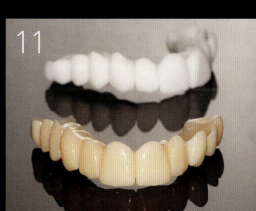

Esthetic and functional validation provisional partial denture and its radiopaque duplicate partial denture. Both partial dentures were milled in the Dentitek Laboratory and the provisional partial denture was made from polymethylmethacrelate (PMMA) (Ivotion Dent Multi, Ivoclar Vivadent).

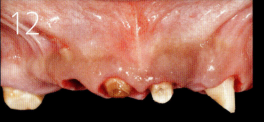

12 Frontal view of the maxilla and teeth trimmed for implant planning and placement of the provisional partial denture for esthetic and functional validation. The porcelain-fused-to-metal crowns and inlays were removed and the teeth were trimmed to remove all undercuts.

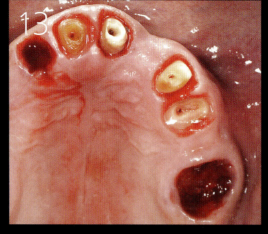

13 Occlusal view of the maxilla prepared for implant planning. Teeth 12 and 26 were extracted because they were future implant sites and a healing socket was desired to increase the primary stability of these implants during implant surgery. The remaining teeth were retained to provide sufficient dental support for the future surgical guide and stability for the esthetic and functional validation partial denture.

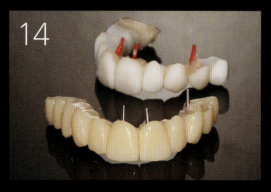

14 Visualization of the esthetically and functionally validated temporary partial denture and its radiopaque duplicate, relined and fitted. The provisional partial denture was fitted to the vital teeth using a self-curing resin reline and to the non-vital teeth using metal posts. For the radiopaque partial denture, the posts were temporary made of plastic to limit the presence of metal artefacts with the CBCT.

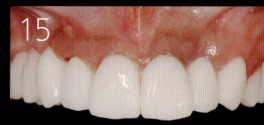

15 Frontal view of the radiopaque partial denture adapted and kept in the mouth while the information was gathered for implant planning.

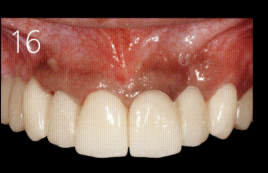

16 Frontal view of the esthetic and functional validation temporary partial denture fitted and cemented in the mouth with a self-curing temporary cement made from zinc oxide and eugenol (Temp-Bond, Kerr Dental, Brea, CA, USA).

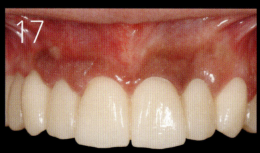

17 Photograph at 15 days after placement of the temporary partial denture. Note the gingival healing of the extraction areas and the good periodontal integration of the temporary partial denture.

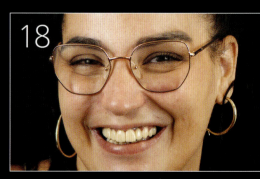

18 Facial photograph of the patient with the esthetic and functional validation provisional partial denture to assess its esthetic integration. The patient validated the esthetic setup.

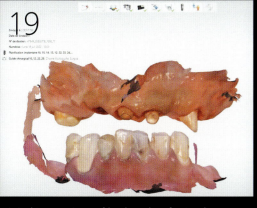

Digital impressions of both arches for implant planning, taken using a Trios 4.

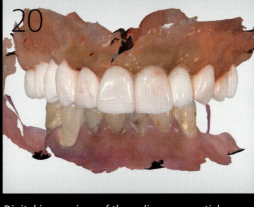

Digital impressions of the radiopaque partial denture and the antagonist arch in occlusion.

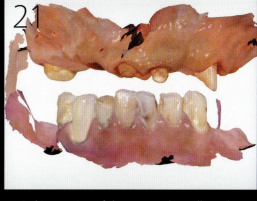

Digital impression of the prepared maxilla with gingival healing of the first-line extraction areas. The interarch relationship without the radiopaque partial denture and the antagonist arch were preserved by the software. Thus, the dental technician had all the information necessary to create the temporary partial denture for instant loading.

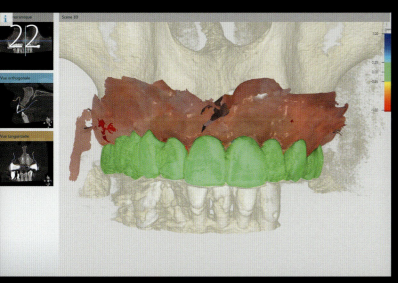

Implant Studio software window in the surfacing step between the stereolithography (STL) file of the optical impression with the radiopaque partial denture in place and the DICOM file of the CBCT acquisition.

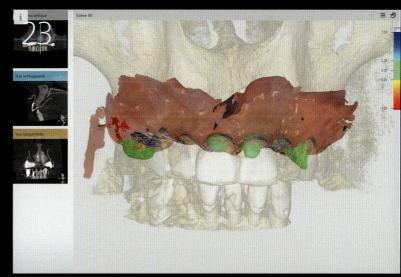

Validation of the surfacing between the STL file of the optical impression without the radiopaque partial denture and the DICOM file of the CBCT acquisition. The few remaining teeth and their low coronal height made it essential to use the radiopaque partial denture to obtain accurate and

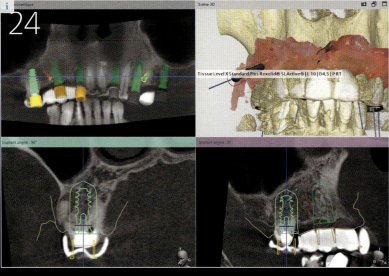

Planning for the implant in zone 16 in Implant Studio software: Straumann SP TLX RT 4.5 x 10.0 mm (Basel, Switzerland). The planning complied with the 3D positioning rules for an extraction and immediate implantation situation.

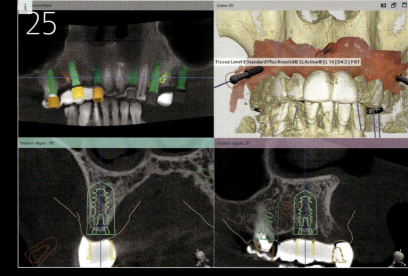

Planning for the implant in zone 14 in Implant Studio software: Straumann SP TLX RT 4.5 x 10.0 mm.

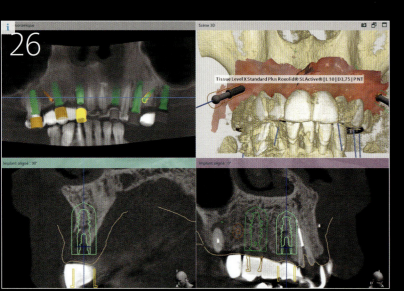

Planning for the implant in zone 12 in Implant Studio software: Straumann SP TLX NT 3.75 x 10.00 mm. Note the planning of buccal GBR to be performed during implant surgery at an early implant site with developing osteoid tissue.

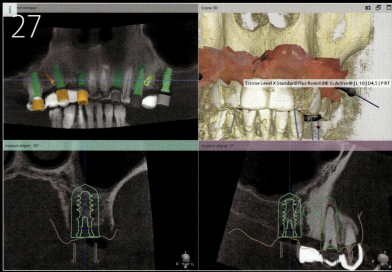

Planning for the implant in zone 26 in Implant Studio software: Straumann SP TLX RT 4.5 x 10.0 mm.

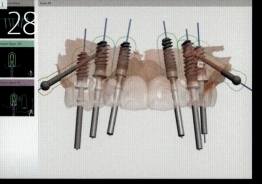

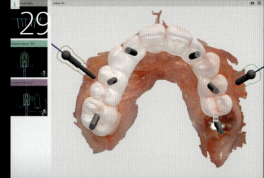

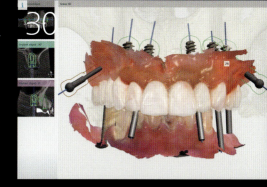

Planning for the six implants as well as the stabilization wedges for the surgical guide.

Visualization of the implant axes in occlusal view. The implant axis, and thus the future screw holes, respected the prosthetic project and were centered on its occlusal surface.

Visualization of the planning of the six implants, their implant axes, the prosthetic design, and the antagonist arch in Implant Studio. The design of the surgical guide was performed in the laboratory in Implant Studio.

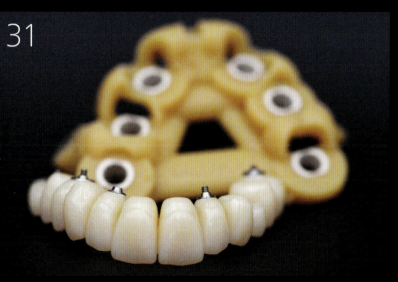

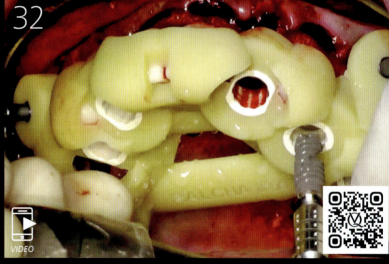

Surgical guide and **immediate loading** partial denture with the Variobases (Straumann) already bonded to the partial denture before surgery (Multilink Hybrid Abutment, Ivoclar Vivadent). The surgical guide was 3D printed while the instant loading partial denture was milled in PMMA (Dentitek Laboratory).

Video of the instant loading surgery. Guided drilling and placement of the implant in 24, vertical positionning at H4. Note the use of self-locking T-sockets made of polyetheretherketone (PEEK), but also the employment of spoons or drilling handles for Straumann TL implants to reduce retention between spoons and sockets (drilling handles for TLX implants are also self-locking). In guided implant surgery, we do not want any mechanical stress or deformation of the surgical guide, so the drilling handles must be stable in the sockets, but without self-locking retention. Note the implant in the 12-zone that had too little primary stability to be loaded and therefore connected to the instant loading partial denture.

The Quokka protocol

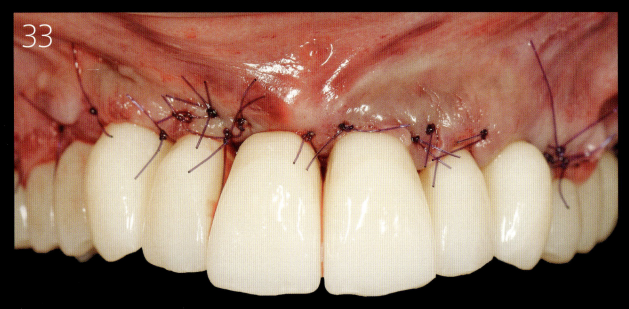

Frontal view of the postoperative situation, ASAF sutures with 6/0 monofilament.

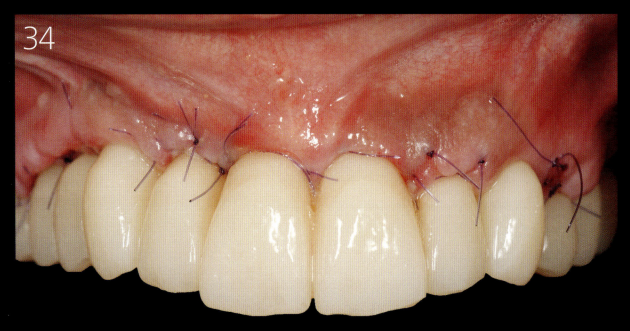

Photograph taken at 7 days post-surgery.

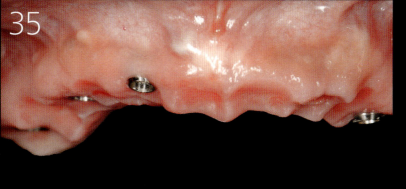

Three-month postoperative photograph. Vestibular view of gingival healing after removal of the instantaneous loading partial denture.

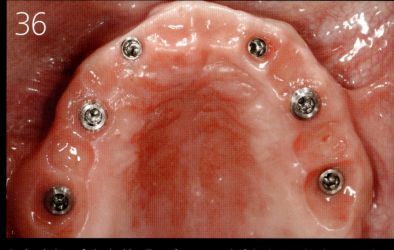

Occlusal view of gingival healing after removal of the instant loading partial denture. Note the implant and pontic beds and their absence of gingival inflammation, and the reconstruction of the vestibular volume in the 22 zone, restoring harmonious vestibular arch rounding.

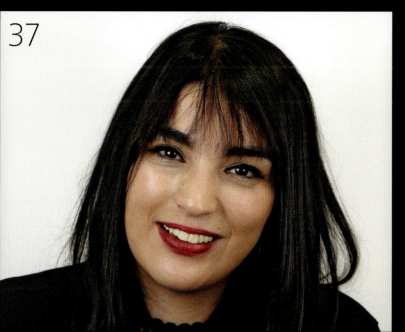

Esthetic integration of the instantaneous loading prosthesis with the face.

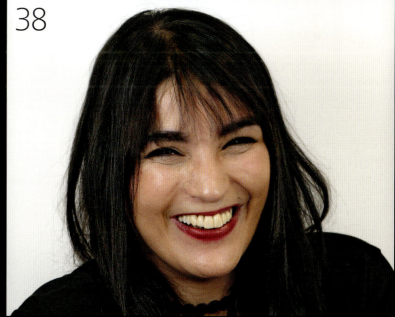

Esthetic integration of the instantaneous loading prosthesis with the face with a forced smile.

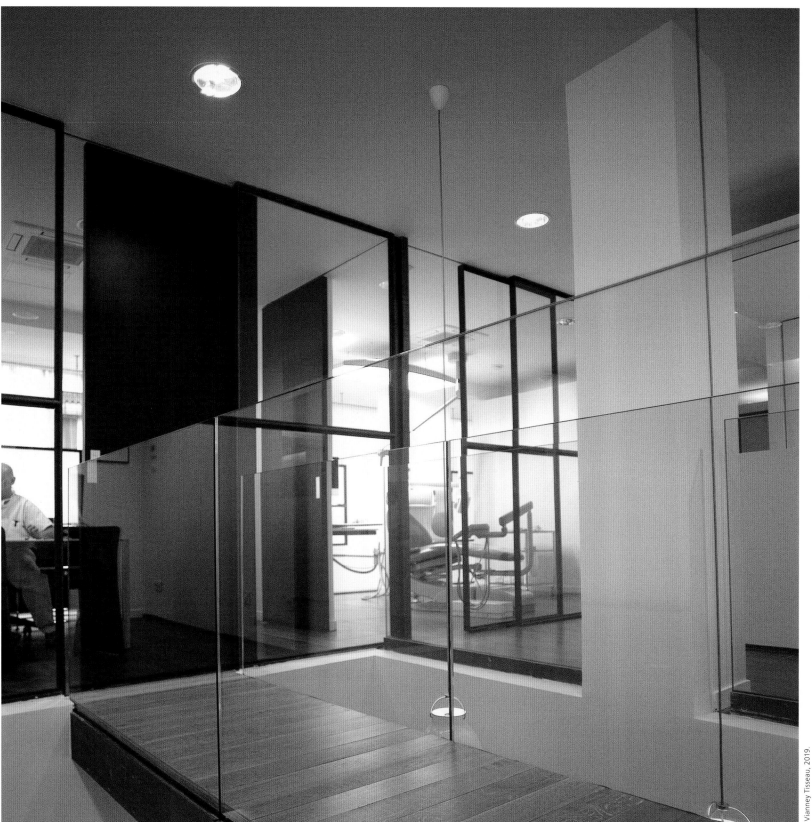

© Vianney Tisseau, 2019.

Full-arch clinical case 34

59-year-old man.

Clinical data

- This patient wanted a fixed maxillary solution to replace his removable partial denture that he had been wearing for 15 years and that he could no longer stand. Indeed, the teeth supporting the brackets of the appliance displayed terminal mobility, which made chewing painful and compromised the effective performance of his appliance.
- First consultation at the office in September 2021.
- Significant vertical bone loss observed in the upper right posterior area due to teeth mobility.
- Correct mucogingival architecture. Hygiene to be modified.

Presurgical treatments

- Optical impression taken using a Trios 4 and 3D examination performed using a 3Shape X1.
- Planning using Implant Studio.
- Placement of Straumann TLX SP RT implants in sites 15, 13, 11, 21, 23, and 25.
- 3D printing of the guide designed in Implant Studio (Dentitek Laboratory).
- Straumann T-socket, self-locking.
- Temporary partial denture milled in PMMA (Dentitek Laboratory) on an A3 shade base.

Assessment of the intervention

- Case treated in the office in **three appointments** (esthetic analysis, placement of a temporary partial denture for esthetic and functional validation, implant surgery). The appointment to validate the provisional partial denture for esthetic and functional performance and to check the implant osseointegration were not counted.
- The patient consulted us to consider a complete implant-supported maxillary rehabilitation. All the remaining teeth had terminal mobility, so we opted for a complete implant-prosthetic rehabilitation with six implants for twelve teeth.
- Since the patient was born hard of hearing, his diction was also slightly altered and his upper lip was slightly hypotonic and therefore drooping. As such, lengthening of the incisal free edges was performed between the temporary partial denture for esthetic and functional validation and the partial denture for instant loading.
- In this case, a radiopaque partial denture was not required to perform surfacing between the digital impression and the 3D examination, but given the change in the prosthetic project, it had to be validated prior to the immediate loading surgery.

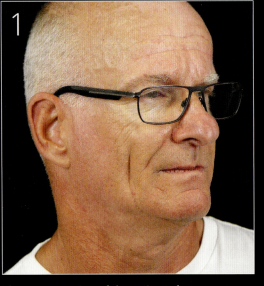

Three-quarter view of the patient's face at rest.

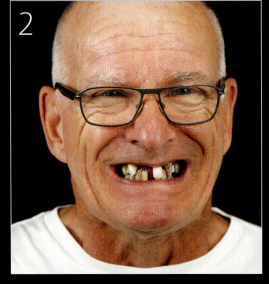

Facial photograph of the patient when smiling.

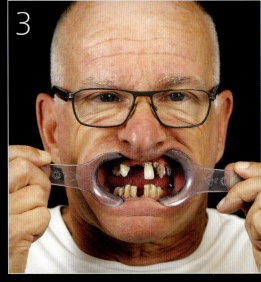

Frontal facial photograph of the patient with a retractor.

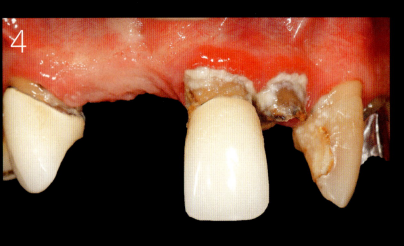

Frontal view of the maxilla. Hygiene instructions as well as scaling and polishing of the teeth were performed.

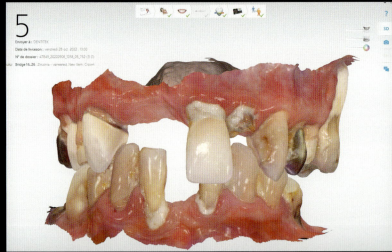

Visualization of the maxillary and mandibular digital impressions in occlusion corresponding to the initial clinical situation. The digital impressions were taken with a Trios 4 optical camera.

Chapter 6 - Full-arch clinical applications

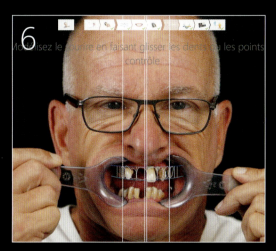

Digital smile design in Smile Design software with the frontal view of the patient with a retractor. The digital dental contours corresponded to the prosthetic design.

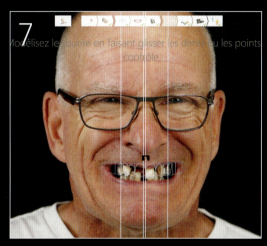

Digital smile design in Smile Design software with the frontal photograph of the patient smiling.

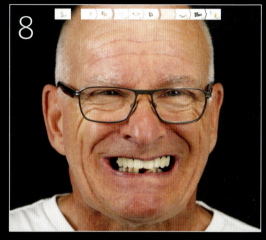

Visualization of the simulation of the prosthetic project in RealView mode in Smile Design software.

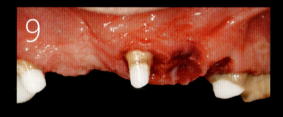

Frontal view of the maxilla and the teeth cut for implant planning and placement of the provisional partial denture for esthetic and functional validation. The porcelain-fused-to-metal crowns and inlays were removed, and a coronal reconstruction with a fiberglass post was performed on teeth 16, 13, 21, and 24 (core-X flow, Denstply Sirona, Charlotte, NC, USA), and tooth 26 was trimmed to support the partial denture.

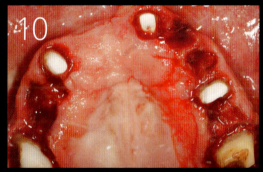

Occlusal view of the maxilla prepared for implant planning. Teeth 14, 15, 22, 23, and 25 were extracted. The remaining teeth were retained to provide sufficient dental support for the future surgical guide and stability for the esthetic and functional validation partial denture. Note the concavity of the maxilla in the area of 11.

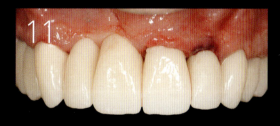

Vestibular view of the provisional esthetic and functional validation partial denture relined and fitted in the mouth.

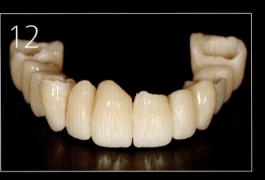

Frontal view of the esthetic and functional validation temporary partial denture, milled and fabricated in PMMA in the Dentitek Laboratory.

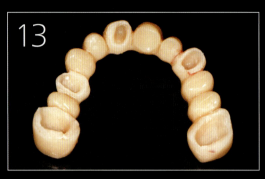

Intrados view of the esthetic and functional validation temporary partial denture with the areas of succinct relining with autopolymerizing resin (Unifast TRAD, GC Europe, Leuven, Belgium).

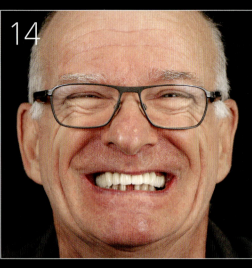

Facial photograph of the patient with the provisional partial denture for esthetic and functional validation to assess its esthetic integration. The patient wished to extend the length of his incisors, which he considered too discreet during phonation due to the hypotonicity of the upper lip.

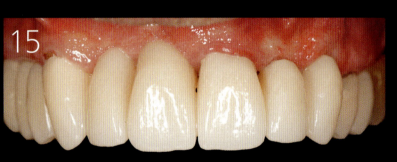

Photograph at 7 days after placement of the temporary partial denture. Note the gingival healing of the extraction areas, the good periodontal integration of the temporary partial denture, and the patient's good compliance with the brushing instructions given.

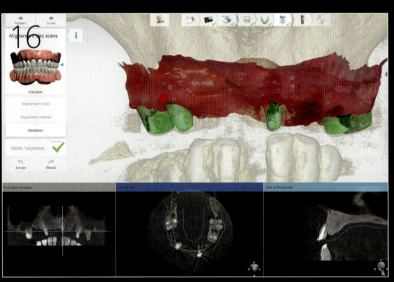

Surfacing step between the STL file of the optical impression of the maxilla in place and the DICOM file of the CBCT acquisition in Implant Studio.

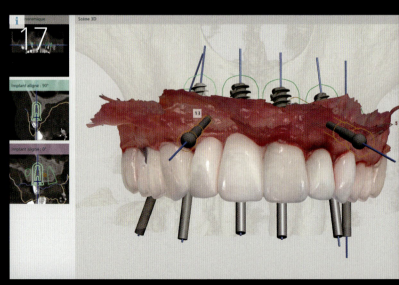

Overall visualization of implant planning and the modified prosthetic project (1-mm increase in the height of the clinical crown of the incisivocanine block).

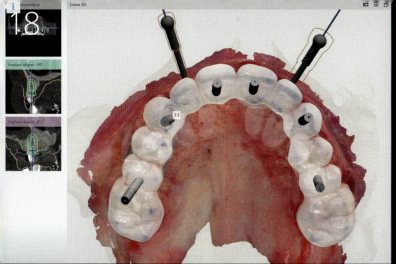

Visualization of the implant axes in occlusal view. The implant axis respected the prosthetic plan and the future screw holes were centered on the occlusal surface.

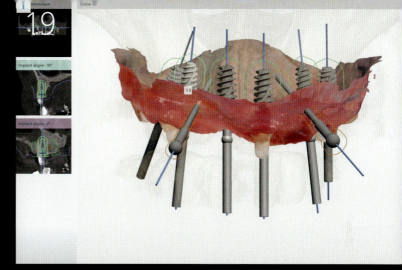

Planning of the six implants as well as the stabilization wedges for the surgical guide.

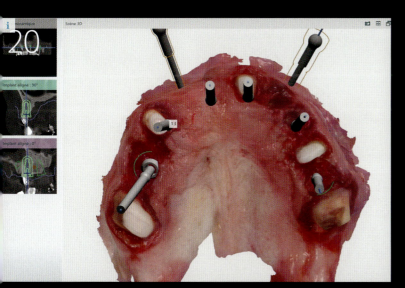

Occlusal view of the six implants and the stabilizing wedges for the surgical guide without the prosthetic design tracing. Teeth 13 and 21 were extracted during instant loading surgery as they were future implant sites. These teeth were not extracted earlier because there was not enough dental support for the stability of the provisional partial denture for esthetic and functional validation

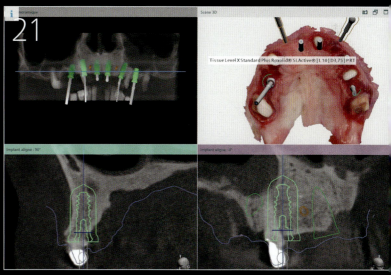

Planning for the implant in zone 13 in Implant Studio: Straumann SP TLX RT 3.75 x 10.00 mm.

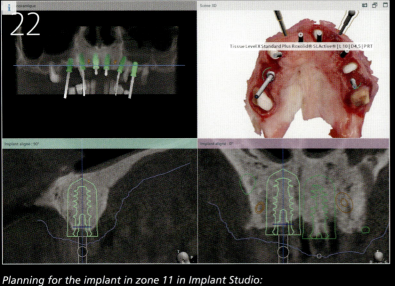

Planning for the implant in zone 11 in Implant Studio: Straumann SP TLX RT 4.5 x 10.0 mm. Note the very high bone density in the maxilla.

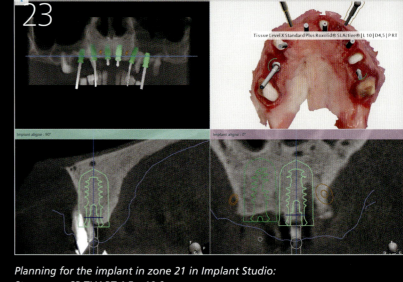

Planning for the implant in zone 21 in Implant Studio: Straumann SP TLX RT 4.5 x 10.0 mm.

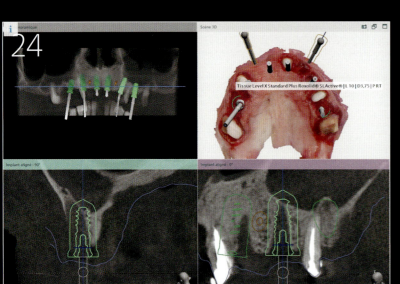

Planning for the implant in zone 23 in Implant Studio: Straumann SP TLX RT 3.75 x 10.00 mm.

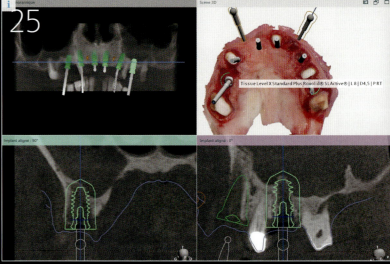

Planning for the implant in zone 25 in Implant Studio: Straumann SP TLX RT 4.5 x 8.0 mm.

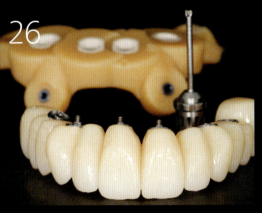

Surgical guide and **immediate loading** partial denture with the Variobases already bonded to the partial denture before surgery (Multilink Hybrid Abutment). The surgical guide was 3D printed and the instant loading partial denture was milled in PMMA (Dentitek Laboratory).

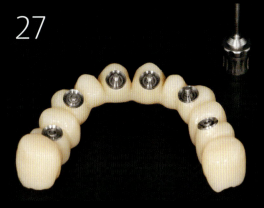

View of the pontic supports and the screw-retained implant abutments bonded to the provisional **immediate loading** partial denture before implant surgery.

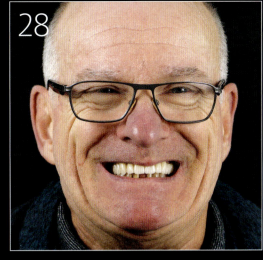

Facial photograph of the patient taken just before immediate loading surgery.

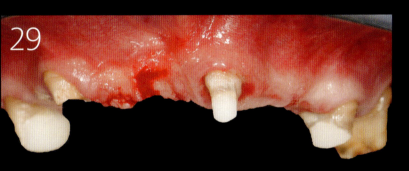

Frontal view of the maxilla after removal of the temporary partial denture.

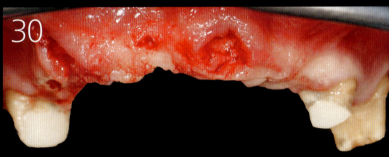

Frontal view of the maxilla and extractions of teeth 13 and 21.

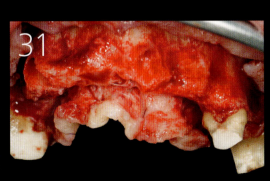

Frontal view of the maxillary bone situation after the vestibular and palatal flaps were removed. The remaining teeth 16, 24, and 26 were used to support the surgical guide.

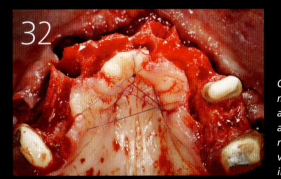

Occlusal view of the maxillary bone situation after the vestibular and palatal flaps were removed. Note the vestibular bone concavity in the area of 11.

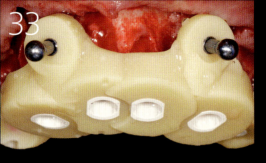

Frontal view of the surgical guide positioned on the supporting teeth and stabilized by the two wedges.

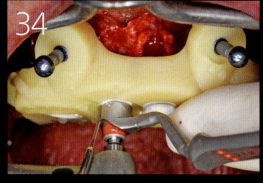

Guided drilling in the 11 zone using a 3-mm reduction drill handle and a 3.5-mm diameter guided drill bit.

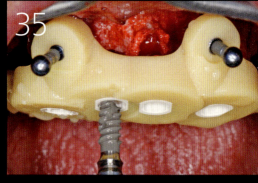

Visualization of the Straumann SP TLX RT 4.5 x 10.0 mm implant and its guided gripper.

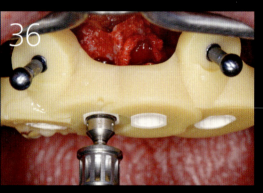

Visualization of the vertical burial of the guided implant. The vertical positioning was determined by the H6 mark on the guided gripper.

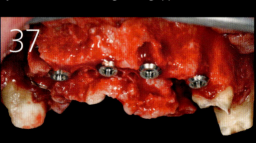

Frontal view of the six guided implants. Note the good vertical burial of the implants based on the existing bone crest and the implant planning.

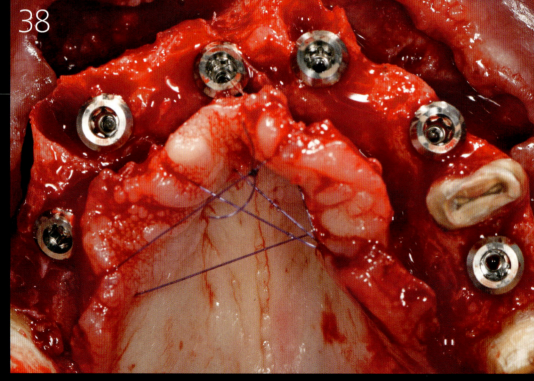

Occlusal view of the six guided implants. Note the vestibular bone concavity opposite 11.

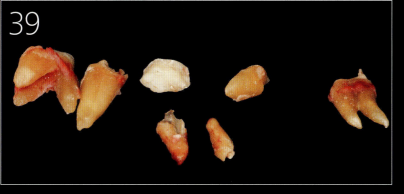

Photograph of the final teeth extracted.

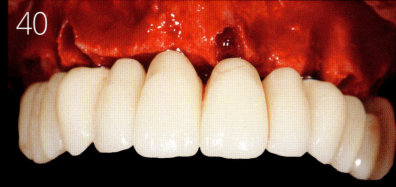

Frontal view of the **immediate loading** temporary partial denture screwed onto the six implants.

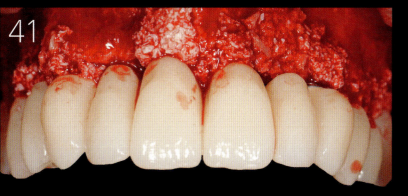

Compensatory GBR on extraction hiatuses around implants and ridge preservation in pontic alveoli. DBBM (Bio-Oss with fine particles, Geistlich) incubated in the F2 fraction of plasma (plasma rich in growth factors [PRGF], Endoret BTI).

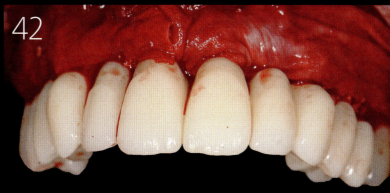

Covering of vestibular bone fillings with a resorbable collagen membrane (Bio-Gide, Geistlich).

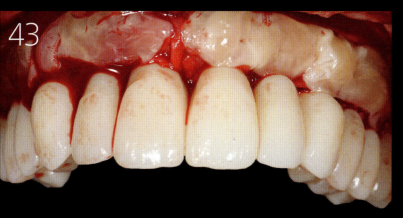

Covering of the assembly with a fibrin membrane from the F1 fraction of the plasma.

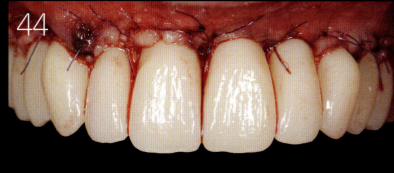

Postoperative photograph. Prosthesis-guided flap suture using ASAF sutures.

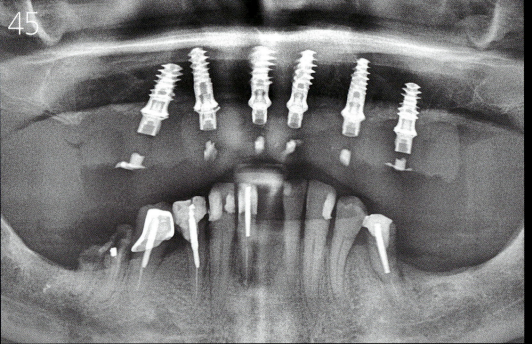

Postoperative panoramic radiograph. Note the offset between the implant neck and the abutment in 13, which was due to the high bone density that caused the implate to deviate slightly in the postextraction socket in 13. This discrepancy had no consequence or clinical significance on implant osseointegration or gingival maturation compared to the comfort and benefit of **immediate loading**. Tightening was performed on the other five implants.

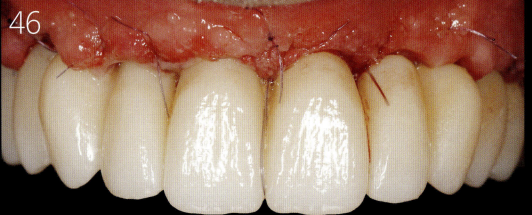

Photograph at 7 days after implant surgery.

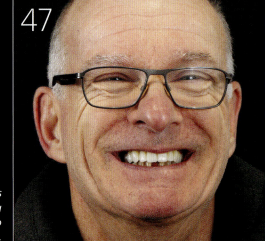

Photograph of the patient's smile 7 days after implant surgery. Note the lengthening of the free incisor edges compared to the initial prosthetic plan.

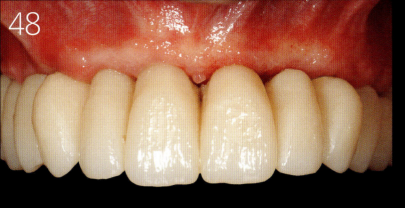

Clinical situation 3 months after the implant surgery with immediate loading. This photograph was taken after maintenance with EMS Airflow Powder Plus. Oral hygiene instructions were given.

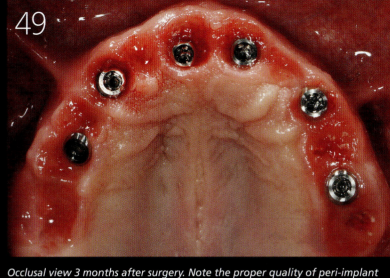

Occlusal view 3 months after surgery. Note the proper quality of peri-implant tissues with very limited inflammation.

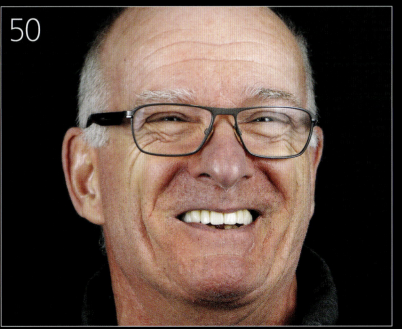

Correct esthetic integration of the immediately loaded bridge.

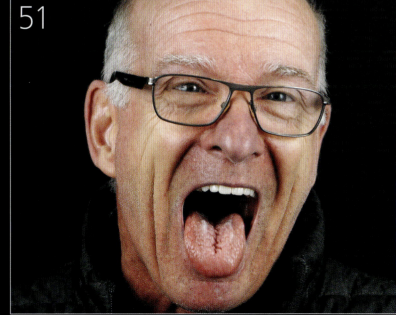

Relaxed patient during the photo session.

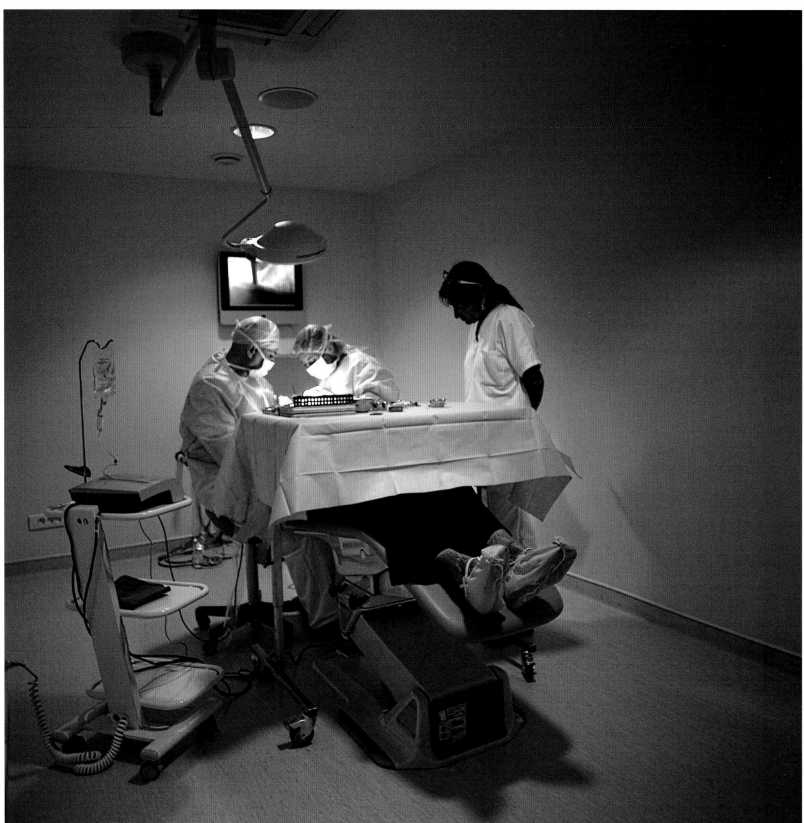

© Vianney Tisseau, 2019.

Full-arch clinical case 35

58-year-old woman.

Clinical data

- This patient was referred to the practice for fixed maxillary and mandibular implant supported rehabilitations.
- Case treated in September 2022.
- Suitable bone context (vertical but homogeneous loss, horizontal loss that was compensable during GBR surgery).
- Favorable mucogingival architecture.

Presurgical treatments

- Optical impression taken using a Trios 4 and 3D examination performed using a 3Shape X1.
- Planning using Implant Studio.
- Placement of Straumann TLX NT 3.75 x 12.00 mm implants in 32 and 42, NT 3.75 x 10.00 mm implant in 34, RT 3.75 x 10.00 mm implant in 44, and RT 4.5 x 10.00 mm implants in 36 and 46.
- 3D printing of the guide designed in Implant Studio, printed in the office on a NextDent 5100 (Soesterberg, The Netherlands) with NextDent SG resin and polymerized in an LC-3D 3D polymerization unit.
- Straumann T-sockets.
- Temporary partial denture milled in PMMA (Dentitek Laboratory) on a shade A2 base.

Assessment of the intervention

- Case treated in the office in **five appointments** (esthetic analysis, partial denture for validation, planning elements after validation, implant surgery, implant control at 3 months).
- The patient came to the office considering a complete maxillary and mandibular r implant-supported rehabilitation. She had suffered from significant edentulism the last 4 years; however, the neuromuscular pattern was good, but she needed to be re-educated to simply having proper teeth volumes and neuromuscular deprogramming had to be performed. We began with **immediate** loading in the mandible to remove the partial denture. Three days after loading, we placed a nocturnal muscle deprogramming splint to help the patient integrate the fixed mandibular denture. The **immediate loading of** the maxillary denture is due to be performed in summer 2023. The final prostheses can be made separately in time for financial reasons.

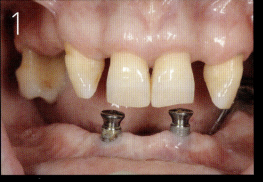
Initial clinical frontal view.

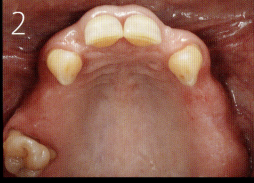
Clinical occlusal view of the maxilla.

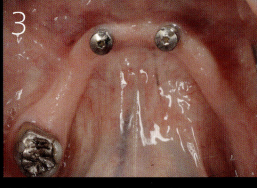
Clinical occlusal view of the mandible.

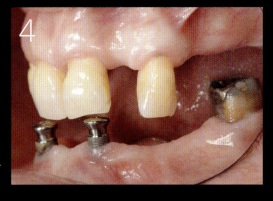
Clinical view of the left lateral bite.

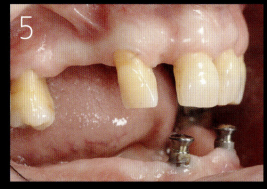
Clinical view of the right lateral bite.

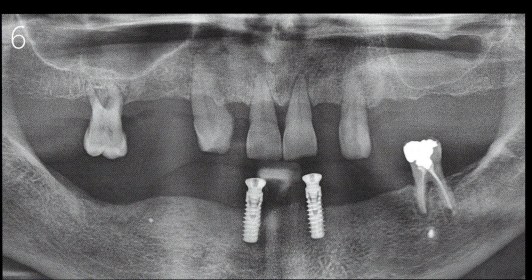
Panoramic radiograph of the initial clinical situation.

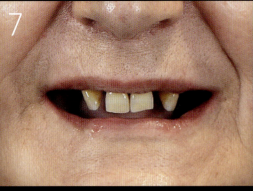

Photograph of the face required for esthetic analysis: the smile.

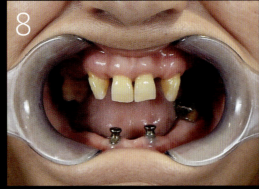

Photograph required for esthetic analysis: the view with retractor.

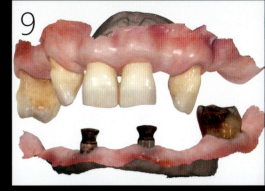

Intraoral digital impression taken with a Trios 4 in addition to the esthetic analysis.

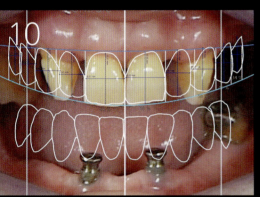

Smile design in the Smile Design module of Trios 4.

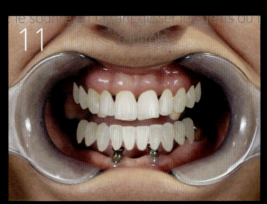

Esthetic simulation in the Smile Design module.

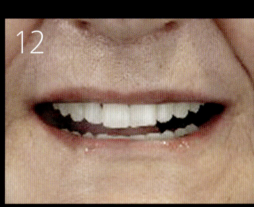

Esthetic rendering in RealView in the software.

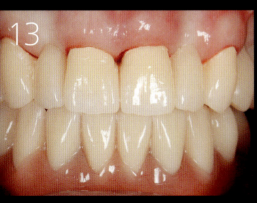

Esthetic and functional validation temporary partial denture in place in the maxilla combined with a validation RPD in the mandible.

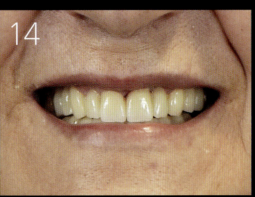

Analysis and validation photograph of the proposed esthetic project.

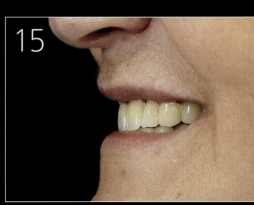

Profile picture for esthetic analysis of the proposed project.

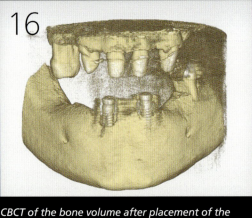

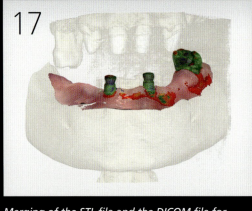

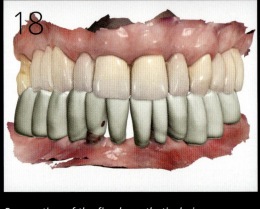

CBCT of the bone volume after placement of the esthetic and functional validation partial denture. One session was dedicated to performing the 3D examination and taking an intraoral digital impression of the situation created with the provisional partial denture to carry out planning. This remote session allowed us to ensure the patient was satisfied with the proposed prosthetic project.

Merging of the STL file and the DICOM file for implant planning in Implant Studio. The existing dental and implant surfaces in the mandible were sufficient for merging the files without using a radiopaque partial denture. Note the colorimetric index for assessing the accuracy of the mergers.

Preparation of the fixed prosthetic design in Implant Studio for implant planning.

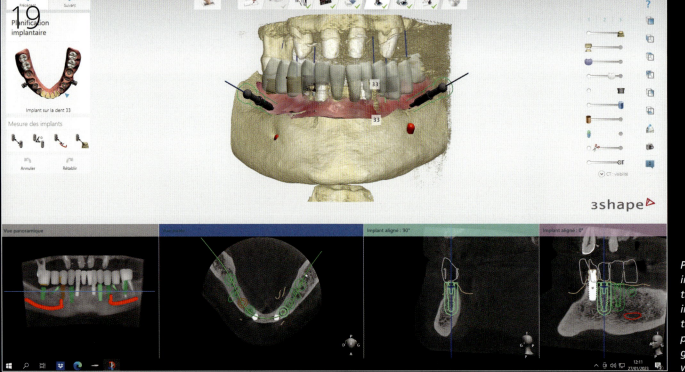

Planning of the six implants based on the prosthetic project in accordance with the bone volume, and planning of two lateral guide stabilization wedges.

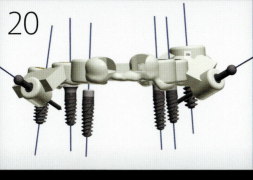

Preparation of the guide after planning and presentation of the guide without the bone and gingival filter.

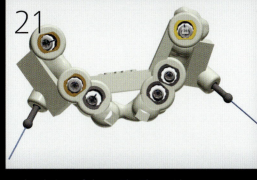

Occlusal view of the guide. The guide was to be supported by the two implant screws before the removal of these implants and by the two lateral wedges.

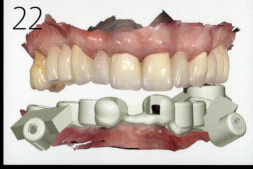

Frontal view of the guide with the two inspection windows on the implant screws.

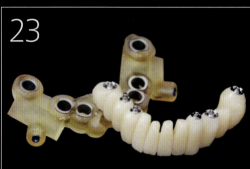

Printed surgical guide and immediate loading partial denture milled before surgery.

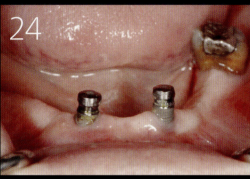

Clinical situation at the beginning of surgery.

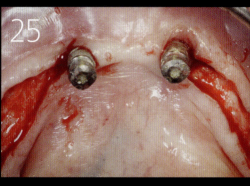

Posterior incision of the full-thickness implants to expose the bony crests. The crestal support was retained between the two implants to stabilize the guide.

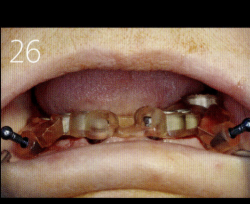

The guide in place stabilized by mucosal support and support on the countersunk screw heads and the two posterior wedges.

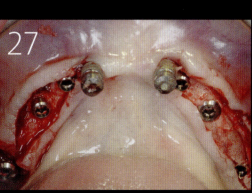

Occlusal view of placement of the six implants after removal of the guide.

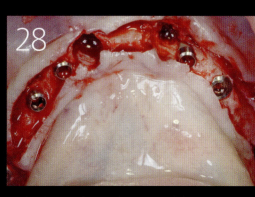

Occlusal view after explantation of the two implants and removal of the full-thickness flap in the anterior region.

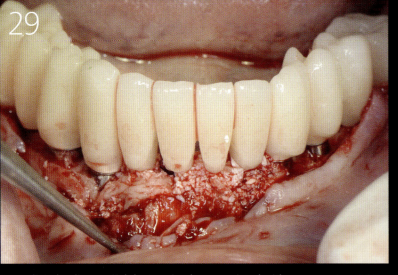

Immediate loading partial denture in place associated with compensatory GBR in the implant placement sites and around the implant emergence profiles. The GBR was performed with DBBM (Bio-Oss) incubated in the F2 fraction of plasma.

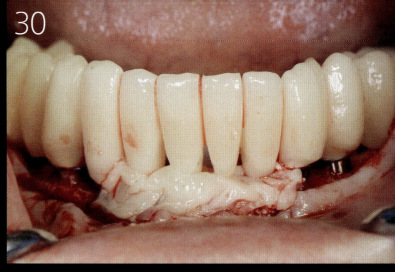

Covering with a fibrin membrane made from PRGF.

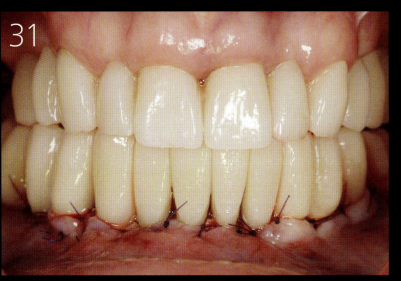

Clinical view at the end of surgery with the flaps sutured with ASAF sutures guided by the prosthesis. Note the precise occlusion of the instant partial denture fabricated made before surgery.

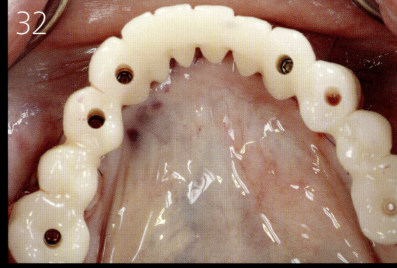

Clinical occlusal view of the screw-retained partial denture in place.

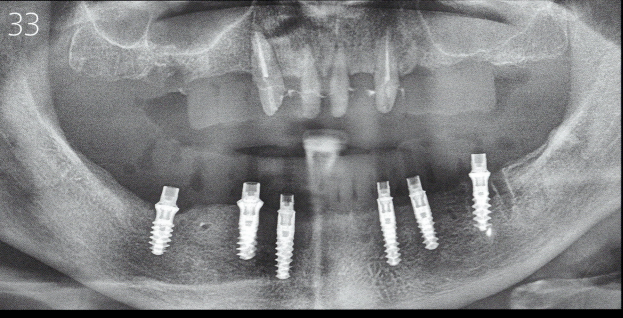

Postoperative panoramic radiograph.

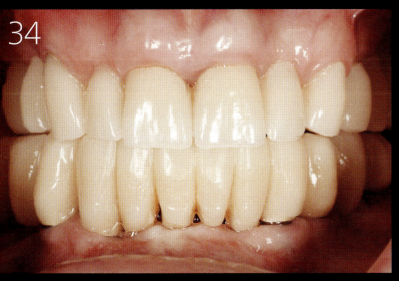

Clinical situation at 3 months postoperatively.

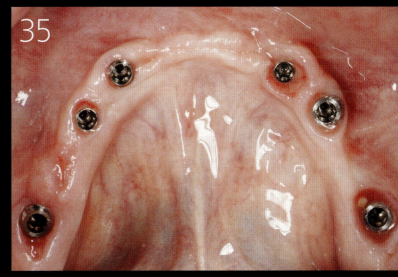

Clinical occlusal view of the implant emergence profiles after removal of the immediate loading partial denture.

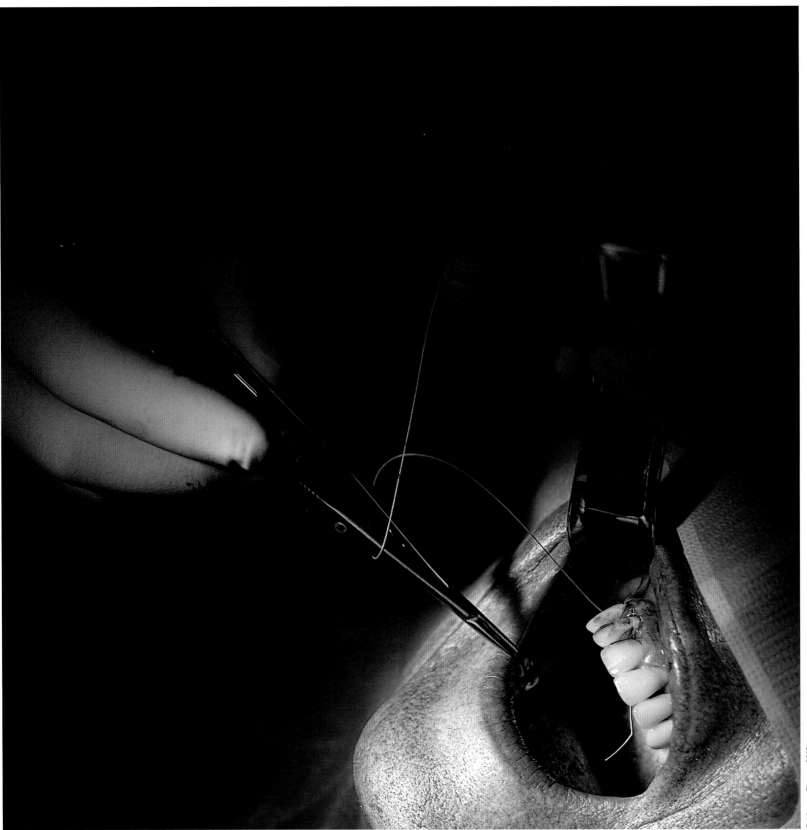

© Vianney Tisseau, 2019.

Full-arch clinical case 36

55-year-old man.

Clinical data

- This patient was referred to the office by a colleague for a fixed maxillary rehabilitation using the Quokka protocol. The colleague will deliver the final prosthesis and take care of the mandibular implant-prosthetic rehabilitation.
- Case treated in October 2022.
- Complex bone context (heterogeneous vertical loss, voluminous sinus).
- Complex mucogingival architecture because heterogeneous in a context of poor initial hygiene.

Presurgical treatments

- Optical impression taken using Trios 4 and 3D examination performed using a 3Shape X1.
- Planning carried out in coDiagnostiX (Dental Wings, Montreal, Canada).
- Placement of Straumann BLX RB 12-mm implants in 13, 12, 22, and 23, and RB 10-mm implants in 15 and 25. Placement of straight 1.5-mm SRA abutments in 12, 22, and 23, 17-degree 3.5-mm SRA abutments in 23 and 25, and 30-degree 3.5-mm SRA abutment in 15.
- 3D printing of the guide designed in coDiagnostiX and printed in the office on a NextDent 5100 with NextDent SG resin and polymerized in a LC-3D 3D polymerization unit.
- Straumann T-sockets.
- Temporary partial denture milled from 15 to 25 PMMA (Dentitek Laboratory) on an A2 shade base and connected to a 4.6-mm SRA Variobase.

Assessment of the intervention

- Case treated in the office in **four appointments** (esthetic analysis, validation partial denture and planning elements, implant surgery, implant control at 3 months).
- The patient consulted the practice for a fixed maxillary solution, aware that the need for multiple extractions had become unavoidable.

The patient was referred by his referring dentist, a general practitioner practicing implantology, for an **immediate loading** protocol. The patient did not want to have a removable prosthesis at any time and was afraid of the operation. Since his sinuses were very large, we opted for an antesinus implant angulation solution to avoid the need for a bone grafting procedure. We used coDiagnostiX software to maintain a fully digital workflow while no longer working directly on TL and TLX implants, but on SRA abutments on BLX implants in order to be able to correct the angulations. Implant Studio does not allow this type of work and forces us to remain in direct connexion to the implants on TL and TLX within the framework of the **immediate** partial denture. coDiagnostiX allows us to apply the Quokka protocol on TL and TLX implants as well as on BL and BLX implants in the full arch. The final partial denture was for 12 teeth, from 16 to 26, so 16 and 26 will be extended.

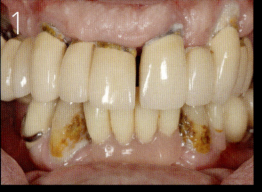
Initial clinical situation in occlusion.

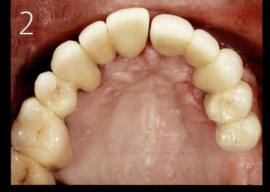
Maxillary occlusal view.

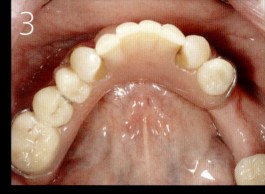
Mandibular occlusal view.

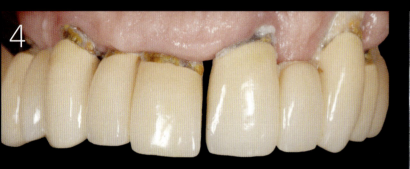
Isolated view of the maxilla showing bone and gingival heterogeneities and the state of dental decay.

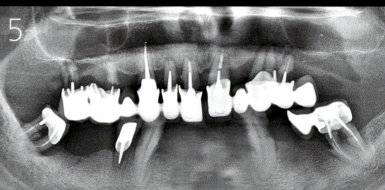
Panoramic radiograph of the initial situation showing the terminal state of the teeth in the maxilla and mandible.

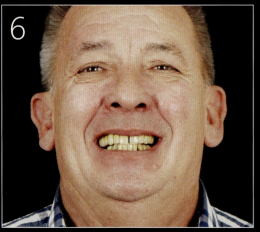
Facial photograph when smiling as part of the esthetic analysis.

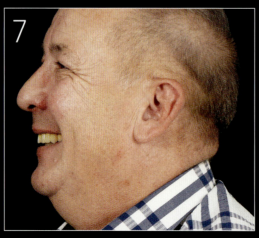
Profile photograph.

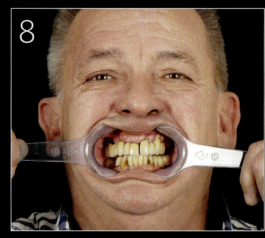
Photograph with a retractor for esthetic analysis.

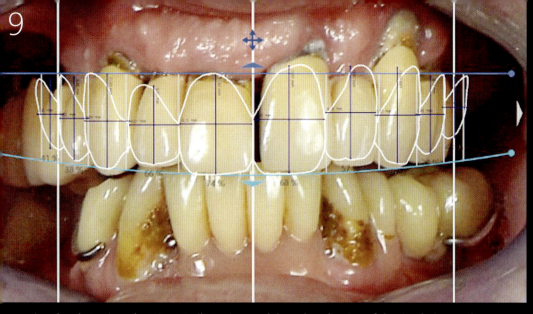

Importing the photos into the Trios 4 Smile Design module and application of the simulation masks.

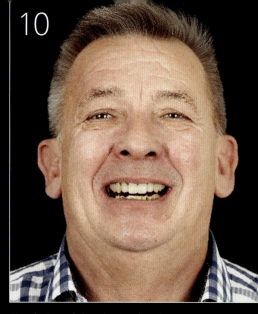

Simulation of the obtained smile.

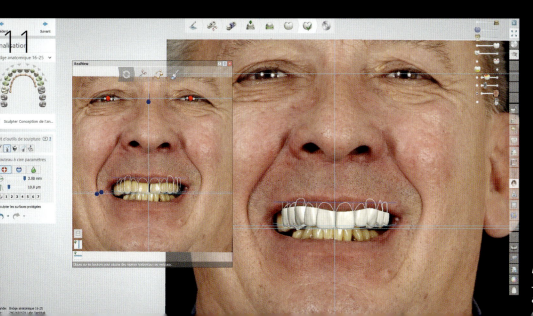

Exporting the module to Dental System, 3Shape laboratory software for esthetic and functional validation partial denture design (Dentitek Laboratory).

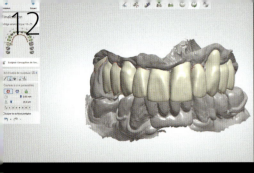

Design for the partial denture on the initial fingerprints.

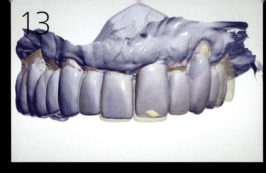

Superposition of the two volumes before and after to analyze the changes.

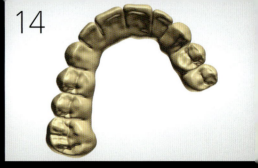

STL file of the esthetic and functional validation temporary partial denture.

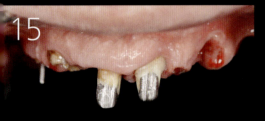

Clinical appearance after removal of the partial denture and extraction of teeth 12 and 23. Tooth 24 was retained as a decayed root to provide minimal support for the esthetically and functionally validated partial denture.

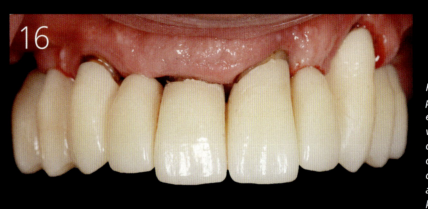

Relining and placement of the esthetic and functional validation partial denture. Extraction of 23 allowed gingival closure and thus achieved a gain of keratinized tissue.

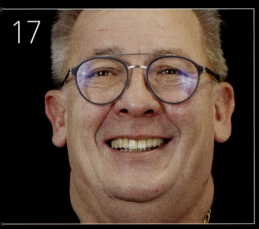

Facial photograph taken a while after placement of the partial denture to evaluate the esthetic integration of the proposed result. The patient was very satisfied with the result. Only slight incisal retouching of 11 and 21 was required to shorten these teeth in response to a request from his wife

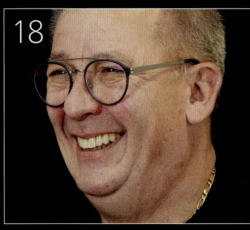

Three-quarter view of the photographic plate.

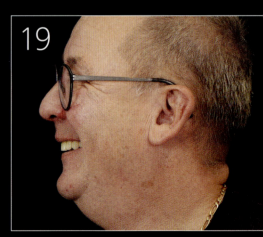

Profile photograph. The patient's comfort was already improved compared to the initial situation for implant surgery.

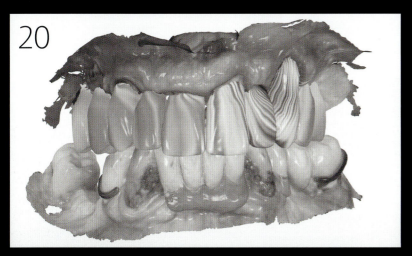

In the same session, we took an intraoral digital impression of the validation partial denture in pre-preparation mode, an impression of the maxilla with the stumps and the antagonist impression associated with the occlusion. This allowed us to create, with the acquisition of the CBCT, the implant plan based on the prosthetic project and the design for the surgical guide on the prepared arch. The STL files were exported to coDiagnostiX (Dental Wings, Montreal, Canada).

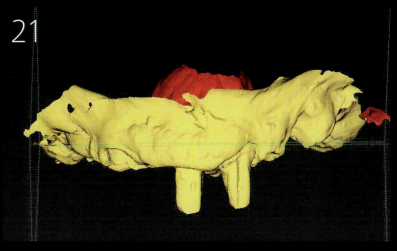

Importation of the STL file of the prepared arch into coDiagnostiX.

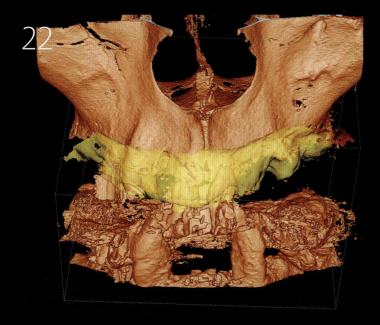

Merging of this STL file with the DICOM file in coDiagnostiX.

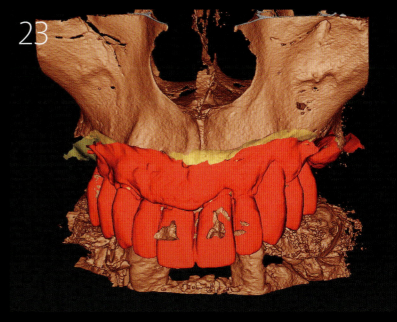

Merging of the pre-preparation STL file representing the prosthetic project with the STL file of the prepared arch and the DICOM bone file.

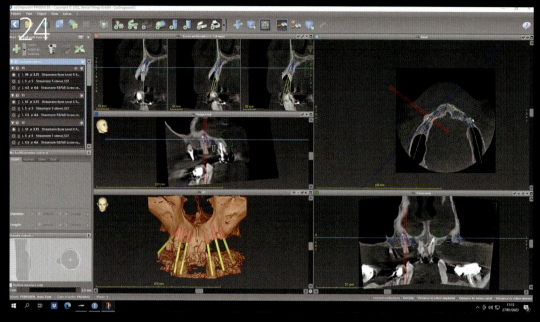

Planning for the six BLX implants in coDiagnostiX.

Enlarged view of the plan for the six implants with their bone ratios.

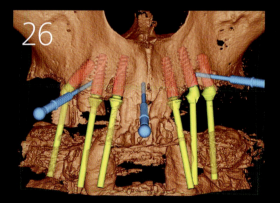

Planning for the three guide stabilization wedges and for the six SRA abutments for axis straightening. This option in coDiagnostiX makes it possible to plan implants with intermediate abutments while remaining in a fully digital workflow. This is not possible in the 3Shape environment.

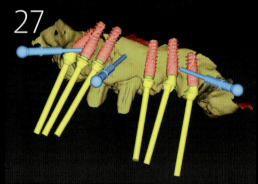

Enlarged view of the SRA abutment planning without the bone filter.

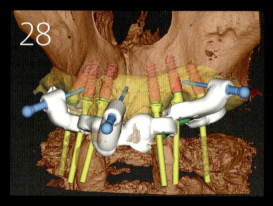

Preparation of the surgical guide after implant planning on the prepared arch file. Fusion view of the guide with SRA abutments, implant planning, and bone volume.

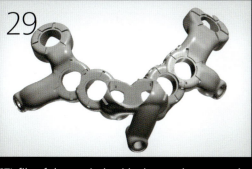

STL file of the surgical guide that can be exported from the Dental Wings ecosystem for printing.

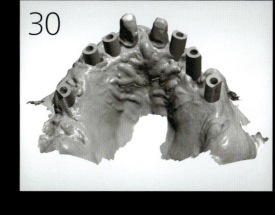

STL file of the model with the scan bodies for Variobase abutment on SRA that can be exported to Dental Wings software. This file can be imported along with the STL files of the antagonist arch and the occlusion into Dental System to design the immediate loading partial denture.

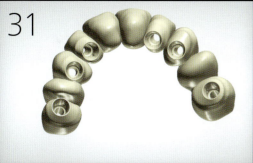

STL file of the instant loading partial denture developed in-house.

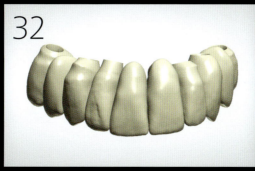

Vestibular view of the STL file to be sent to the Dentitek Laboratory for PMMA milling.

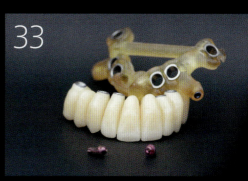

In-office printed surgical guide and the immediate loading partial denture connected to Variobase and SRA abutments before surgery.

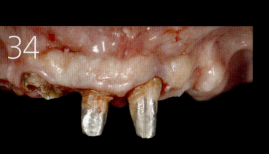

Initial clinical view at the beginning of surgery after removal of the validation partial denture.

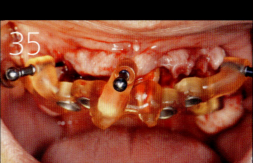

The surgical guide in place on the tooth stumps and stabilized by the three wedges.

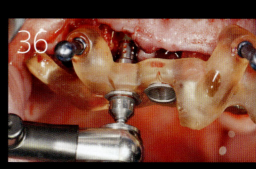

After the guided drilling sequence, guided placement of the BLX implant in 12.

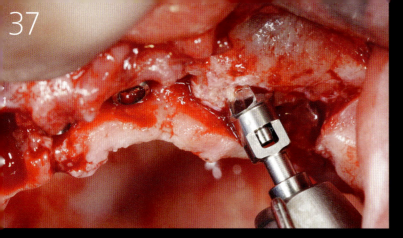

37 After placement of the six implants, flaring of the implant emergence profiles to allow placement of the angled SRA abutments.

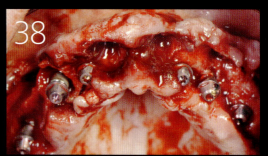

38 Occlusal view of the six implants with their SRA abutments in place. The implant in 25 was not loaded due to poor rotational stability (mobility when the SRA abutment was tightened).

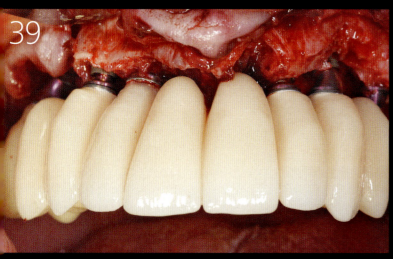

39 View of the immediate loading partial denture in place on the five implants, with the unloaded tooth 25 removed.

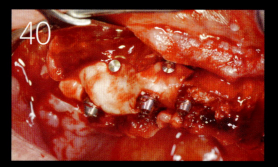

40 Compensatory GBR performed on the right side both in the extraction sites and in the implant hiatuses and ridge irregularities with DBBM (Bio-Oss) incubated in the F2 fraction of plasma, covered with a resorbable collagen membrane (Bio-Gide) stabilized by pins.

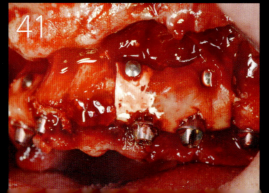

41 Compensatory GBR performed in the same manner on the left side.

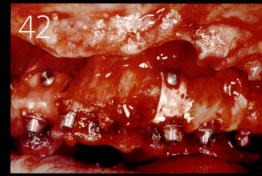

42 Frontal view of the compensatory GBR assembly.

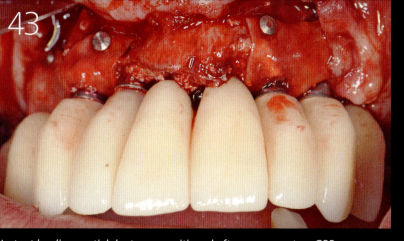

Instant loading partial denture repositioned after compensatory GBR for better palatal access.

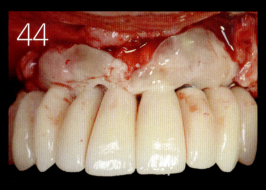

Positioning of a fibrin membrane from PRGF before suturing the flaps. A half-thickness incision was made at the back of the vestibule from 14 to 24 to obtain good flap laxity.

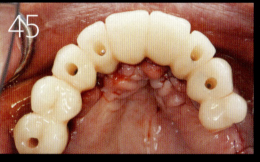

Occlusal view of the instant loading partial denture screwed onto the SRA abutments after flap suturing.

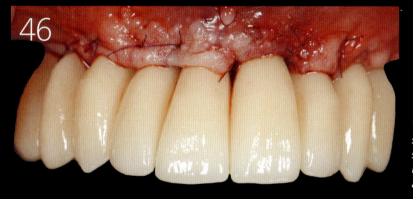

Vestibular view of flaps sutured with ASAF sutures around the implant emergences and pontic areas.

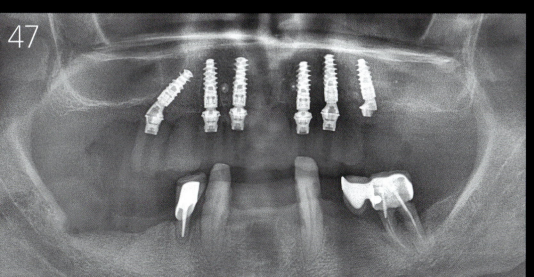

Panoramic radiograph taken at the end of surgery.

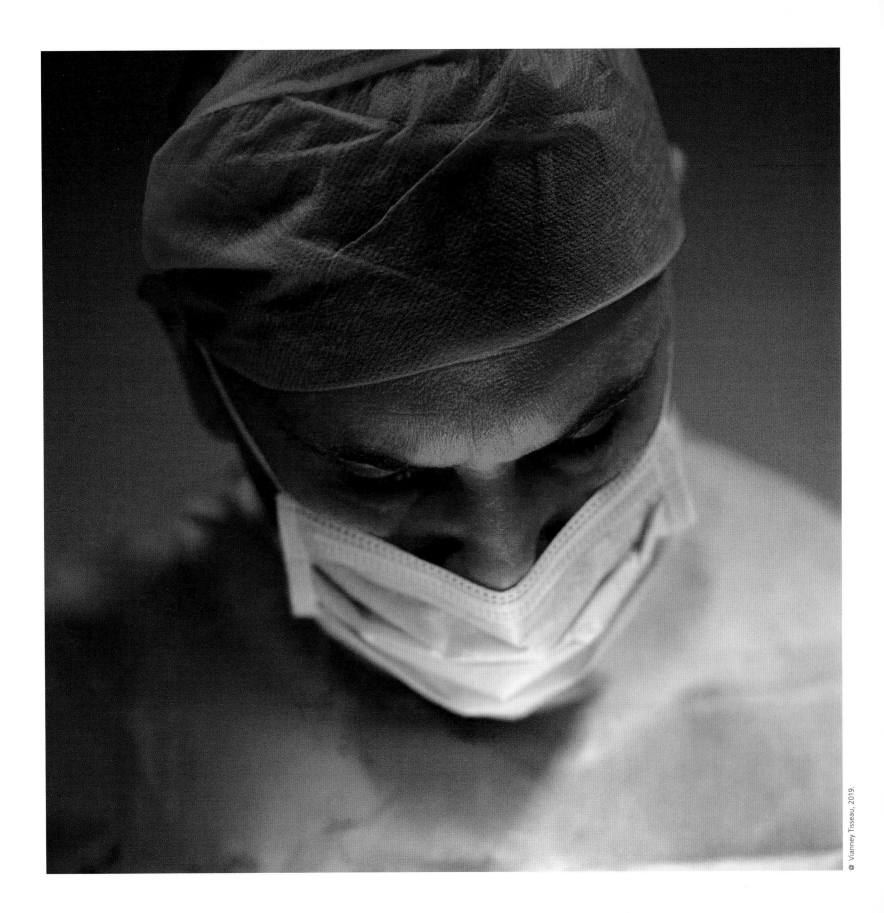

© Vianney Tisseau, 2019.

Full-arch clinical case 37

62-year-old woman.

Clinical data

- The patient attended the office for removal of her two maxillary and mandibular removable partial dentures. In the maxilla, two sinus grafts were needed to create two partial dentures with two implants for three teeth. In the mandible, major bone loss in the posterior region led to the requirement for an all-on-four rehabilitation.
- Case treated in January 2023.
- Simple bone context (homogeneous vertical loss).
- Simple mucogingival architecture.

Presurgical treatments

- Optical impression taken with a Trios 4 (3Shape, Copenhagen, Denmark) and 3D examination performed with a 3Shape X1.
- Planning performed in coDiagnostiX (Dental Wings, Montreal, Canada).
- Placement of Straumann BLX RB 3.75 x 12.00 mm implants in 35, 32, 42, and 45 combined with 1.5-mm straight SRA abutments in 32 and 42 and 3.5-mm 30-degree SRA abutments in 35 and 45 (all Basel, Switzerland).
- 3D printing of the guide designed in coDiagnostiX, printed in the office on a NextDent 5100 printer with NextDent SG resin (both Soesterberg, The Netherlands) and cured in an LC-3D 3D curing unit.
- Straumann T-sockets.
- Temporary partial denture milled in polymethylmethylacrylate (PMMA) 35 to 45 (Ivotion Dent Multi, Ivoclar Vivadent, Schaan, Liechtenstein) (Dentitek Laboratory) on an A3 shade base and connected to the 4.6-mm Variobase for SRA.

Assessment of the intervention

- Case treated in the office in **three appointments** for the mandible (gathering information or planning, implant surgery, 3-month control).
- Final prosthesis to be placed after insertion of the 16 and 26 implants, 6 months after placement of the sinus graft.
- The patient opted for a short arch and extraction of the anterior block, which was condemned in the medium term anyway (pocket of 6 mm and more, but with bleeding on probing BOP lower than 0) to avoid posterior vertical bone grafts which were, in her case, invasive and had a more limited success rate. We will therefore place a partial denture from 35 to 45. As in the previous case, the planning in coDiagnostiX allowed us to keep to a fully digital workflow by planning the most suitable SRA implant abutments on BLX implants for angulations.

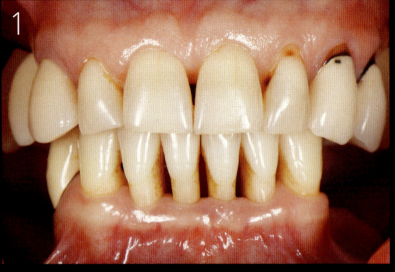

Initial clinical view after placement of the implants in 14 and 25 and of the delayed loading fixed provisional prostheses in 14, 15, and 25 to allow the patient to remove the maxillary partial denture.

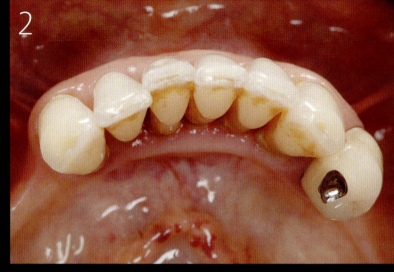

Occlusal view of the mandible.

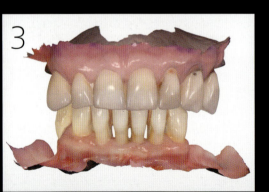

Intraoral optical impression taken during the appointment to gather information for planning in addition to the CBCT.

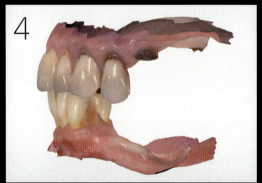

Lateral view of the fingerprint in occlusion.

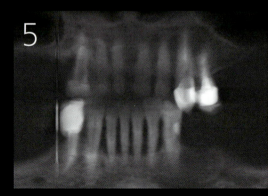

CBCT scout view of the initial situation. Note the very low height of the bony crests opposite the inferior dental nerve on the left and right, posterior to the chin emergence.

Chapter 6 - Full-arch clinical applications

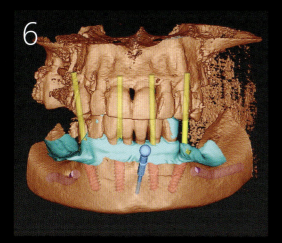

After importing the CBCT and the mandibular STL file into coDiagnostiX, the four implants were planned. The presence of the patient's natural teeth served as the prosthetic plan in the absence of esthetic and functional malpositioning.

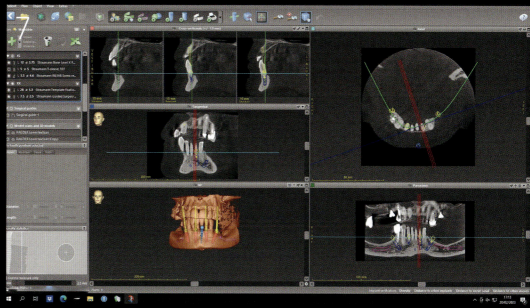

Complete view of the working window in coDiagnostiX (Dental Wings, Montreal, Canada).

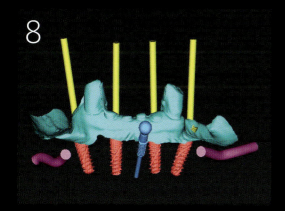

View of the planning of the four implants with the mandibular STL file modified by the virtual extractions of the four incisors and premolars, keeping teeth 33 and 43, future supports of the surgical guide.

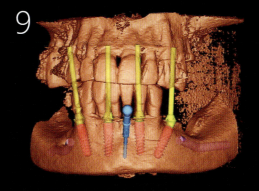

Vestibular view of the planning without the mandibular STL file, but with the bone DICOM file and placement of the SRA abutments on the four implants. In 35 and 45, 30-degree SRA abutments were used to straighten the axis of angulation required to bypass the chin emergence.

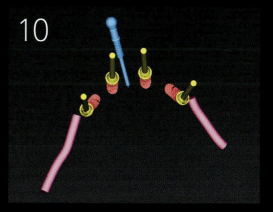

*Occlusal view of the planning with 30-degree SRA abutments in 35 and 45 and straight SRA abutments in 32 and 42, thus simplifying the insertion axis of the **immediate** partial denture.*

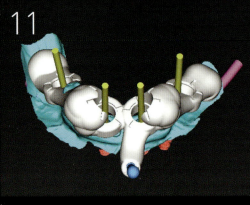

Occlusal view of the surgical guide drawn in coDiagnostiX. Note the presence of mucosal supports in the area of teeth 6 and 7 on the two posterior sectors associated with an anterior stabilization key.

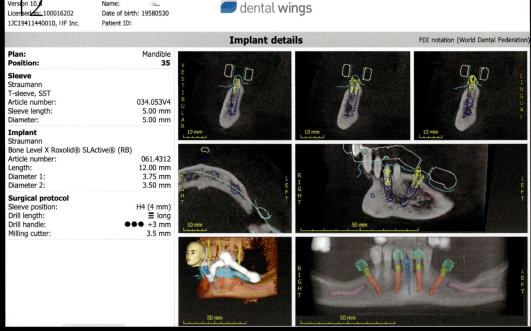

Summary file in PDF format of the drilling protocol, the surgical report, and the components to be ordered (implants, abutments, sockets).

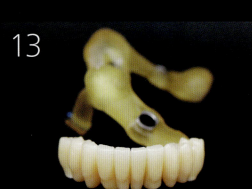

Instant loading temporary partial denture connected to the Variobase for SRA abutment before surgery.

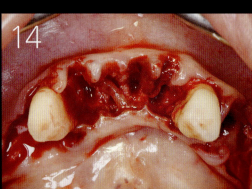

Clinical situation after extraction of the incisors and premolars, 33 and 43, used as supports for the surgical guide.

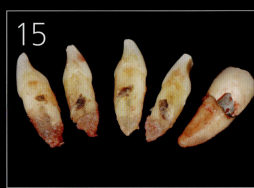

Extracted teeth with the presence of serous calculus on the apical third of the roots, confirming their medium-term condemnation.

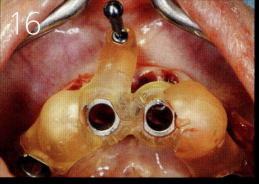

Occlusal view of the surgical guide in place at 33 and 43 and keyed in the medial sagittal plane. Note the presence of two mucosal supports posteriorly.

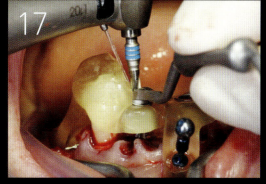

Guided drilling sequence; 2.2-mm drill.

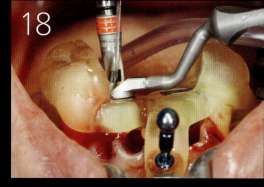

Guided drilling sequence; 3.5-mm drill.

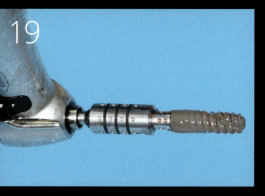

Straumann BLX 3.75 x 12.00 mm implant in Roxolid SLActive on the guided implant holder.

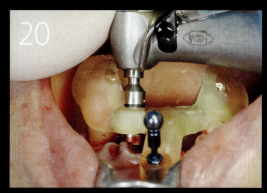

Guided implant placement in 42.

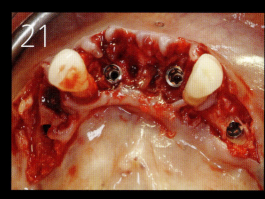

Clinical situation after placement of the four implants and removal of the surgical guide.

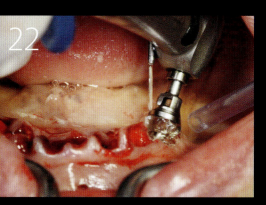

After extraction of the two canines, the bone profiles opposite the angled BLX implants were flared for insertion of the SRA abutments.

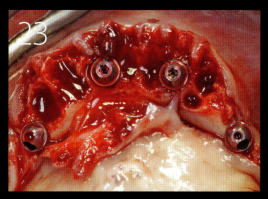

Occlusal view of the clinical situation with implants and SRA abutments in place.

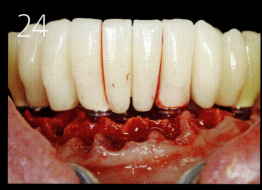

Trying in of the instant loading temporary partial denture positioned optimally on the four abutments.

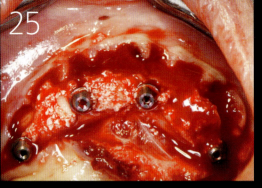

Compensatory GBR at both extraction sites and peri-implant hiatuses with DBBM (Bio-Oss with fine particles, Geistlich Pharma) incubated in the plasma F2 fraction (PRGF, Endoret BTI).

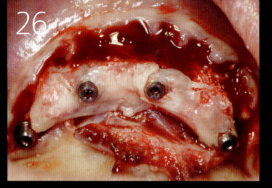

Ridge preservation with a fibrin membrane from the plasma F1 fraction.

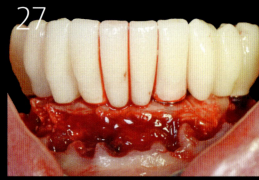

Placement of the instant loading partial denture to stabilize the fibrin membrane on the GBR. Note the bone profiles that match the prosthetic profiles.

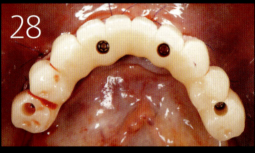

Occlusal view of the instant loading partial denture screwed onto the four implants.

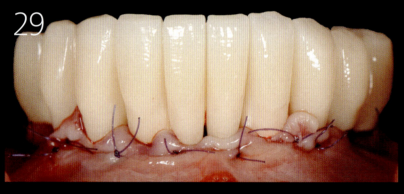

Vestibular view of the partial denture after prosthesis-guided flap suturing with ASAF sutures.

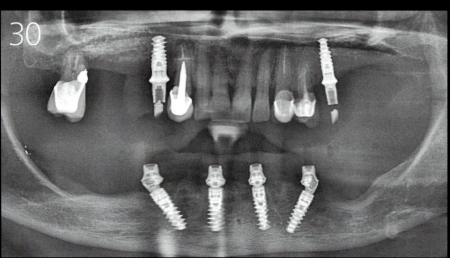

Postoperative panoramic radiograph confirming the optimal fit of the partial denture on the four implants.

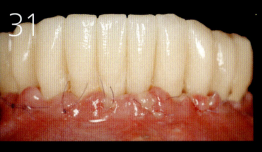

Clinical view at 8 days. Note the optimal tissue integration around the prosthetic emergence profiles.

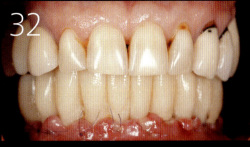

Vestibular view in occlusion. Note the precision of the 3D positioning of a partial denture made before surgery thanks to the complete digital flow.

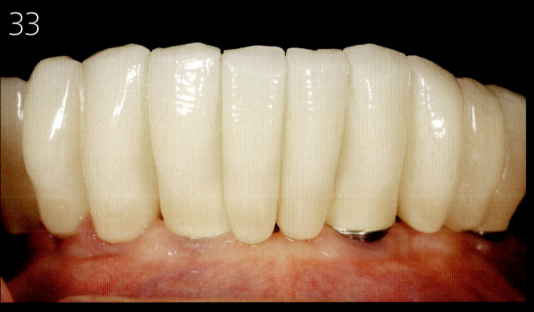

Clinical situation at 3 months after surgery. Note the supragingival position of the SRA abutments. The two anterior abutments could be removed in the final partial denture and used for a direct implant connection. The two posterior SRA abutments, correcting the 30-degree angulation, will be left in place for periodontal reasons.

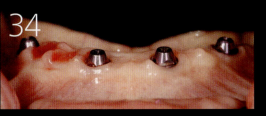

Vestibular view after removal of the provisional instant-loading partial denture.

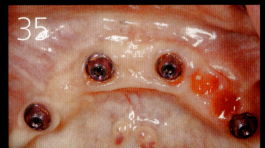

Occlusal view after removal of the instant loading partial denture.

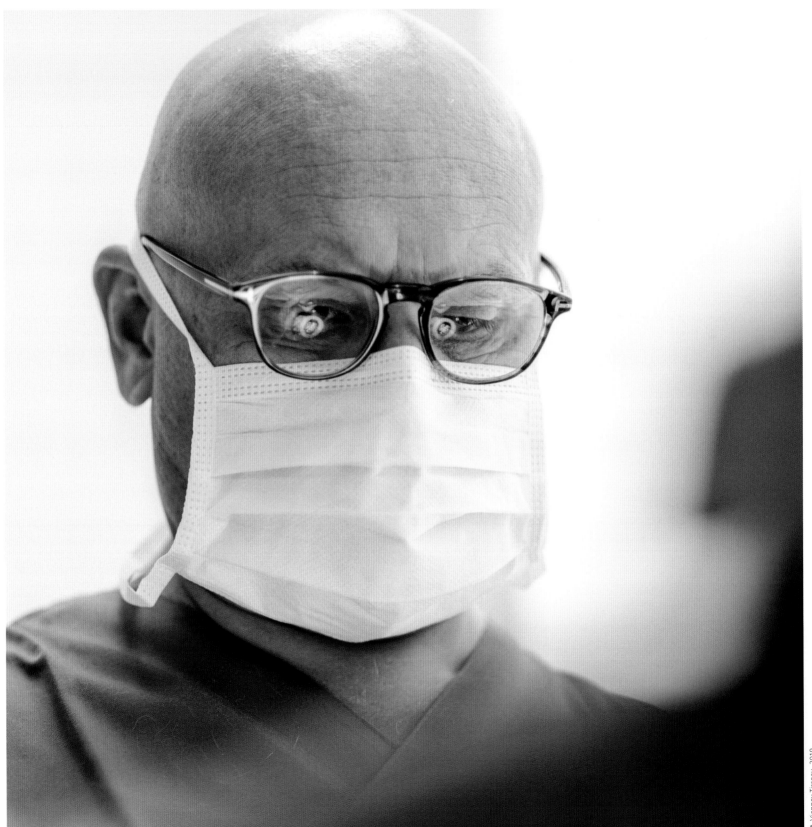

© Vianney Tisseau, 2019.

Full-arch clinical case 38

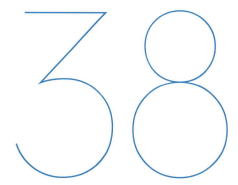

53-year-old woman.

Clinical data

- The patient wished to have a fixed maxillary implant solution and get rid of her immediate complete removable appliance. The maxillary tooth extractions were performed in February 2020 at another dental office.
- Case treated in November 2020.
- Simple bone context (homogeneous vertical loss and significant ridge width).
- Simple mucogingival architecture.

Presurgical treatments

- Optical impression taken with Trios 4 and 3D examination performed using a 3Shape X1.
- Planning performed in Implant Studio (3Shape).
- Placement of Straumann TL SP RN 3.3 mm implants in 12 and 22, and TL SP RN 4.1-mm implants in 14, 16, 24, and 26.
- 3D printing of the guide designed in Implant Studio (Dentitek Laboratory).
- First-generation Straumann socket.
- Temporary partial denture milled in PMMA (Dentitek Laboratory) on a shade B2 base.
- Final partial denture made from stratified zirconia (JC Allègre Laboratory).

Assessment of the intervention

- Case treated in the office in **six appointments** (esthetic analysis, validation of the prosthetic project and information gathering, implant surgery, digital impression, validation of the impression and the CAD/CAM model, placement of the final partial denture).
- **Immediate** loading surgery was performed with a temporary partial denture connected to the Variobases without any relining. Parallelization of the implant axes and the use of a non-engaging implant platform made it possible to perform a surgical procedure that facilitated management of the instant loading prosthesis.
- The lack of relining of the **immediate loading** prosthesis offers two advantages:
  – an ultra-smooth surface of the prosthetic emergence profiles, which induces better peri-implant tissue healing;
  – a unity of mass in the partial denture without areas of fragility (most often the relining areas), truly acting as a framework and thus securing implant osseointegration.

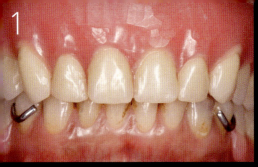

Frontal view of the initial situation with the two arches in occlusion (an immediate maxillary complete removable appliance and a mandibular partial removable appliance).

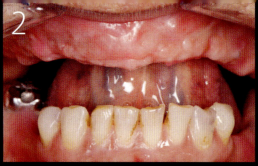

Frontal view of the initial situation after removal of the immediate maxillary complete removable appliance.

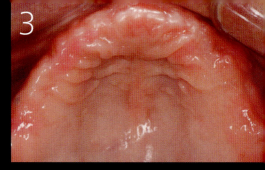

Occlusal view of the edentulous maxilla.

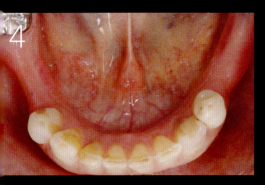

Occlusal view of the mandible after removal of the partial denture.

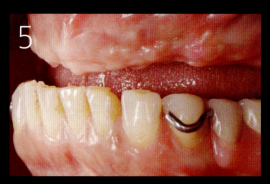

Left three-quarter view of the initial situation.

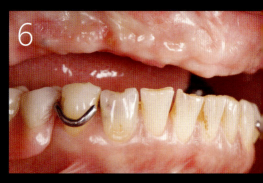

Right three-quarter view of the initial situation.

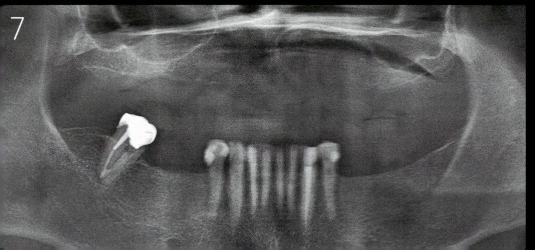

Panoramic radiograph of the initial situation.

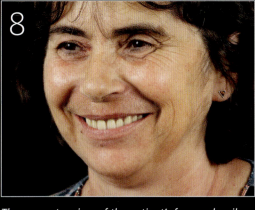
Three-quarter view of the patient's face and smile.

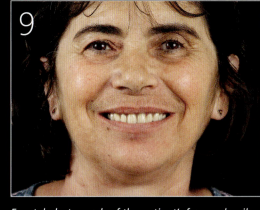
Frontal photograph of the patient's face and smile.

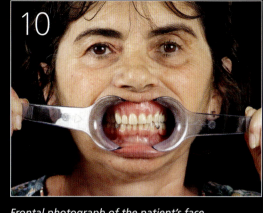
Frontal photograph of the patient's face with a retractor.

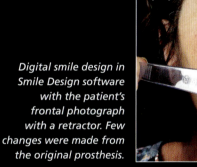
Digital smile design in Smile Design software with the patient's frontal photograph with a retractor. Few changes were made from the original prosthesis.

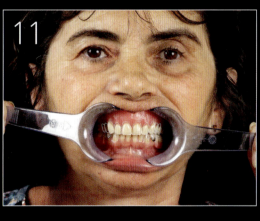

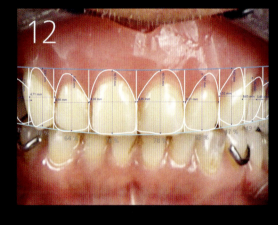
Smile Design software window with the width–height ratio. The height of the digital crowns was increased in favor of the false gingiva to achieve a better ratio.

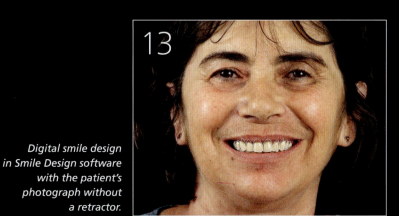
Digital smile design in Smile Design software with the patient's photograph without a retractor.

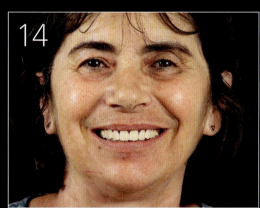
Visualization of the simulation of the prosthetic project in the RealView function in Smile Design software.

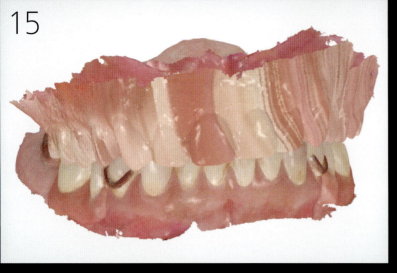

Digital impressions of the maxillary immediate complete removable appliance in occlusion with the antagonist arch (Trios 4).

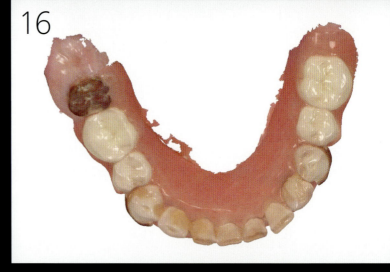

Digital impression of the antagonist arch.

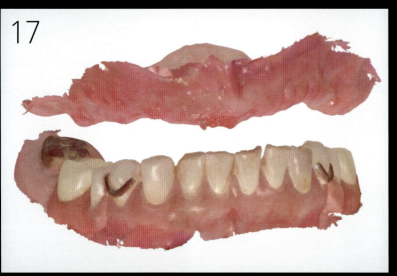

Digital impressions of the maxilla without appliances and the antagonist arch at the vertical dimension of occlusion.

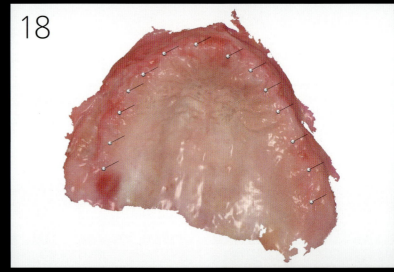

Digital impression of the edentulous maxilla.

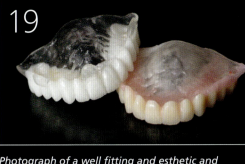

Photograph of a well fitting and esthetic and functional validation model, made according to the digital smile design, and its radiopaque duplicate (Dentitek Laboratory).

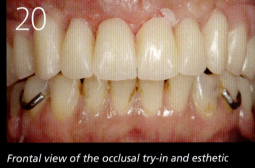

Frontal view of the occlusal try-in and esthetic and functional validation mock-up. The mock-up was glued to obtain more stability (Fixodent, Procter & Gamble, Cincinnati, OH, USA).

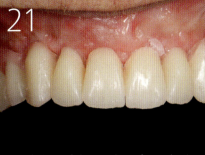

Frontal view of the mock-up for esthetic and functional validation. Note the absence of gingival volume in the anterior area. It is important to correct the support of the lip.

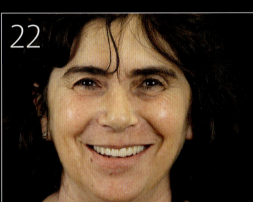

Frontal photograph of the patient with the model for fitting and esthetic and functional validation in the mouth.

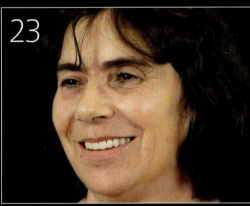

Three-quarter view of the patient with the mock-up for try-in and esthetic and functional validation in the mouth.

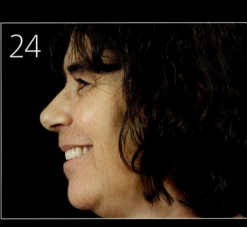

Profile photograph of the patient with the mock-up for try-in and esthetic and functional validation in the mouth. The nasolabial angle was correct. The prosthetic project was validated.

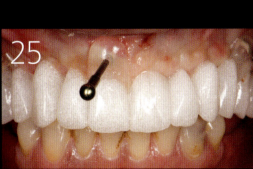

Frontal view of the radiopaque duplicate of the mock-up for esthetic and functional validation in occlusion.

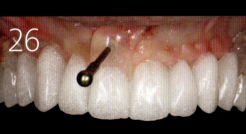

Frontal view of the radiopaque duplicate. As the information required for implant planning is gathered with this duplicate, it was keyed for greater stability.

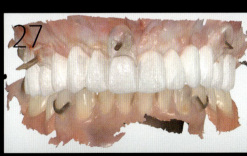

Digital impressions of both arches for implant planning, taken using a Trios 4.

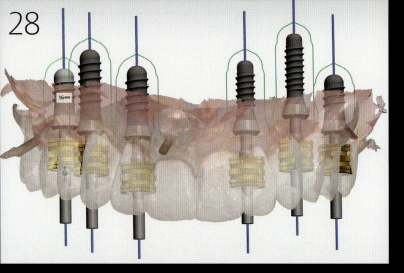

Planning of the six implants and stabilization pins for the surgical guide. The bone volume made it possible to parallelize the axis of the six implants.

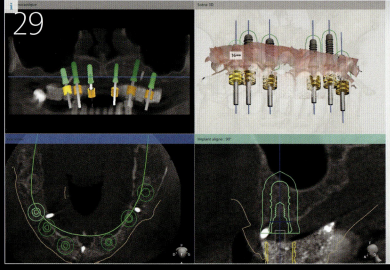

Visualization of the planning of the six implants, their implant axis, and the prosthetic project in Implant Studio. The design of the surgical guide was performed in the laboratory in Implant Studio.

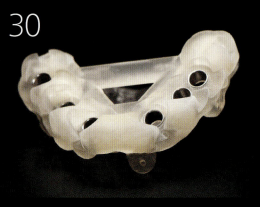

Visualization of the surgical guide made according to the radiopaque duplicate. 3D printing (Dentitek Laboratory).

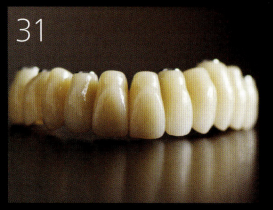

Visualization of the **immediate loading** partial denture with the Variobase already bonded to the partial denture before surgery (Multilink Hybrid Abutment, Ivoclar Vivadent, Schaan, Liechtenstein). It was milled in polymethylmethacrylate (PMMA) (Ivotion Dent Multi, Ivoclar Vivadent) (Dentitek Laboratory).

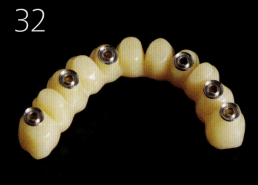

Visualization of the prosthetic emergence profiles and the pontic areas. Note their surface condition.

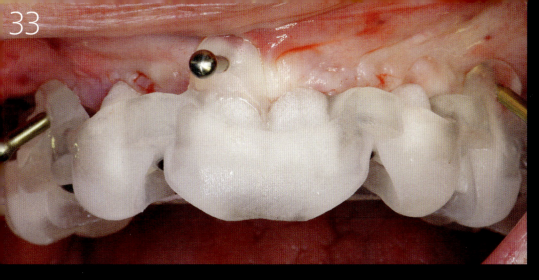

Frontal view of the keyed surgical guide.

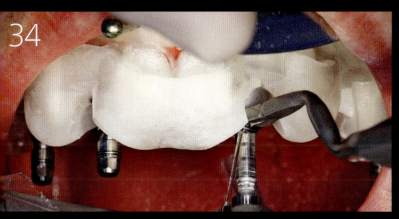

Visualization of guided drilling in the 22 zone.

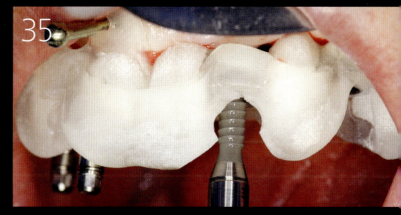

Guided placement of a Straumann TL SP RN 3.3 x 10.0 mm implant.

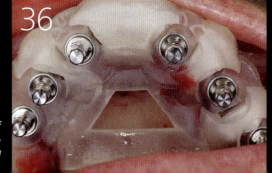

Occlusal view of the surgical guide and the six guided implants placed with their grippers.

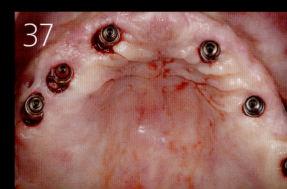

Occlusal view of the six implants placed. A gingival punch was used before drilling and implant placement.

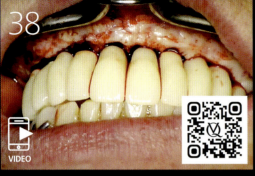

QR code of the video of the screwing of the provisional *immediate loading* partial denture onto the implants. Note the alignment of the interincisal spaces.

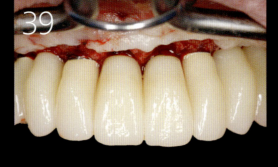

Frontal view of the provisional *immediate loading* partial denture screwed onto the six implants without relining.

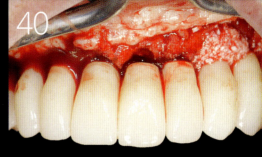

Compensatory GBR in extraction gaps around implants and ridge preservation in pontic alveoli with placement of DBBM (Bio-Oss) incubated in F2 fraction plasma.

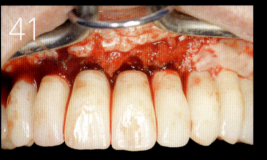

Vestibular bone fillings were covered with a fibrin membrane from the F1 fraction of the plasma. A resorbable collagen membrane was then applied (Bio-Gide, Geistlich Pharma).

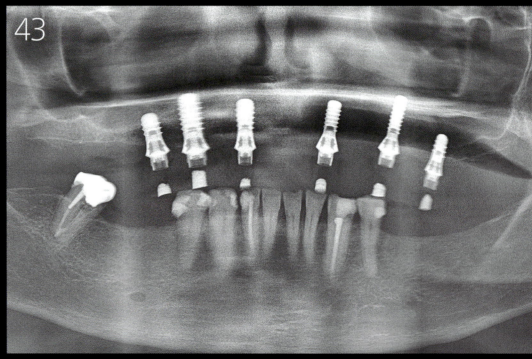

Postoperative photograph. Prosthesis-guided flap suture using ASAF sutures and double-crossed sutures.

Postoperative panoramic radiograph. Note the optimal fit of the implant abutments with the six implants.

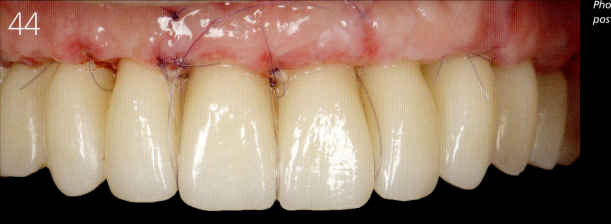

44 Photograph taken 7 days post-surgery.

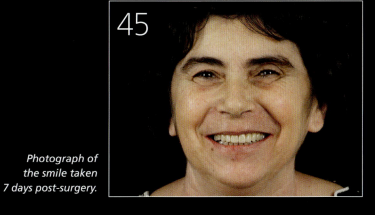

45 Photograph of the smile taken 7 days post-surgery.

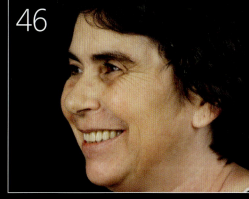

46 Three-quarter view of the patient 7 days post-implant surgery.

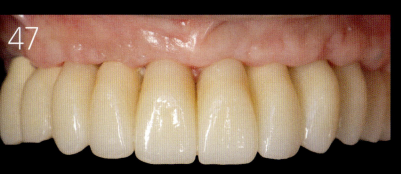

47 Photograph taken 3 months post-surgery.

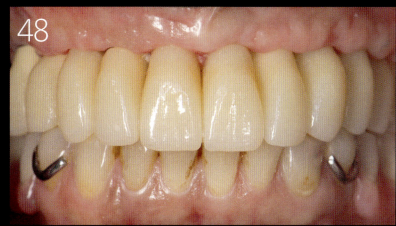

48 Frontal view of the partial denture in occlusion after 3 months of healing.

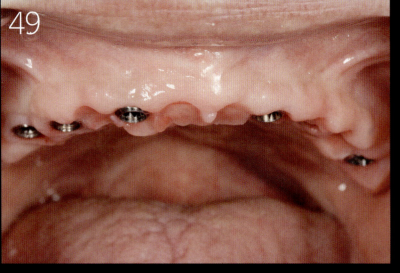
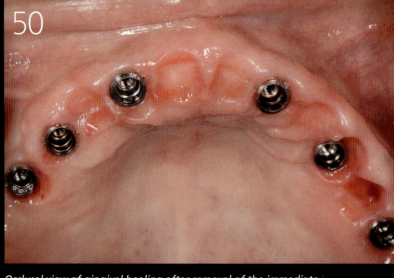

Vestibular view of gingival healing after removal of the immediate loading partial denture. The height of the gingival areas of the pontics allowed for gingival sculpting and the creation of pseudopapillae.

Occlusal view of gingival healing after removal of the immediate loading partial denture.

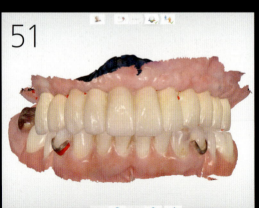
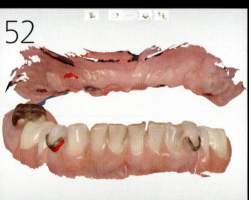
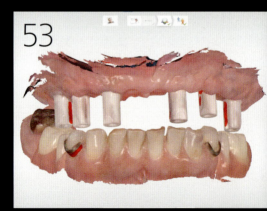

Digital impressions of the provisional **immediate loading** partial denture and the antagonist arch in occlusion taken using a Trios 4.

Digital impressions of the maxilla without the temporary partial denture and of the antagonist arch at the vertical occlusal dimension. The implant emergence profiles were therefore digitized and sent to the dental technician.

Digital impressions of the maxilla with digital impression transfers (scan body for the RN implant) and of the antagonist arch at the vertical occlusal dimension.

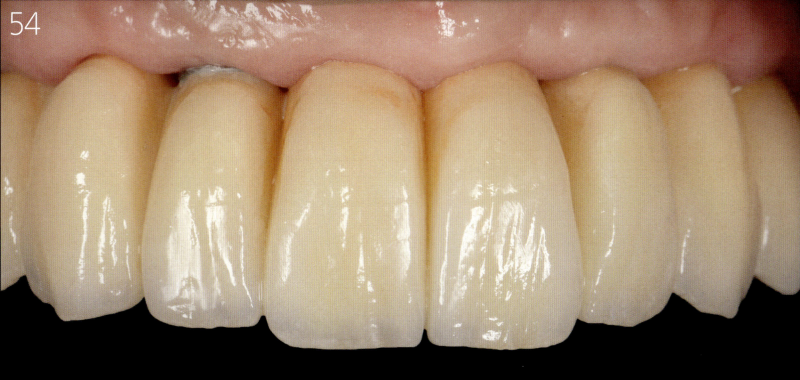

Photograph of the final partial denture (JC Allègre Laboratory). A slight lack of gingival reconstruction during implant surgery left the implant neck slightly visible in the 12-zone.

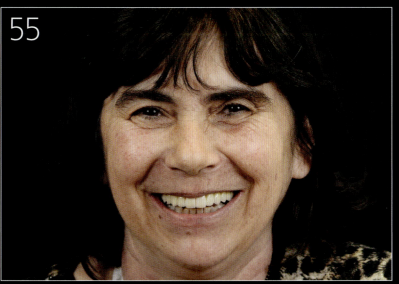

Final facial photograph of the patient.

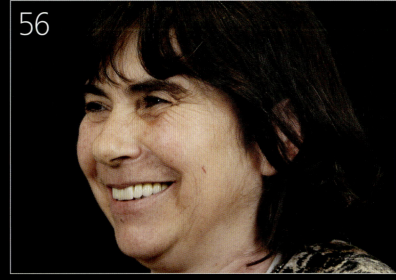

Final facial photograph of the patient (side view).

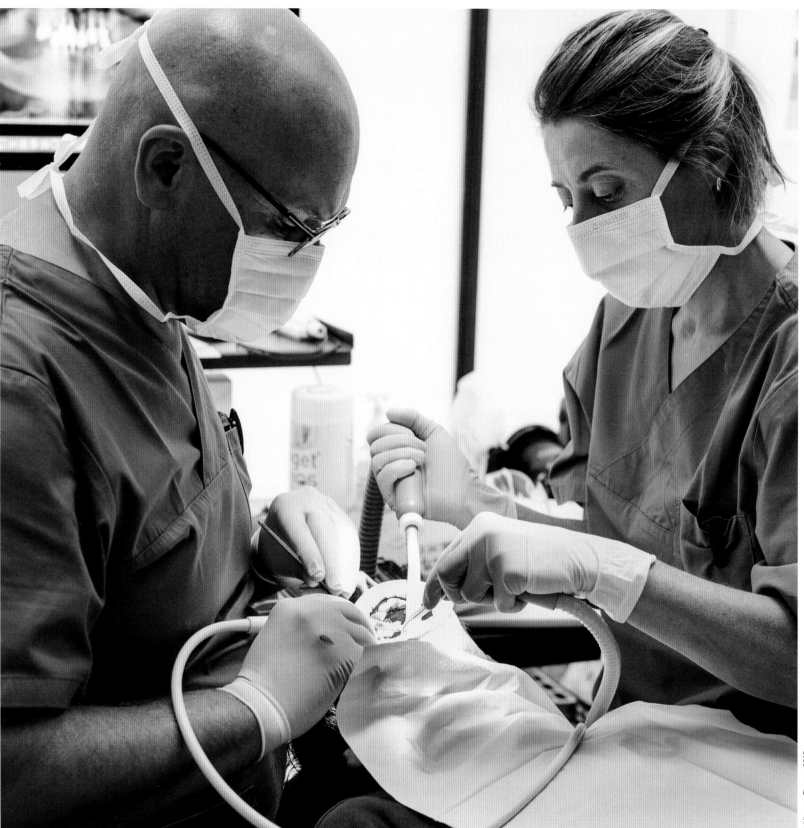

© Vianney Tisseau, 2019.

Full-arch clinical case 39

69-year-old woman.

Clinical data

- The patient wished to have a fixed solution and get rid of her removable maxillary and mandibular appliances.
- She had complete maxillary edentulism and was missing mandibular posterior sectors.
- Case treated in November 2021.
- Maxillary anterior horizontal bone loss. Sub-sinus vertical bone loss.
- Peri-implantitis presents on mandibular implants with absence of keratinized gingiva and exposed threads.
- In the maxilla, two sinus grafts as well as an anterior lateral apposition graft were required before implant surgery. In the mandible, the significant vertical bone loss and thus the proximity of the bone crest to the lingual floor led us to use a complete implant-supported fixed prosthesis.
- Correct maxillary mucogingival architecture.

Presurgical treatments

- Optical impression taken with Trios 4 and 3D examination performed using a 3Shape X1.
- Planning performed using Implant Studio.
- Placement of Straumann TL SP RN implants in 16, 14, 12, 22, 24, and 26.
- 3D printing of the guide designed in Implant Studio (Dentitek Laboratory).
- Second-generation Straumann T-socket.
- Temporary partial denture milled in PMMA (Dentitek Laboratory) on a shade A3 base.
- Laminated zirconia partial denture milled from Metoxit discs at Createch Medical (Dental Art Technology, Richard Demange).

Assessment of the intervention

- Case treated in the office in **six appointments** (esthetic analysis, provisional esthetic and functional validation appliance, implant surgery, digital impression, validation of the impression and the CAD/CAM model, final placement of the partial denture).
- The patient wished to have a maxillary and mandibular implant solution. She came to the office for her first consultation in February 2021 and her mandibular implants were removed in April 2021. A maxillary lateral apposition bone graft and subsinusal grafts were performed in June 2021, and mandibular implants were placed in August 2021.
- **Immediate loading** surgery was performed in November 2021, and the stabilized mandibular appliance on the four mandibular implants was placed in February 2022 before insertion of the final partial denture took place in March 2022.

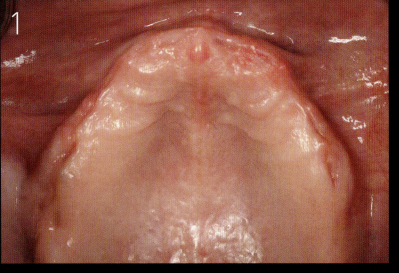

Occlusal view of the edentulous maxilla.

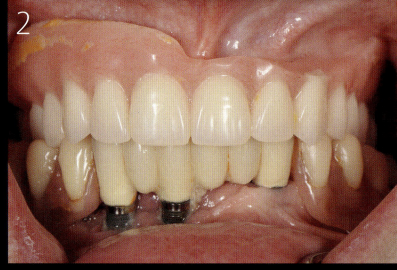

Frontal view of the initial situation with both arches in occlusion. The patient wore a maxillary complete removable appliance and a mandibular partial removable appliance.

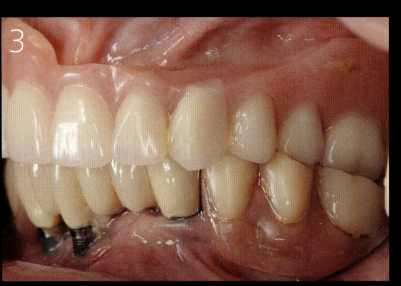

Three-quarter view of the left occlusion.

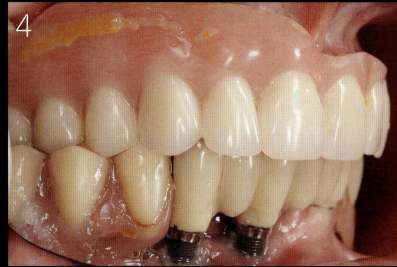

Three-quarter view of the right occlusion. The mandibular implants, which were outside the mandibular bone corridor, had to be removed to make a mandibular complete removable appliance stabilized on implants.

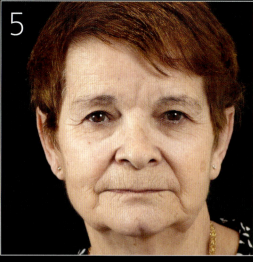

Frontal facial photograph of the patient at rest.

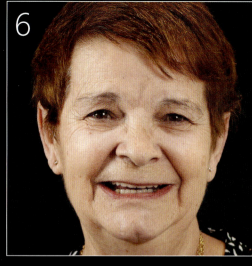

Frontal photograph of the patient's face and smile.

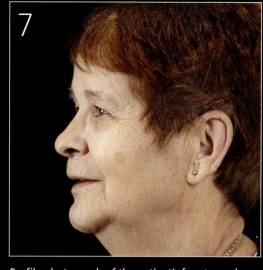

Profile photograph of the patient's face to analyze the upper lip support. The nasolabial angle was correct with the maxillary appliance worn; the same upper lip support needed to be reproduced with the maxillary implant rehabilitation.

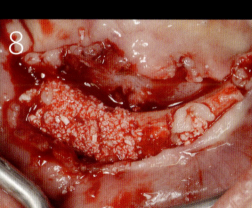

Occlusal view of GBR with DBBM (Bio-Oss) incubated in the F2 plasma fraction after the mandibular implants were placed.

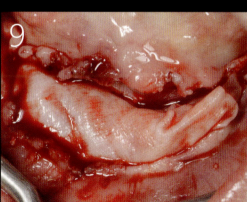

Occlusal view of the mandibular bone fillings covered with a resorbable collagen membrane (Bio-Gide). Four months of healing were required before implants could be placed in the mandible again.

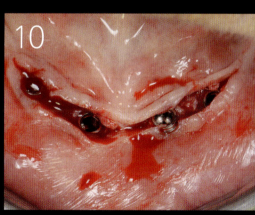

Occlusal view of placement of four Element RC implants (Thommen Medical, Grenchen, Switzerland) in positions 34, 32, 42, and 44 to stabilize a mandibular complete removable appliance with Locator attachments. The implants were placed 4 months after the first implant removal procedure.

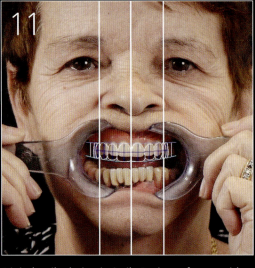

Digital smile design in Smile Design software with the patient's frontal photograph with a retractor. The height of the maxillary clinical crowns was increased to achieve a better width–height ratio.

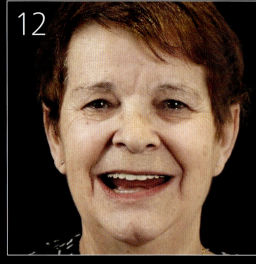

Visualization of the simulation of the prosthetic project using the RealView function in Smile Design software. The patient validated the esthetic setup.

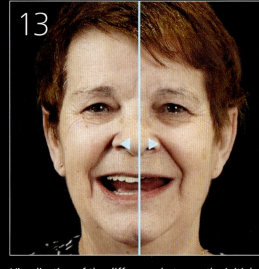

Visualization of the difference between the initial clinical situation on the right and the simulation of the prosthetic project on the left of the blue line.

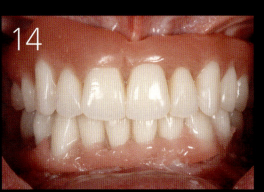

Frontal view of the two temporary esthetic and functional validation removable appliances made according to the digital smile design. Relining with Silagum Comfort (DMG Dental, Birchwood, UK) was performed to increase the retention of the appliances (Dentitek Laboratory).

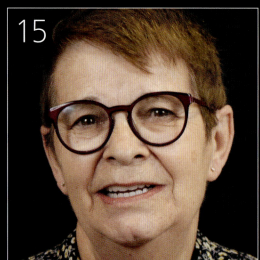

Frontal facial photograph of the patient wearing the temporary appliances for esthetic and functional validation.

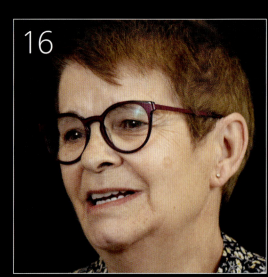

Three-quarter view of the patient's face. The patient validated the esthetic and functional setup.

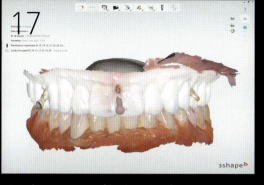

Digital impressions of both arches for implant planning. A radiopaque duplicate of the temporary esthetic and functional validation appliance was clamped in the mouth to gather information (digital impression and 3D scan). Impressions were taken using a Trios 4.

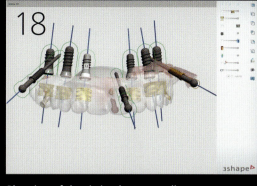

Planning of the six implants as well as the stabilization wedges of the surgical guide.

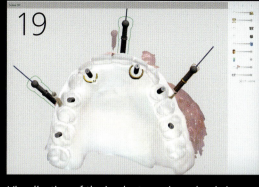

Visualization of the implant axes in occlusal view.

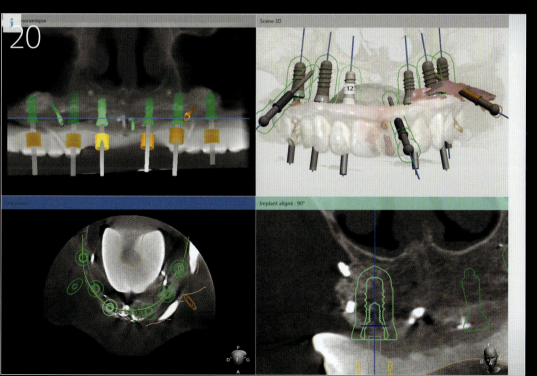

Visualization of the planning of the six implants, their implant axis, and the prosthetic project in Implant Studio software. The design of the surgical guide was performed in the laboratory in Implant Studio.

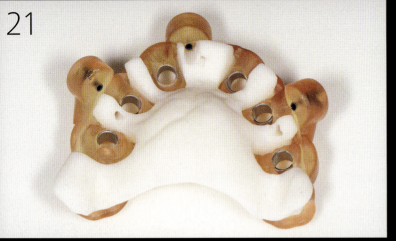

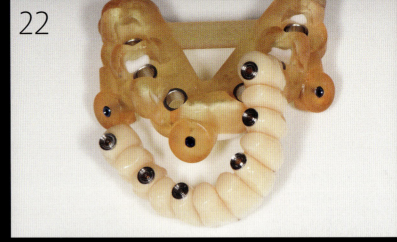

Visualization of the surgical guide made with the radiopaque device. The surgical guide had been hollowed out in the implantation area, but the palatal support, maxillary tuberosities, and wedge areas were preserved to place the surgical guide in the same position as during implant planning.

*Visualization of the **immediate loading** partial denture with the Variobases already bonded to the denture before surgery. The surgical guide was 3D printed while the immediate loading partial denture was milled from PMMA (Dentitek Laboratory).*

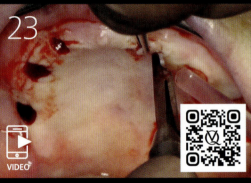

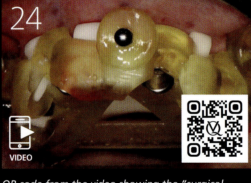

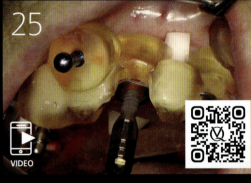

QR code from the video of circular gingivectomies in the implantation zone performed with the "mucosa punch" drill and finalized with blade 15.

QR code from the video showing the "surgical guide and radiopaque plate" assembly positioned in the mouth, keyed and having good stability.

QR code from the video showing guided drilling and guided placement of a Straumann TL RN implant in zone 21.

QR code from the video showing the six maxillary implants placed and the beginning of the vestibular flap elevation.

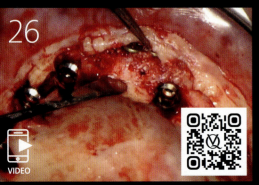

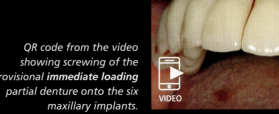

QR code from the video showing screwing of the provisional **immediate loading** partial denture onto the six maxillary implants.

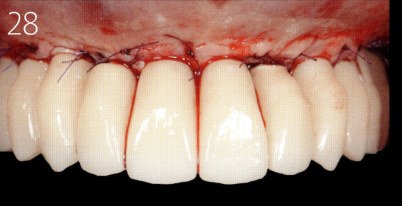

Frontal view of the postoperative situation with ASAF 6/0 sutures.

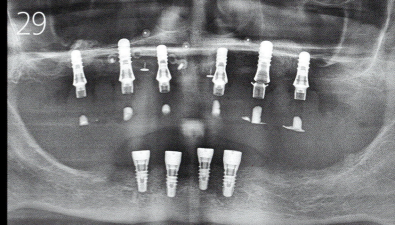

Postoperative panoramic radiograph. Note the mismatch between the implant and the Variobase in zone 24 due to interference from an osteosynthesis screw during implant placement. Tightening was performed on the other five implants.

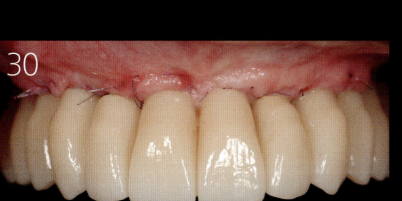

Photograph taken 7 days post-surgery.

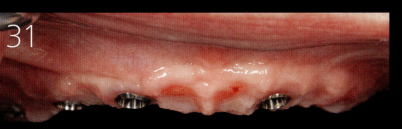

Photo taken 3 months post-surgery. Vestibular view of gingival healing after removal of the immediate loading partial denture.

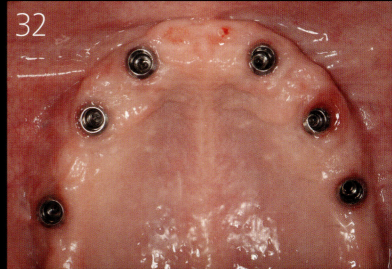

Occlusal view of gingival healing after removal of the instant loading partial denture. The lack of adaptation in zone 24 had no consequence or clinical significance on implant osseointegration or gingival maturation compared to the comfort and benefit of **immediate loading**.

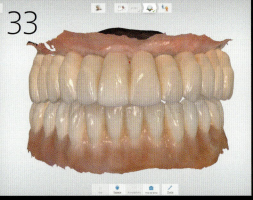

Digital impressions of the provisional **immediate loading** partial denture and the antagonist arch in occlusion taken using a Trios 4.

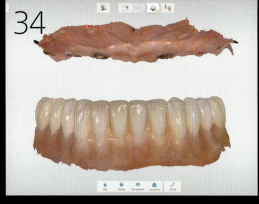

Digital impressions of the maxilla without the temporary partial denture and the antagonist arch at the vertical occlusal dimension.

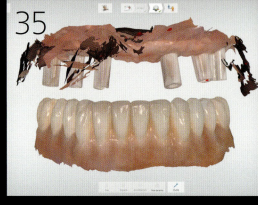

Digital impressions of the maxilla with digital impression transfers (scan body for RN implant) and the antagonist arch at the vertical occlusal dimension. The STL files were ready to be sent to the prosthetic laboratory (outside the 3Shape ecosystem).

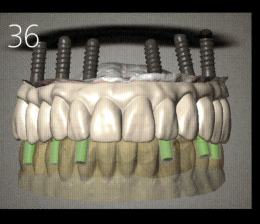

Dental Wings laboratory software window with the final prosthetic volume modeled from the STL files. From this design, a CAD/CAM model was milled to correct the identified esthetic details and validate the occlusion (Dental Art Technology Laboratory, Richard Demange).

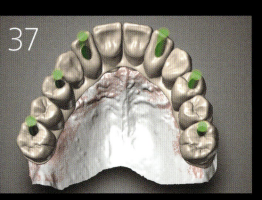

Occlusal view of the final prosthesis design and the emergence profile of the screw holes.

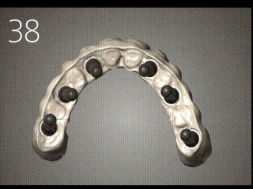

Visualization of the emergence profiles and pontic areas of the final prosthesis.

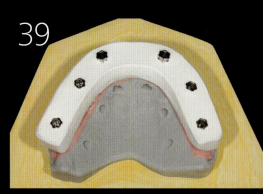

Photograph of the printed model and the plaster key for validation of the impression.

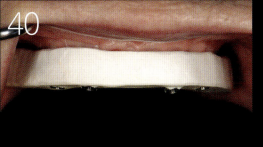

40 Photograph of the validation plaster key screwed onto the implants. The intact key validated the digital implant impression.

41 Frontal view of the CAD/CAM model. This model was placed on the same day as the fitting of the plaster key to validate the impression and volumes (Dental Art Technology Laboratory, Richard Demange).

42 View of the prosthetic emergence profiles and pontic areas of the CAD/CAM model.

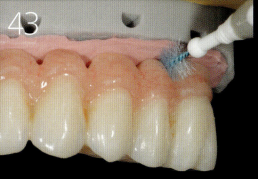

43 Checking the spaces for the use of interdental brushes.

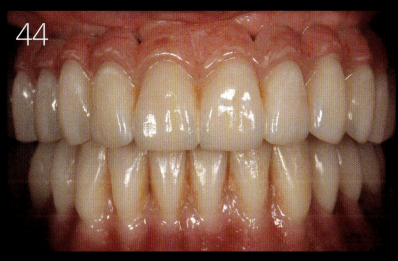

44 Frontal view of the CAD/CAM model in occlusion.

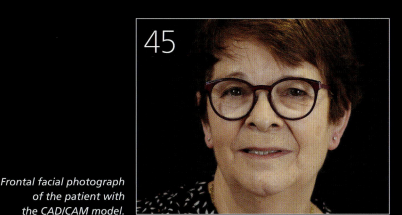

45 Frontal facial photograph of the patient with the CAD/CAM model.

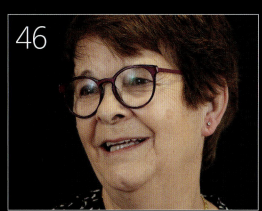

46 Three-quarter view of the patient's face with the CAD/CAM model.

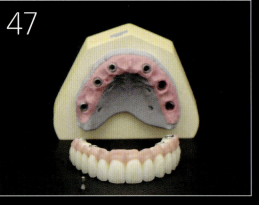

Frontal view of the final zirconia laminate partial denture milled from Metoxit discs (Createch Medical) (Dental Art Technology Laboratory, Richard Demange).

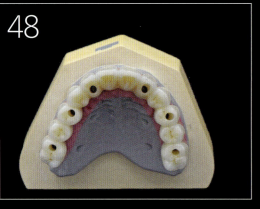

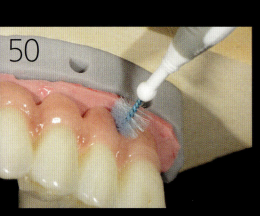

Checking the spaces for the use of interdental brushes.

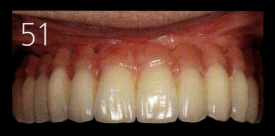

Photograph of the final partial denture (Dental Art Technology, Richard Demange).

View of the screw holes in the partial denture, the location of which did not interfere with the installation of the ceramic.

Final screw-retained partial denture.

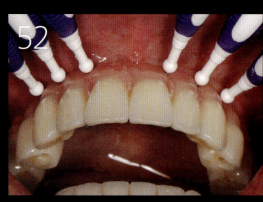

Visualization of the access for dental hygiene for interdental brushes.

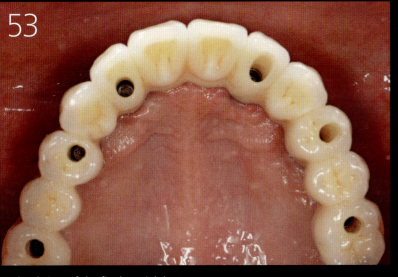
Occlusal view of the final partial denture.

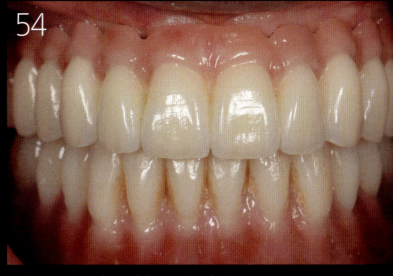
Final screw-retained partial denture in occlusion.

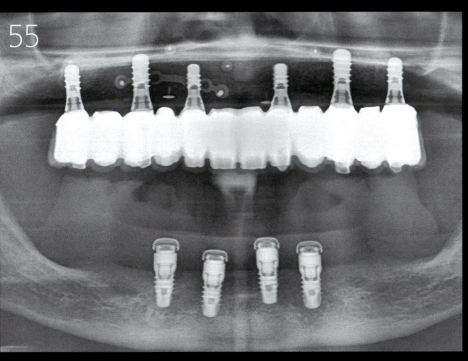
Panoramic radiograph of the final screw-retained partial denture.

Final facial photograph of the patient.

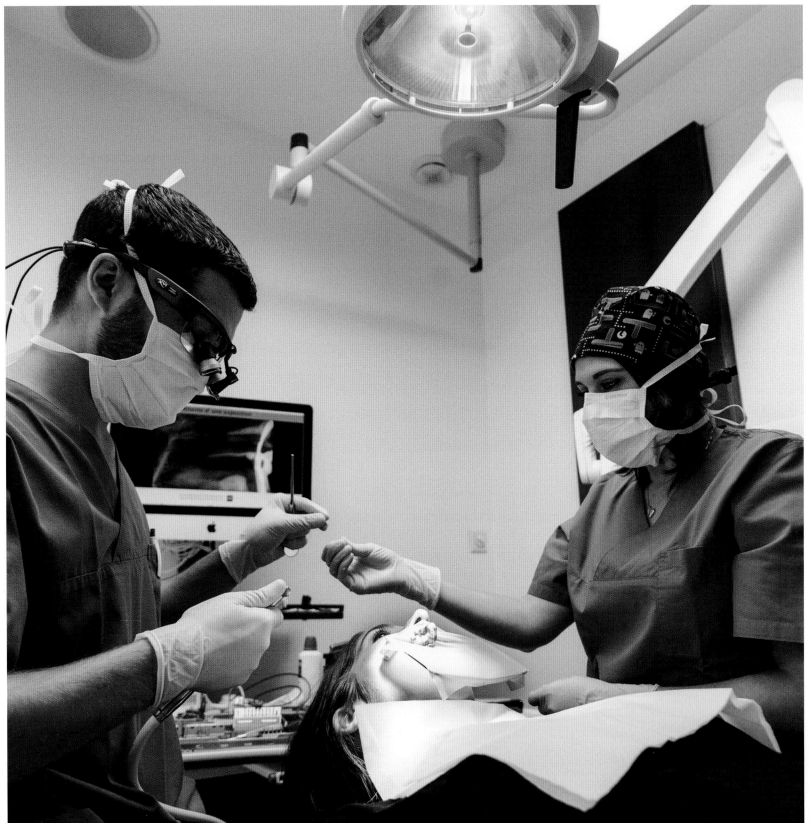

© Vianney Tisseau, 2019.

Full-arch clinical case 40

57-year-old man.

Clinical data

- The patient was referred by his referring dentist in Savoie. He attended the office to find an esthetic and durable solution to his fixed prostheses which regularly loosened at the top and caused him functional and esthetic discomfort.
- Case treated in June 2020.
- Simple bone context (homogeneous vertical loss).
- Simple mucogingival architecture.

Presurgical treatments

- Optical impression taken with a Trios 4 and 3D examination performed using a 3Shape X1.
- Planning performed using Implant Studio.
- Placement of Straumann TL SP RN 10-mm implants in 16, 14, 24, and 25, RN 12-mm in 12 and 22, and RN 12-mm in 33 and 43 in a second phase.
- 3D printing of the guide designed in Implant Studio and printed at the Dentitek Laboratory.
- Straumann T-sockets.
- Provisional partial denture milled in PMMA 16 to 26 (Dentitek Laboratory) on a shade A3 base and connected to the Variobase direct implant for RN.

Assessment of the intervention

- Case treated in live surgery during a session of the CampusHB full arch treatment.
- Case treated in the office in **five appointments** for the maxilla (esthetic analysis, placement of the esthetic and functional validation partial denture, gathering of information for planning, implant surgery, 3-month check-up) and in four additional sessions for the mandible (placement of implants in 33 and 43, impression taken at 3 months, placement of complete temporary partial denture, 3-month check-up).
- The patient still wears his temporary partial denture. He attends regular follow-ups with his referring dentist in Savoie for maintenance.
- The patient already had four Straumann implants in the mandibular posterior region placed 6 years earlier by one of our colleagues from Savoie. A mix of already osseointegrated implants and planning of new implants is currently difficult to treat as an **immediate** full denture (see clinical case 30). We are working on merging the STL scan file of the existing implants with the STL implant planning file ("scan with implant info") to obtain a single file to design and connect a complete instant partial denture. In this case, we placed the two implants in 33 and 43 while maintaining the anterior partial esthetic and functional validation partial denture and took a digital impression of all six implants after osseointegration to place a complete denture on the day of extractions and implant placement.

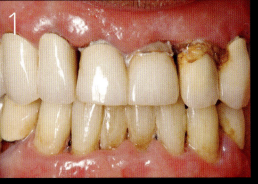
Vestibular view of the initial clinical situation.

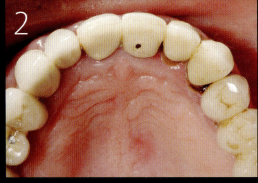
Occlusal view of the maxilla.

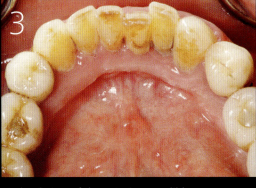
Occlusal view of the anterior mandible.

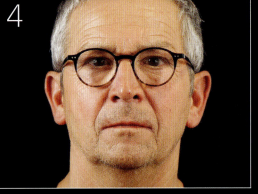
Photograph of the face at rest for esthetic analysis.

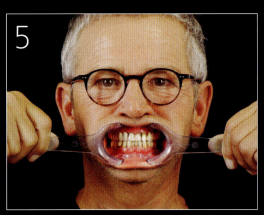
Photograph of the face with retractors.

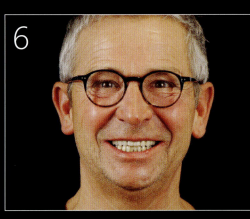
Photograph of the face when smiling.

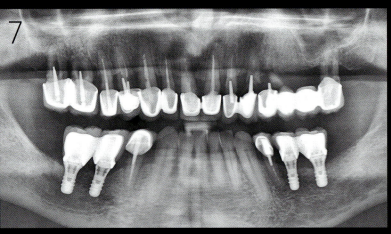
Panoramic radiograph of the initial situation.

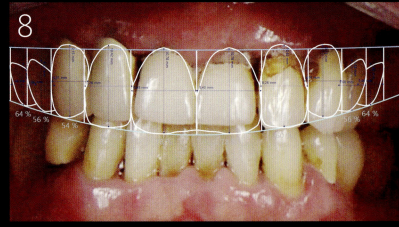
Development of the new smile design in the Smile Design module in Trios 4.

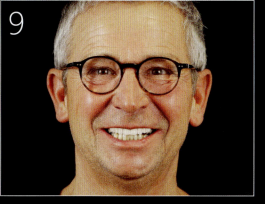
Simulation of the assembly in situation.

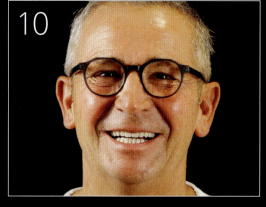
Facial photograph when smiling, incorporating the esthetic and functional validation partial denture.

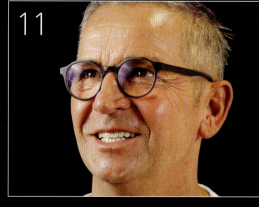
Photograph in three-quarter view incorporating the esthetic and functional validation partial denture.

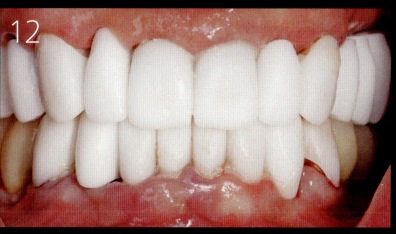
Placement of the radiopaque maxillary and mandibular anterior partial denture.

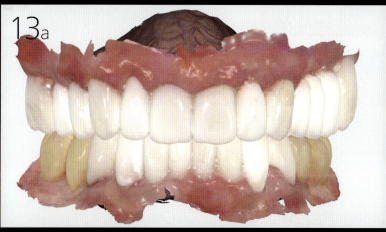
Intraoral digital impression of the situation with radiopaque partial dentures in place, in occlusion for implant planning.

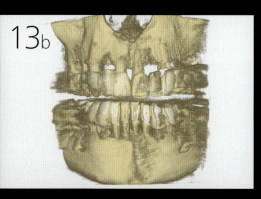
CBCT examination with radiopaque partial dentures in place.

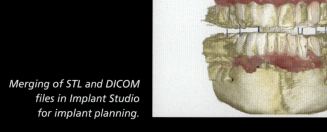
Merging of STL and DICOM files in Implant Studio for implant planning.

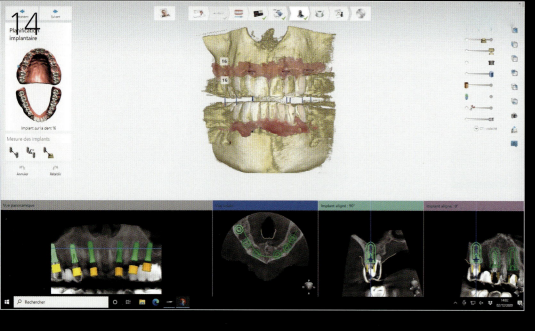

Planning of the six maxillary implants.

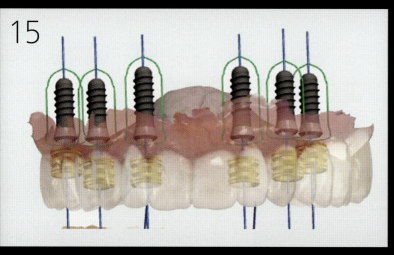

Enlarged view of the planning without the DICOM file to understand the relationship between the implant necks, prosthetic project, and gingival environment.

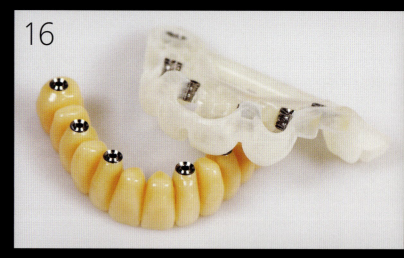

Surgical guide and instant loading partial denture before surgery.

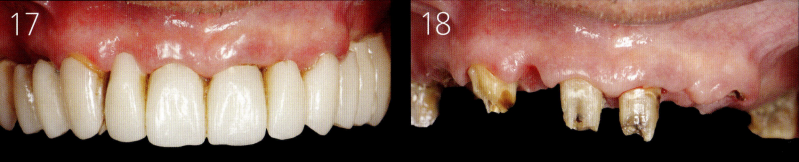

17 Clinical situation at the beginning of surgery with the esthetic and functional validation partial denture that the patient kept for 3 months.

18 Removal of the partial denture at the beginning of surgery to place the radiopaque supports for the surgical guide.

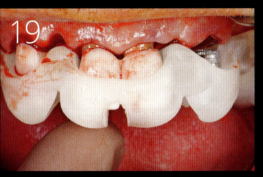
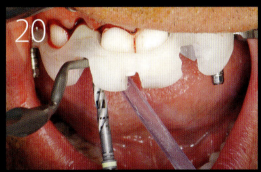
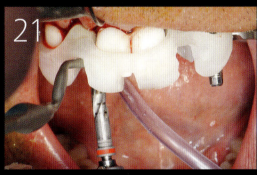

19 Surgical guide in place on radiopaque teeth, guide supports after sulcal incisions and minimal flap removal.

20 Guided drilling.

21 Passage of the guided drills with increasing diameters.

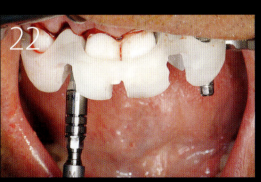
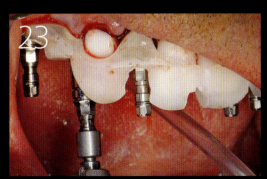
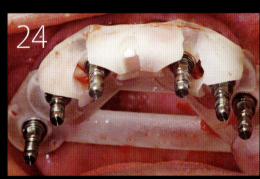

22 Guided implant placement in 12.

23 Guided placement of the sixth and final maxillary implant.

24 Overall view of the six first-generation implants placed with the supplied implant grippers already connected to the implants and serving as locking wedges for the surgical guide throughout surgery.

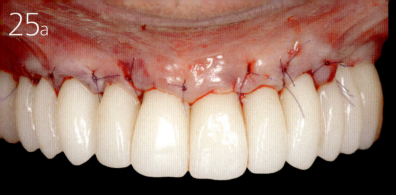

25a Instant loading partial denture screwed onto the implants and prosthesis-guided flap suture with ASAF sutures. Compensatory GBR was performed in the ridge-preserving extraction sites and around the implants.

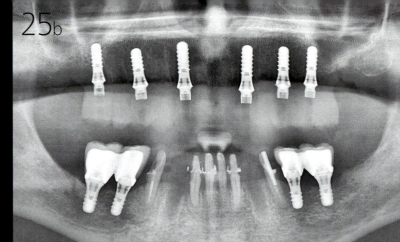

25b Panoramic radiograph at the end of the procedure, confirming the optimal fit of the instant loading partial denture on the six implants and RN placed.

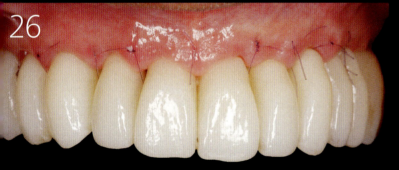

26 Clinical situation 8 days postoperatively.

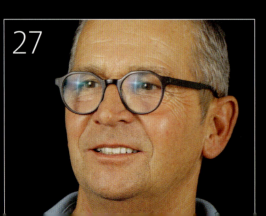

27 Facial photograph confirming the proper integration and replication of the instant loading partial denture in accordance with the esthetic validation done with the initial validation partial denture.

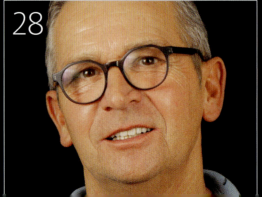

28 Frontal photograph

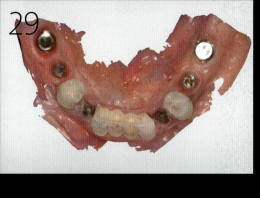

Three months after the maxillary instant loading surgery and 2 months after placement of the two implants in 33 and 43, digital impressions were taken of the six mandibular implants after unscrewing the four existing crowns on the posterior implants. The validation denture in front of 33 to 43 was sectioned to allow an implant impression with the validated prosthetic volumes.

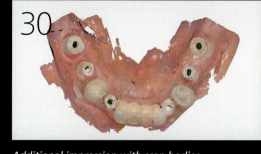

Additional impression with scan bodies.

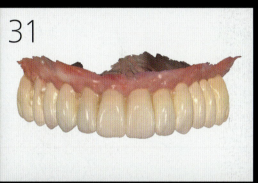

Antagonist impression with the instant loading partial denture.

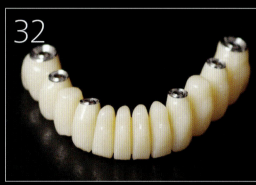

Using these STL files, the provisional full denture was fabricated by CAD/CAM on the lower part of the mouth, supported by the six implants. The pontic areas were worked on with an adapted design that made it possible to induce esthetic pontic beds after gingival healing guided by the prosthesis.

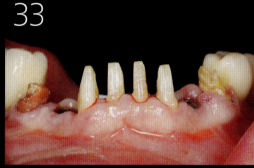

Clinical situation after removal of the provisional partial denture for initial esthetic and functional validation.

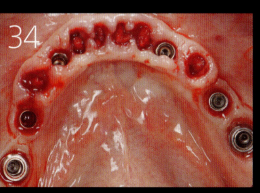

Occlusal view of the clinical situation after extraction of the anterior teeth and removal of the screw-retained crowns on the posterior implants.

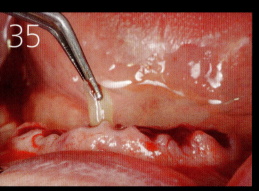

Preservation of extraction sockets with PRGF.

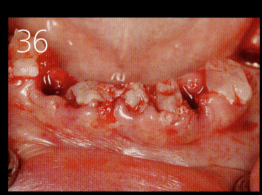

Closure of the extraction sockets with the fibrin membrane from the PRGF.

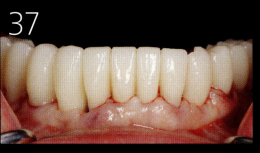

Temporary partial denture screwed in at the end of surgery.

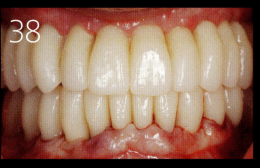

Vestibular view of the intermaxillary situation confirming the optimal transfer of the maxillomandibular relationship by the precision of the impression.

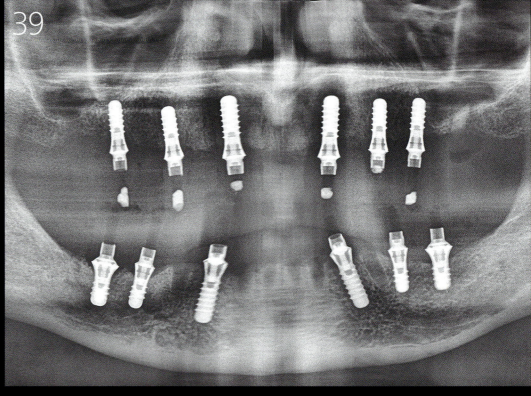

Panoramic radiograph confirming the optimal fit of the mandibular temporary partial denture on the six implants.

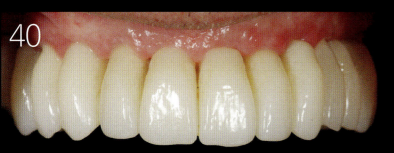

The maxilla with the temporary partial denture in place after 3 months.

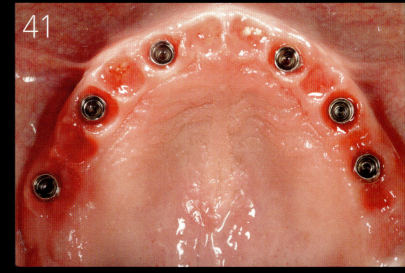

Occlusal view of the maxilla after removal of the temporary partial denture. Note the quality of the implant emergence profiles and pontic beds.

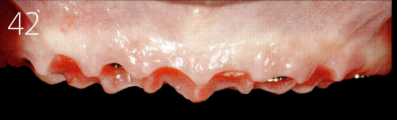

42 Vestibular view of the gingival scalloping obtained.

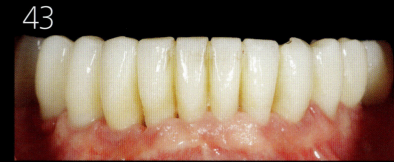

43 Vestibular view of the situation at 3 months in the mandible before removal of the temporary partial denture.

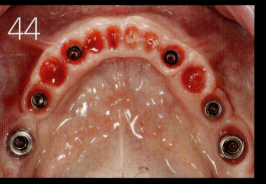

44 Occlusal view of the mandibular situation. Note the quality of the implant emergence profiles and the quality of the pontic beds.

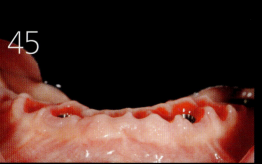

45 Vestibular view of gingival healing in the mandible.

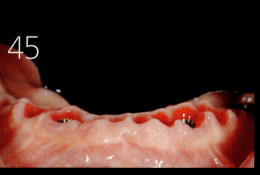

46 Global view under the temporary partial denture pending the final prosthesis.

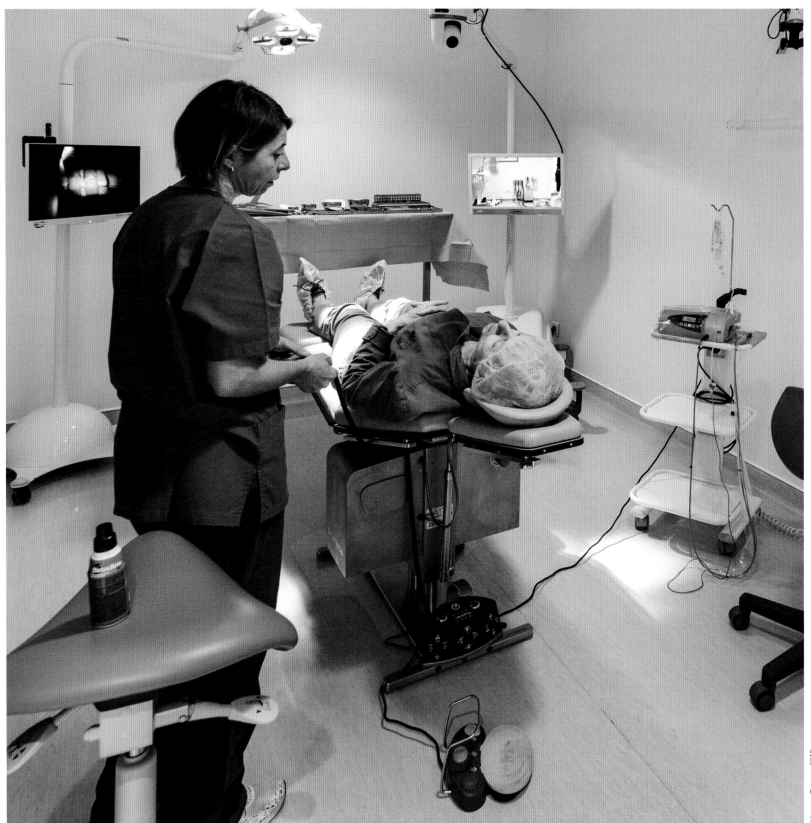

© Vianney Tisseau, 2019.

Full-arch clinical case 41

57-year-old man.

Clinical data

- The patient was referred by his wife, who we had previously treated with a Quokka full-arch procedure. The patient had two removable partial dentures and terminally mobile supporting teeth. He had serious anxiety relating to dental care, associated with a complex medical history with a history of aortic artery dissection.
- Case treated in July 2020.
- Complex bone context (heterogeneous horizontal vertical loss in both arches).
- Complex mucogingival architecture related to the bone architecture, but with a favorable amount of keratinized gingiva.

Presurgical treatments

- Optical impression taken with a Trios 4 and 3D examination performed using a 3Shape X1.
- Planning performed using Implant Studio.
- Placement of Straumann TL SP RN 10-mm implants in 14, 24, and 25 and 3.3 x 12.0 mm RN implants in 12 and 22 for the maxilla for a fixed partial denture for 10 teeth. Placement of a Straumann TL SP RN 12-mm implant in 44 and three 3.3 x 12.0 mm RNs in 42, 32, and 34 for a fixed partial denture for 10 teeth.
- 3D printing of the guides designed in Implant Studio and printed at the Dentitek Laboratory.
- Straumann T-sockets.
- The two provisional partial dentures were milled in PMMA (Dentitek Laboratory) on a shade A3 base and connected to the Variobase for RN in direct connection to the implants.

Assessment of the intervention

- Case treated in the office in **10 appointments** (esthetic analysis and planning elements, maxillary implant surgery, mandibular implant surgery, 3-month control, maxillary optical impression, validation key, placement, mandibular optical impression, validation key, placement).
- Final prosthesis placed in the office: two screw retained resin partial dentures replacing 10 teeth on a PEEK framework (JC Allègre Laboratory).
- To reduce costs and simplify the sessions for the patient, we made a virtual digital wax-up based on the esthetic analysis. This allowed us to save on the management and cost of the esthetic and functional validation of the partial denture. The patient trusted that the esthetic outcome would be good (following his wife's experience at our office) and primarily requested a comfortable result. To reduce costs, we made two all-on-four implants from resin on PEEK. The two arches were planned and designed at the same time in CAD/CAM. Placement was performed in two sessions 2 weeks apart to limit the duration of the sessions (2 hours each) and the amount of anesthesia with adrenaline in this context, which was stressful for the patient.

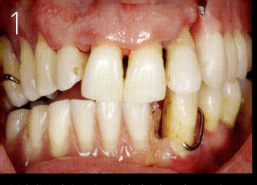
Initial clinical situation with the dental egressions and the two removable partial dentures present.

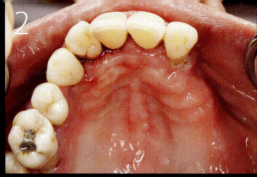
Occlusal view of the maxilla.

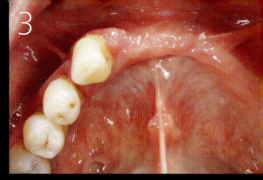
Occlusal view of the mandible.

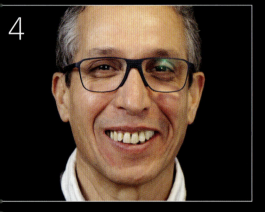
Facial photograph when smiling for esthetic analysis.

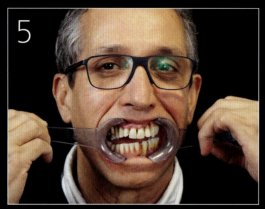
Frontal photograph with retractors for esthetic analysis.

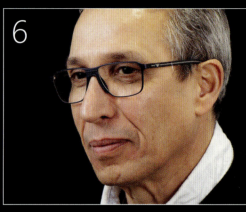
Three-quarter view for analysis of the lip volume and support.

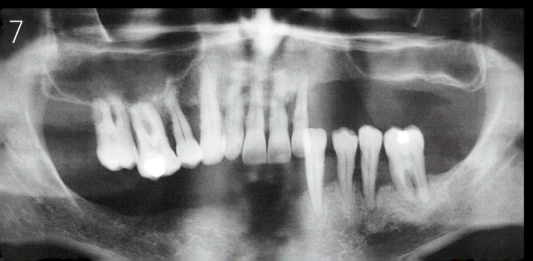
Panoramic radiograph of the initial situation.

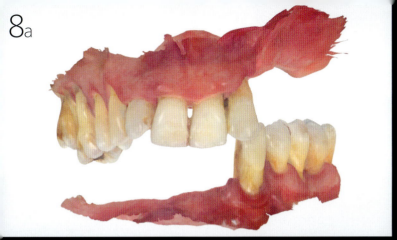

Intraoral optical impression taken during the same esthetic analysis appointment.

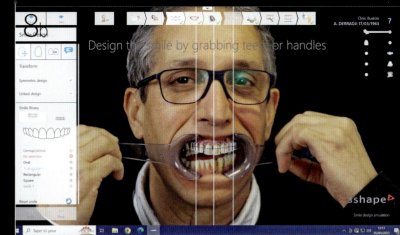

Importing the facial photos into the Trios 4 Smile Design module and designing the dental montage.

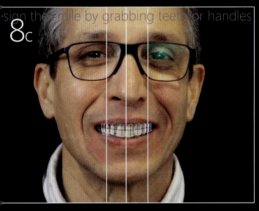

Selection of the morphology, length, and width of teeth.

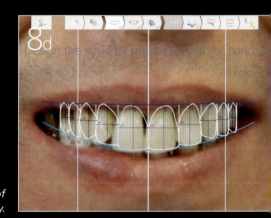

Enlarged view of the conceptualized assembly.

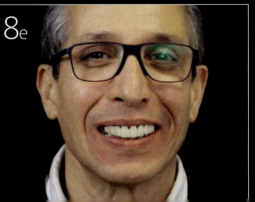

Simulation of the volume and shade of the teeth based on the design selected.

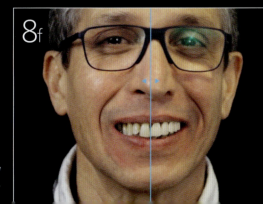

Comparison cursor before and after, highlighting the difference between the two setups

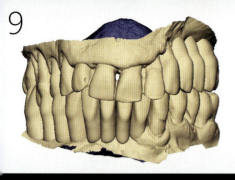

Virtual assembly of the missing teeth while keeping the teeth currently present to merge the STL files of the situation in the mouth and the STL file of the virtual assembly situation in order to best plan the implant positions to replace the missing teeth.

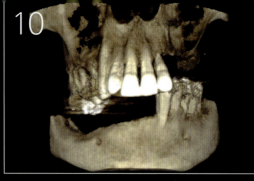

DICOM file acquired during the esthetic analysis session.

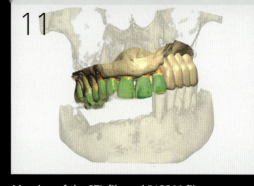

Merging of the STL file and DICOM file. The preservation in the file of the digital wax-up of the natural teeth allowed a fusion with the DICOM file. This same STL file could be merged with the native STL file of the teeth since they both came from the same coordinate system.

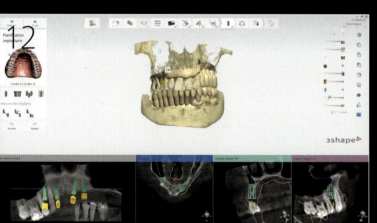

Planning window in Implant Studio with maxillary implant planning prior to mandibular implant planning.

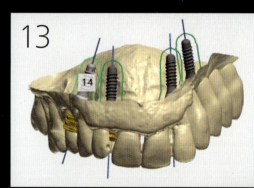

The four planned maxillary implants with the STL file of the digital wax-up without the bone DICOM file.

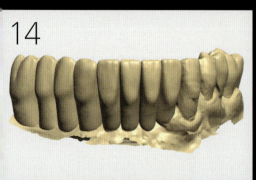

STL file of the mandibular digital wax-up.

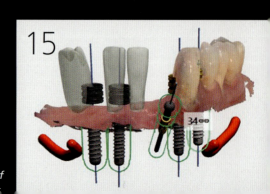

Planning of mandibular implants

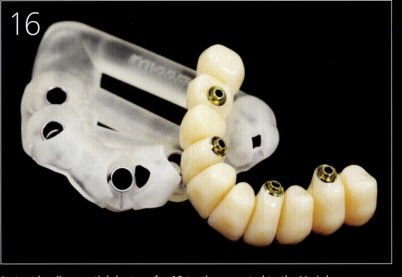

Instant loading partial denture for 10 teeth connected to the Variobase for the maxilla and the surgical guide before surgery.

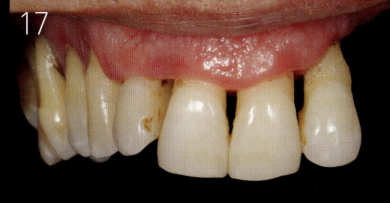

Maxillary situation at the beginning of surgery.

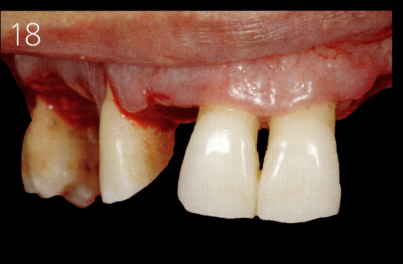

Extraction of teeth 12 and 14, which are future implant sites and preservation of the other teeth, future supports of the surgical guide.

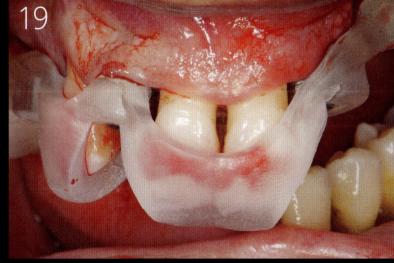

Surgical guide in place on the supporting teeth.

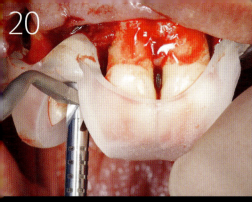

Passing a first drill, a "milling cutter", that was adapted to the terminal diameter of the drill in the extraction socket to create a horizontal flat to prevent deviation of the first guided drill.

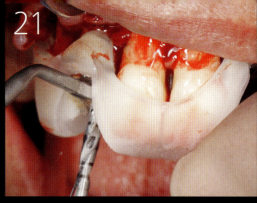

Passage of the first guided drill.

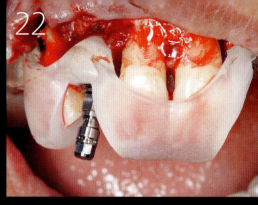

Guided implant placement in 12.

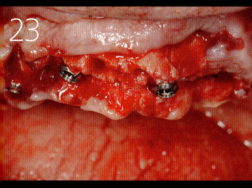

Vestibular view of the four implants placed after removal of the surgical guide and extraction of the residual support teeth.

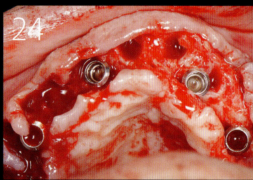

Occlusal view of the four placed implants and the extraction sites as well as the bone defects to be corrected.

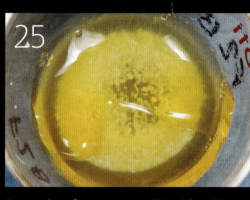

Preparation of compensatory GBR with PRGF in which the DBBM was incubated.

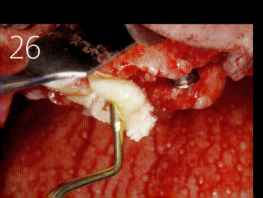

Placement of sticky bone in the extraction sockets to preserve the sites, future seats of the pontic supports.

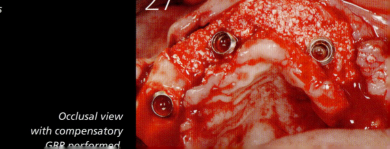

Occlusal view with compensatory GBR performed

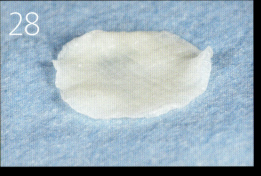

28 Fibrin membrane from the exuded PRGF.

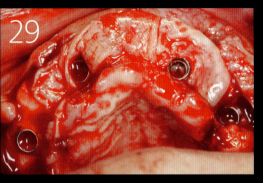

29 Covering of the compensatory GBR material with fibrin membranes from the PRGF. A resorbable collagen membrane covered the whole based on the principles of GBR.

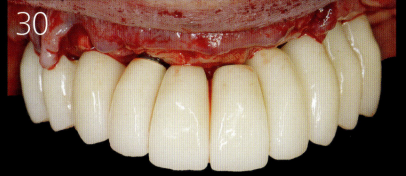

30 Placement of the instant loading bridge and control of compensatory GBR in relation to the prosthesis. Note the optimal fit of the denture on the implants.

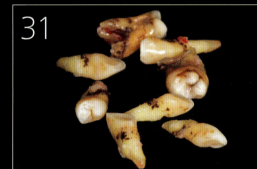

31 Teeth extracted during surgery, as opposed to fixed partial dentures already in place.

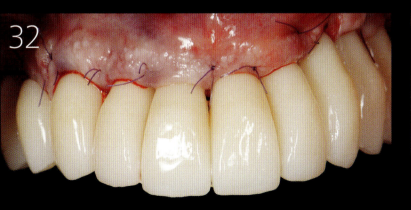

32 After a half-thickness incision was made at the back of the vestibule, coronal traction of the vestibular flap and stabilization with ASAF sutures were performed.

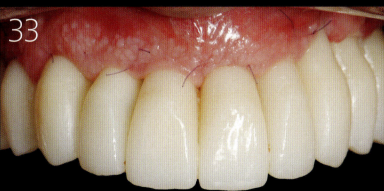

33 Clinical appearance at 8 days.

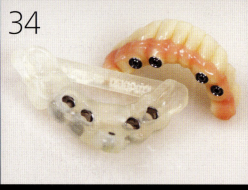

Fifteen days after the first surgery, surgical guide and instant loading partial denture in the mandible at the beginning of mandibular surgery. Note the presence of a dental support in sector 3, a mucosal support in sector 4, and a stabilization key in the medial sagittal plane.

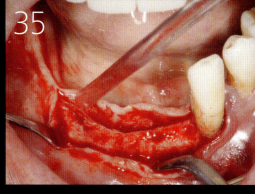

Preparation of full-thickness flaps from 44 to 34. Strategic extractions had not yet been performed.

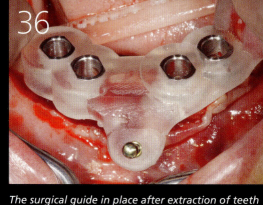

The surgical guide in place after extraction of teeth from implant sites and with no guide supports.

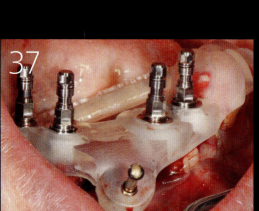

The four guided implants in place.

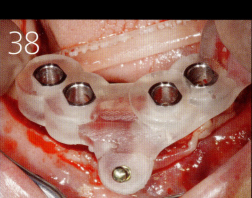

Removal of the screwed grippers on the guided implants prior to removal of the surgical guide.

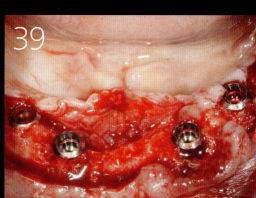

Clinical appearance after removal of the surgical guide. Note the minor defects to be corrected by compensatory GBR in addition to the placement of the instant loading partial denture.

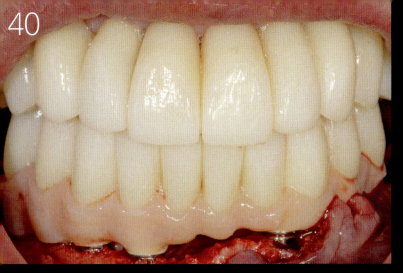

Instant loading partial denture screwed onto implants and guide for compensatory GBR.

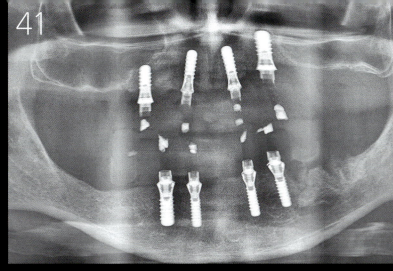

Panoramic control radiograph showing the adaptation of the two provisional partial dentures on the eight implants. Note the slight divergence of the Variobase in 34, which had no esthetic or functional impact.

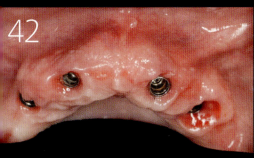

Clinical situation in the maxilla at 3 months post-surgery after removal of the instant loading partial denture.

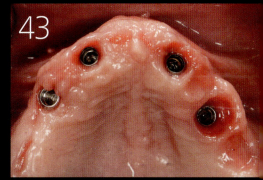

Occlusal view of the maxilla.

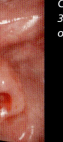

Occlusal view of the mandibular situation 3 months after removal of the instantaneous loading partial denture.

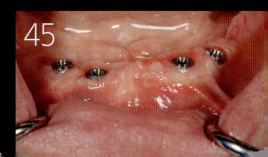

Vestibular view

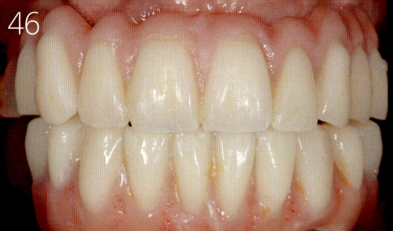
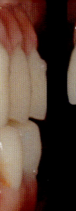

46 The two final prostheses in place: two resin partial dentures on a PEEK framework screwed in directly on the implant.

47 Frontal view of the maxillary rehabilitation.

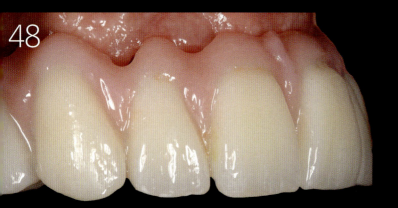

48 View of the right profile.

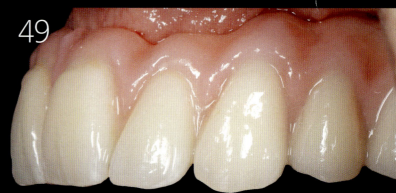

49 View of the left profile.

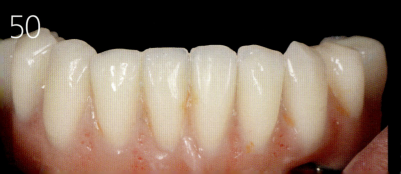

50 Front view of the mandibular prosthesis

Chapter 6 - Full-arch clinical applications

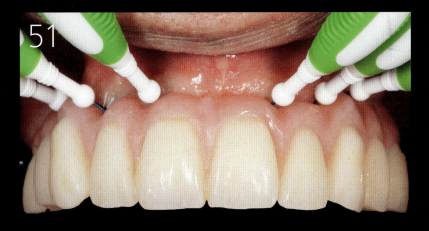

The pontics were calibrated for the passage of similar standardized interdental brushes at the maxilla.

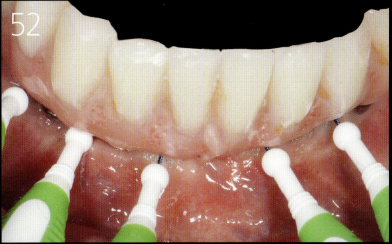

The pontics were calibrated for the passage of similar standardized interdental brushes at the mandible.

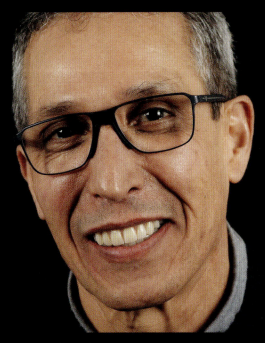

Facial photograph when smiling, showing the optimal integration of the final prostheses.

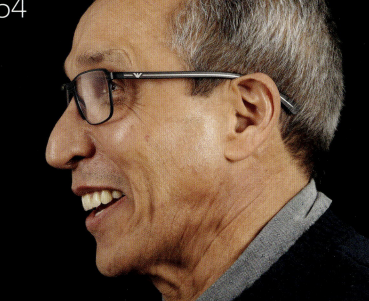

Profile photograph showing the optimal anteroposterior integration of the rehabilitations.

CAMPUS HB
Sharing and exchanging knowledge

IMPLANTOLOGY TRAINING CENTER

Production and design: Quintessence International, France
Illustrations: Laurent Baudchon
Printing: GRAFIČKI ZAVOD HRVATSKE d.o.o., Croatia
Legal deposit: October 2023
Printed: October 2023